PRAISE FOR *AYURVEDA MAMA*

"*I've always been fascinated by the ancient wisdom of Ayurveda. Dhyana's book was my go-to for valuable insights throughout my pregnancy—and these age-old principles supported me and my baby tremendously. I'm sure you'll gain just as much from it as I did.*"
—Miranda Kerr, model and CEO of KORA Organics

"Ayurveda Mama *is a must-have guide for every parent seeking to offer the best physical, mental, emotional, and spiritual care to their child. Dhyana Masla exemplifies how to transform the primordial needs of conception, pregnancy, and childcare into sacred practices that will also evolve the consciousness of both parents and children. Thank you, Dhyana, for sharing your most intimate journey of motherhood so eloquently and cheerfully.*"
—Divya Alter, Ayurvedic chef, culinary educator, and author of *What to Eat for How You Feel*

"*Dhyana makes integrating Ayurveda into your life so easy. I could not put this book down and feel every female, whether you want to have children now or way in the future, needs to read this wisdom.*"
—Melissa Ambrosini, podcaster and author of *Mastering Your Mean Girl*

"*Dhyana beautifully guides those looking to conceive consciously through her book* Ayurveda Mama. *Conception, pregnancy, and birth are such powerful experiences, and this book shines a light on the beauty of this stage of life. Dhyana approaches this time in a woman's life from all fronts of yoga, ayurveda, spirituality, and consciousness that truly creates a holistic experience, not overlooking one aspect or overpowering another. This book is a beautiful depiction of how to utilize ancient wisdom as well as the inner-nature and intuition for the modern and divine mama.*"
—Nishita Shah, Certified Ayurvedic Practitioner, C-AIYT, ERYT500

"*This book is sure to be a catalyst for raising the next generation of enlightened, compassionate, and flourishing individuals.*"
—Jay Shetty, author of *Think Like a Monk*, host of the *On Purpose* podcast

Ayurveda Mama

A Comprehensive Guide to Preparing for Pregnancy, Birth, and Postpartum

Dhyana Masla

FOREWORD BY
Radhi Devlukia-Shetty

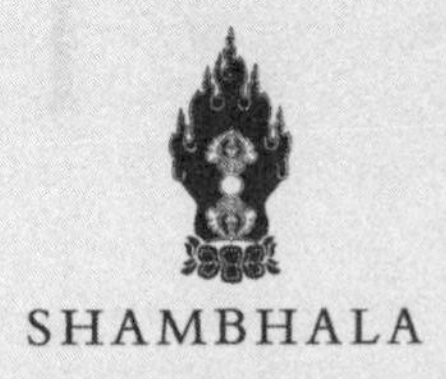

SHAMBHALA

Shambhala Publications, Inc.
2129 13th Street
Boulder, Colorado 80302
www.shambhala.com

Illustrated by Amy Charlotte

Cover art: Amy Charlotte
Cover design: Amy Sly
Interior design: Amy Sly

9 8 7 6 5 4 3 2 1

First Edition
Printed in the United States of America

Shambhala Publications makes every effort to print on acid-free, recycled paper.
Shambhala Publications is distributed worldwide by Penguin Random House, Inc., and its subsidiaries.

Library of Congress Cataloging-in-Publication Data
Names: Masla, Dhyana, author. | Devlukia-Shetty, Radhi, author of foreword.
Title: Ayurveda mama: a comprehensive guide to preparing for pregnancy, birth, and postpartum / Dhyana Masla; foreword by Radhi Devlukia-Shetty.
Description: First edition. | Boulder, Colorado: Shambhala, [2024] | Includes bibliographical references and index.
Identifiers: LCCN 2022056764 | ISBN 9781645471196 (trade paperback)
Subjects: LCSH: Pregnancy—Popular works. | Medicine, Ayurvedic—Popular works. | Prenatal care—Popular works. | Postnatal care—Popular works.
Classification: LCC RG551 .M375 2023 | DDC 618.2—dc23/eng/20230418
LC record available at https://lccn.loc.gov/2022056764

FOR MY MOM AND DAD

who have been the
most loving examples.

♦

FOR MY HUSBAND

who has embarked on the journey
of conscious parenting with me.

♦

& FOR MY LITTLE DARLINGS

who have taught me everything
that I know about being a mama.

Contents

Foreword by Radhi Devlukia-Shetty ix
Preface xi
Note to the Reader xv
Introduction 1

1
Foundations of Ayurveda 7

2
Conscious Conception 31

3
Cultivating the Seed 71

4
Preparing for Birth 115

5
The Birth of Your Babe 141

6
The Sacred Window 171

7
Newborn Mama 223

8
Nutrition and Recipes 267

9
Beneficial Herbs and Essential Oils 301

Epilogue 323
Resources 324
References 326
Index 328
About the Author 345

Foreword

Over the past several years, Dhyana has been in my life in many different ways: as a teacher, as an adviser, and as a friend. Now it gives me much joy to know Dhyana as an author and recommend her book *Ayurveda Mama* for all mothers- and fathers-to-be. Her book is a must-read Ayurvedic guide for conscious living and parenthood, full of helpful insights into how your consciousness plays a role in your child's life even before conception.

As a certified Ayurvedic health counselor, an advanced yoga teacher, and a practicing yogi, Dhyana infuses her life with conscious and intentional living. Inspired by her parents, she has practiced the teachings of Ayurveda from birth. As a teacher herself, Dhyana has a beautiful way of translating the ancient wisdom and vital knowledge of Ayurveda, making it easy to apply in the world we live in today.

My relationship with Dhyana has transformed over time. I started out as her yoga student but we became dear friends, and through the years I have seen firsthand how she weaves Ayurvedic principles into all aspects of her life. I have always been inspired by the way Dhyana consistently practices daily rituals, infuses positive energy into conversations with others, and nourishes her body, which she views as an instrument of God's grace. She transforms a simple interaction or conversation into an entire experience that encourages you to adopt that same lifestyle.

As a mother herself, Dhyana has all the credentials for sharing her experience in this book that simplifies the intricate process of preparing your mind, body, and soul for the magical journey of parenthood. From adopting a specific diet, to supporting conception, to cultivating self-care rituals during pregnancy and postpartum care, her guidance will help you build a strong foundation for your entry into parenthood.

Dhyana has been teaching this Ayurvedic approach to maternal health to small groups for years, and I am delighted that her book will make this precious vital knowledge accessible and available to the world.

With love and gratitude,
Radhi Devlukia-Shetty

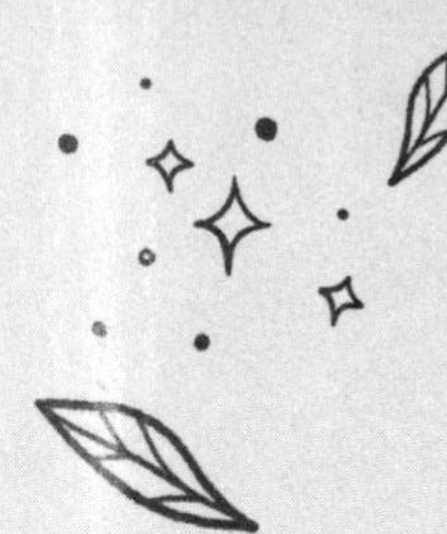

Preface

I remember my mom telling me how much she wanted my sister and me. She and my dad prayed for us, and she told me that on the day we were each conceived, they meditated on the names of the Divine for over ten hours. I have always appreciated the deep intention that my parents brought to the experience of inviting my sister and me into my mama's womb. More than merely a physical act, the act of making love became spiritual; for them, it became a deep service, an offering to the world.

The practices of Bhakti yoga and Ayurveda include an understanding that the consciousness of the parents at the moment of conception invites in a very specific soul. Modern science suggests that the sperm and the egg gather information from both donors moments to hours before conception. Through this interaction, the emotions that both parents are experiencing imprint upon the genes of the fetus as their first embodied experience. Understanding this, in most ancient cultures there would be a time of preparation before conception, during which both parents would create a very clear intention for what they wanted to contribute to their community or tribe. They would prepare their bodies. They would look at emotions that limited them: lust, confusion, greed, anger, envy, and the like, and do the work necessary to heal. They would meditate on the qualities that they wanted this soul to embody and try to see how they, themselves, could embody them more. When couples consummated their love, they would do so with the intention to propagate a species for evolution. In the Vedic times, this was seen as pivotal to the maintenance of the earth and of the future; to bring children into the world who, at the core of their being, felt at-home, welcomed, and wanted.

Ayurveda teaches that a person's core belief systems—beliefs that lay the foundation for how the rest of their lives will be lived—begin to develop at the moment of conception. By the time mama finds out she is pregnant, the heart of the fetus is fully exposed. Whether she is excited, scared, sad, or angry imprints deeply on the little one's sense of "self." Humans are relational beings, and at this very early stage of life, babies develop in response to those they are connected with. Every thought and emotion that mama feels while pregnant is felt by her little one. The mother's blood flow is in constant communication with her babe, and as the mother is experiencing her environmental conditions, the hormones that she is releasing begin to shape and mold even the physical structure of her baby. Babies that develop in the womb under severely stressful conditions—for instance in an environment of acute fear, scarcity, or aggression—are born with a smaller frontal lobe, larger adrenal glands, and a weakened immune system. The thoughts, behaviors, and emotions that a mother experiences are epigenetically passed along to a child in utero—as they are being prepared to be born into the same environmental conditions that surround her—giving the infant a better chance of survival.

That being said, is any parent ever truly "ready"? Yes and no.

Ayurveda teaches us that we can prepare with as much attention and intention as possible—but we cannot control the outcomes. Some of you who are reading this may have been trying to conceive for months or years already and are feeling more ready than you'll ever be! Others may be reading this after finding yourselves unexpectedly pregnant. You may be excited or resentful (or perhaps teetering between the two!), feeling that you're not ready, your career isn't ready, your relationship isn't ready. Perhaps you don't have a partner to parent with. It could be that you've wanted to become pregnant for some time, yet now that it has happened you're grieving the life you'll be leaving behind. Ayurvedic tradition says that the soul of your baby comes when it is time, ready or not. This arrival time is exactly what you need, no matter your situation—you are exactly the parent that your little one needs, for the evolution of both of your souls' journeys. Your life—who you are now and *everything* about you—is what your little one needs to experience. What we can do as conscious mamas is to continue to refine. It is a journey that doesn't end, and I hope this book guides you into becoming more of who you *really* are, more healed and more whole, so that you may hold the loving space for your little one to blossom into their wholeness.

Note: My intention in this book is to be authentic to the ancient tradition of Ayurveda, and I also hope to share the Ayurvedic approach to conception, pregnancy, birth, and postpartum health in a way that feels relevant to readers in our present day. To that end, I strongly encourage everyone who picks up this book to read themselves into the teachings and practices of Ayurveda in whatever way best reflects their own experience. I've embraced the word *mama* for my own experience, and it's a term I have used in this book as a way of labeling the deeply binding and intimate role we embark upon when bringing a tender new life into the world. Please don't hesitate to substitute whatever loving words and appropriate terms are a fit for yourself and your own family.

♦

Years before conceiving my first baby, I began diving into Ayurveda's teachings about preparing for pregnancy. I learned that there were dietary and lifestyle recommendations, cleansing and nourishing routines, mantras for conception, and even details of how to decorate the room. Love is in the details, and I felt in my heart that the most beautiful way to invite a soul into my womb would be to pay attention to all the details that have been passed down for thousands of years through the traditions of yoga and Ayurveda.

While pregnant in 2019, I read every book that offered a holistic approach to pregnancy that I could get my hands on. As a first-time mama, being pregnant and birthing a baby was the greatest mystery, the greatest adventure I had ever embarked upon! I wanted to feel as prepared as possible, as I felt that my preparedness would allow me to trust in the process much more deeply.

I was surprised to find that although many books talk about pregnancy, and some books talk about building physical and mental health postpartum, no books shared wisdom about preparing my mind and body, or guidance about deeply connecting to my spiritual nature, before becoming pregnant. Many books touched on Ayurveda, but none of them overviewed the entirety of Vedic science from preconception to the weeks postpartum.

With my background and deep faith in Ayurveda's holistic approach to health, I wanted more guidance from its ancient (and thus time-tested) perspective. So I reached out to all the teachers I knew, researched online and in books, and then put into practice everything that I learned. My pregnancy was one of the most beautiful and nourishing times of my life! I felt vibrant, like a shining temple that was housing the most special little soul.

I shared my experiences online throughout my pregnancy as well as during my postpartum window. I wrote about the different lifestyle practices I was applying to invite balance; I talked about the different herbs I used to stay nourished; I offered details about why a newly birthed mama stays home for the first forty-two days with her little one. I was surprised by the incredible interest and by the number of mamas who wrote to me saying, "I wish I knew all these things when I was pregnant!" Hearing the response of so many mamas moved me to make this wisdom more widely accessible. All mamas should feel deeply cared for so that they in turn can care for their little ones in such profound ways.

My hope for this book is that it gives parents-to-be the tools to create the ideal environment (internally and externally) to invite a soul into. I hope that it may inspire even one family to nourish their little one with deeper intention, and thus greater love. I pray it gives couples the tools to feel empowered in their lifestyle choices throughout the childbearing year, supporting the health and well-being of themselves and their babe. The book offers Ayurvedic wisdom about how to care for a mama postpartum, so that she may grow, heal, and deepen in ways that she never knew possible, along with guidance for the newborn mama about how to parent with more awareness and how to use practical and natural solutions to correct common newborn imbalances.

I'd like to offer my greatest appreciation to my mom and dad, who have offered such a beautiful example of intention and love in their parenting. My heartfelt gratitude goes out to all the helpful mamas and mamas-to-be who generously read different drafts of this book and offered abundant encouragement and helpful feedback. To Krsna Jivani, whose deep passion about caring for mamas moved her to help me complete this book, I extend thanks for her countless hours of editing, formatting, writing, meeting, and cooking. You will find a beautiful short essay toward the end of chapter 6 with her wisdom regarding the postpartum window, as well as other bits of her knowledge throughout the book. Thank you, Radhi Devlukia-Shetty, whose encouragement while I was pregnant inspired me to start writing, and who lovingly wrote the foreword that makes this book feel complete. And last, my appreciation to all of you reading. Thank you for wanting to live and love with more intention. For wanting to nourish your little babes in ways that will invite them to care more deeply for this world and all beings that live here.

The world needs more little ones who are raised like that . . . who are loved like that.

With love and deep gratitude,
Dhyana Masla

Note to the Reader

This is for all mamas.

To the independent mamas, the single mamas, the mamas with partners who are not involved, or maybe only partly involved. To the surrogate mamas, to the mamas who conceived through methods such as using a sperm donor or with their partners through in-vitro fertilization. To the same-sex and queer mamas and the mamas whose support systems may not include an opposite-sex partner but include parents, siblings, community members, friends, children, doulas, and caregivers. This is for you. This book is for all mamas, no matter what your life may look like, no matter what your relationship may look like, no matter what your family may look like, no matter the country you live in or the resources you have or the color of your skin or the religion you follow. This is for you.

You do not have to have the "perfect" situation in order to implement conscious parenting, or conscious mothering. You do not have to implement *all* or *nothing*. Take the pieces of knowledge in this book and apply what resonates with you, what fits with your life, and what feels right. Use this book as a starting point to dive into your own heart and find the place within you that is full of deep meaning and intention, so that you can approach your motherhood from that place, whatever that may look like for *you*. You can do this with or without a partner, you can do this with a support system of your own making, with whomever it is that you love and cherish. You can do this on your own. The intention to mother with awareness comes from your heart and your heart only. While Ayurveda teaches certain rituals, routines, and recipes to promote health and wellness throughout pregnancy and birth, you don't need permission from anyone else, and you don't need a certain environment to look a certain way. The knowledge and guidelines provided in this book are meant to inspire you to connect more deeply to yourself.

As mamas and pregnant mamas, we can get so wrapped up in wanting everything to be perfect that we become extra hard on ourselves when things don't work out the way we want them to or when our situations turn out different from what we had envisioned. Even in those moments, everything you learn in this book can be applied. Just do your best, mama, and that will be enough for your babe.

According to Vedic philosophy, nothing can occur without the sanction of God (you may also refer to God as your higher power, your Source, the Divine, or whatever word or name resonates with your belief system). Everything that happens in your life, to you and around you, is a co-creation between you and Source. Your life circumstances are created based on your desires, your will and actions, and the sanction of the Creator. In your motherhood journey, there may be circumstances that are challenging, and you may question many aspects of yourself. Just know that these moments, and all moments, are there for your soul evolution.

Vedic philosophy says that in co-creation with the Supreme, a soul chooses its next lifetime before taking birth. The soul knows who its family will be, who its mother will be, and it knows what its major karmic lessons will be in this lifetime. That means *your baby chose you as its mother,* knowing exactly who you are and what life you will provide it in this world. The baby's soul chose *you* because it knows that your relationship with it, and the life you provide for it, is exactly what the baby needs on its own journey of soul evolution.

So, mama, if you find yourself questioning your ability to be an Ayurveda mama based on your external circumstances, your relationship, your family, your lifestyle or home, the circumstances under which you conceived, or any other doubts that come up along your motherhood journey that make you feel "less than," please know and remember that if you picked up this book and are reading this right now, you are already an Ayurveda mama. You are already setting the intention to mother with awareness and consciousness. You are already creating a life of love and good health for your baby, just with your intention and desire to better yourself for them. You are doing a *great* job, and you will always be the perfect mother for your babe.

With love,
Krsna Jivani
Ayurvedic postpartum doula,
clinical herbalist, and mama

What if every child knew that they were wanted?
What if,
from the onset of conception
your child's body was literally built in an environment
enveloped in love, care, and deep, deep nourishment?
. . . their nervous system
built with the *knowing* that they held value and worth
based on who they are.

What if all of the children of the future never had to question
whether they were a burden?
If they knew,
deep down on the cellular level,
that they were prayed for, welcomed, and carried with love.

What if all mamas knew
that once the soul enters in,
she wraps that soul in matter
built by the food she consumes
through her eyes, ears, nose, tongue, and skin?

. . . that this little soul's sense of Self
is built by its environment,
cultured by its surroundings,
including the mind and emotions
of the body that sustains it.

If parents knew that for the first forty-two days after birth,
their little babe still does not yet know themself as separate.
"I am my environment;
the sounds, the temperature, the mood, the emotions
continue to build my nervous system."

What if their nervous systems were built on a foundation of love?
What if love was their North Star,
their "normal,"
that they always strived to come back to
when life seemed to throw them off course?

Our past experiences build our foundation of "normal."
Our early experiences shape what we seek in future relationships.
Whatever energy our nervous system was built on
creates a standard
that we return to again, and again, and again.
Too many nervous systems are built with anxiety,
creating a fundamental experience of fear
that we create,
and re-create,
because it somehow reminds us of home.

What if intention invited us,
love grew us,
and attention sustained us?

What type of leaders would we raise?
What quality of relationships would they experience?
What injustice would they never settle for?
How would they, then, raise their own little ones?

What if we knew that how we speak to them
creates the standard of how they will one day speak to themselves?
What if we knew
that as we heal our past,
we give the opportunity for our little ones
to have a better future?

What if we knew
to see the best in them, always?

If only we knew
that they see themselves
through our eyes.

Ayurveda Mama

Introduction

Birth and infancy are beyond the conscious memory of most people. Yet, as primary experiences, they indirectly pervade every aspect of our being.

—Anodea Judith, *Eastern Body, Western Mind*

There is no single effort more radical in its potential for saving the world than a transformation of the way we raise our children.

—Marianne Williamson

So much of the dysfunction in our world and in our relationships comes from stories that we have built around our earliest experiences. At a young age, we unconsciously created ways to cope with pain and trauma when we did not yet have the skills to adapt. We have taken on shields of armor that have found their home in our bodies and psyches and that now govern the way we *are* in the world. This armor keeps us safe—or so we think. Actually, this armor keeps us from meeting life authentically. It keeps us from being able to love deeply and fully, feel deeply and fully, live deeply and completely, with consciousness and intention.

So much of the work of inviting a child into this world consciously is becoming conscious yourself, healing your past and becoming aware of what's driving you. When you can develop a healthy dialogue with the part of yourself that feels broken, abandoned, or unworthy of love, you begin to heal. As you become more conscious, you can invite a child into the world consciously, and then raise a conscious little being who will not have to spend their whole life healing the wounds from their past, unlearning what they have learned from their unconscious parenting.

I deeply believe that the glory of our future depends on the ways in which we care for our children today, from preconception, to birth, and beyond.

While their first years do not necessarily determine a child's happiness for their entire life, their rapidly growing brain during that time builds a foundation for how they will communicate and interact with the world based on how the world has responded to them. In a baby's first years of life, cries are common signals for a caregiver's nurturing. The cycle completes when the caregiver responds to the baby's crying by feeding them, changing their diaper, or rocking them to sleep. Foundational beliefs such as "the world is safe (or unsafe)," "I will be provided for (or there is not enough to go around)," "I am enough (or I have to prove my worth)," "I am supported (or I must do it all myself)," or "It is okay to ask for what I need (or my needs will never be met)" are all created, subconsciously, based on our environment and how our primary caregivers show up (or do not show up) for us. Investing early in our children means not only giving them food and clothes: it means giving them presence, security, attention, and love.

♦

Yoga and Ayurveda teach us that experiences begin to imprint themselves on the baby's mind and body during pregnancy. Based on the emotional, spiritual, and physical environment within which the child is developing, these impressions will either serve to uplift the child and create patterns of harmony, trust, and connection or they will create patterns that will play themselves out in the future through dysfunctional relationships, addictions, violence, fear, and anxiety.

Some babies are created in the context of challenging circumstances. Perhaps a mama has faced violence while the baby is growing in the womb, or a baby has been unknowingly conceived and not initially wanted, or a mama's needs have not been met. Left unaddressed, these experiences may create a foundation for a baby's future built on the sense that they are not safe, valuable, worthy, or deserving of love. Their nervous systems may be built on a foundation of dis-ease or instability. But if you are reading this book, you are taking the necessary step to invite your little one into your womb on purpose, and with utmost intention; you are demonstrating the desire to establish a deep, fundamental, core belief within your child that they are wanted and not a burden. If you cultivate their presence with love and deep care while they are in your womb, their nervous system will be soft and at ease. Ideally a mama will be nourished and supported throughout pregnancy, which helps assure that the baby's mind and mood will be stable. The more safe and secure you can feel in all aspects of your life, the more your little one will feel that they too are at home.

Although the mind may not remember, our bodies remember everything. All of your past experiences are imprinted onto your nervous system. Those experiences create fundamental belief systems about you and your place in the world. If a child does not feel valued, they will be on the quest to validate their value in their role or position. If they did not feel worthy of love and attention, they may spend their entire life trying to prove their own worth. If they were spoken to in ways that were condescending, they will speak to themselves in the same way and then project that same energy into other relationships in their life. If they do not do the inner work to heal, they will treat their own children in the ways that their parents treated them, thus continuing the cycle of abuse and dysfunction.

In the same way, the love and affection, the attention and intention, that you pour into your little one grows a human being who is emotionally adept. If you raise them with care, they learn how to care for themselves, for others, and for the world. If you speak to them with kindness, they learn to be kind. If you are able to *be* with them when they are feeling big emotions (rather than trying to fix, change, or control), they learn how to not run away from themselves. If you are present with them, offering them your full attention, they learn that they are valuable and worthy of loving attention. If you listen and respond, they become capable of doing the same. If you teach boundaries in a supportive way, they understand that boundaries are not limiting but are important in order to protect what is sacred. By your example, and by the ways that you treat them, they learn how to *be* in the world.

How can you heal your own body so that you can provide this little soul with a healthy and strong vehicle to live in? How can you become more conscious and intentional, and then invite a child into the world with more consciousness and intention? How can you strengthen your own relationship so that you can show your little one what it means to really love? How can you identify your own limiting belief systems so that you do not instill the same beliefs into your child? How can you learn to *feel*, and thus to *heal*, the parts of yourself that you've learned to be unworthy? How can you live a life founded in trust, harmony, and love, so that those are the patterns that build your little one's foundation?

♦

By raising wholesome individuals who feel safe, loved, and cared for, you begin to create a world that is more safe, loving, and caring. By existing in conscious, loving partnerships and intentionally bringing children into this world, you breed a world where each person feels fundamentally important and will thus give what is important back to the world.

This book explores, through the lens of Ayurveda, ways to build a foundation of health before conception; the process of consciously inviting a child into the fertile soil already established; how to maintain balance throughout pregnancy; ways to prepare for birth and labor; the classical yet practical ways to nourish the newborn mama and surround your little one with love and care during the first forty-two days after birth; reflections on mothering with self-awareness; the basics of caring for a newborn; and knowledge about using diet, herbs, and essential oils to support the health of you and your little babe. We will explore the ancient science of Ayurveda as it applies to conceiving, growing, birthing, and caring for this precious soul who has been entrusted to your care.

You are my greatest adventure
and my greatest mystery.
I have never felt so protective over anyone
or anything
in my life.

May my heartbeat sustain you,
little one.
With all the love and care and soul nutrition
that lets you know that you are always safe,
always taken care of,
always at home.

May this foundation give you the strength
for a lifetime of service
so that you may experience
unmotivated
uninterrupted
unconditional
love

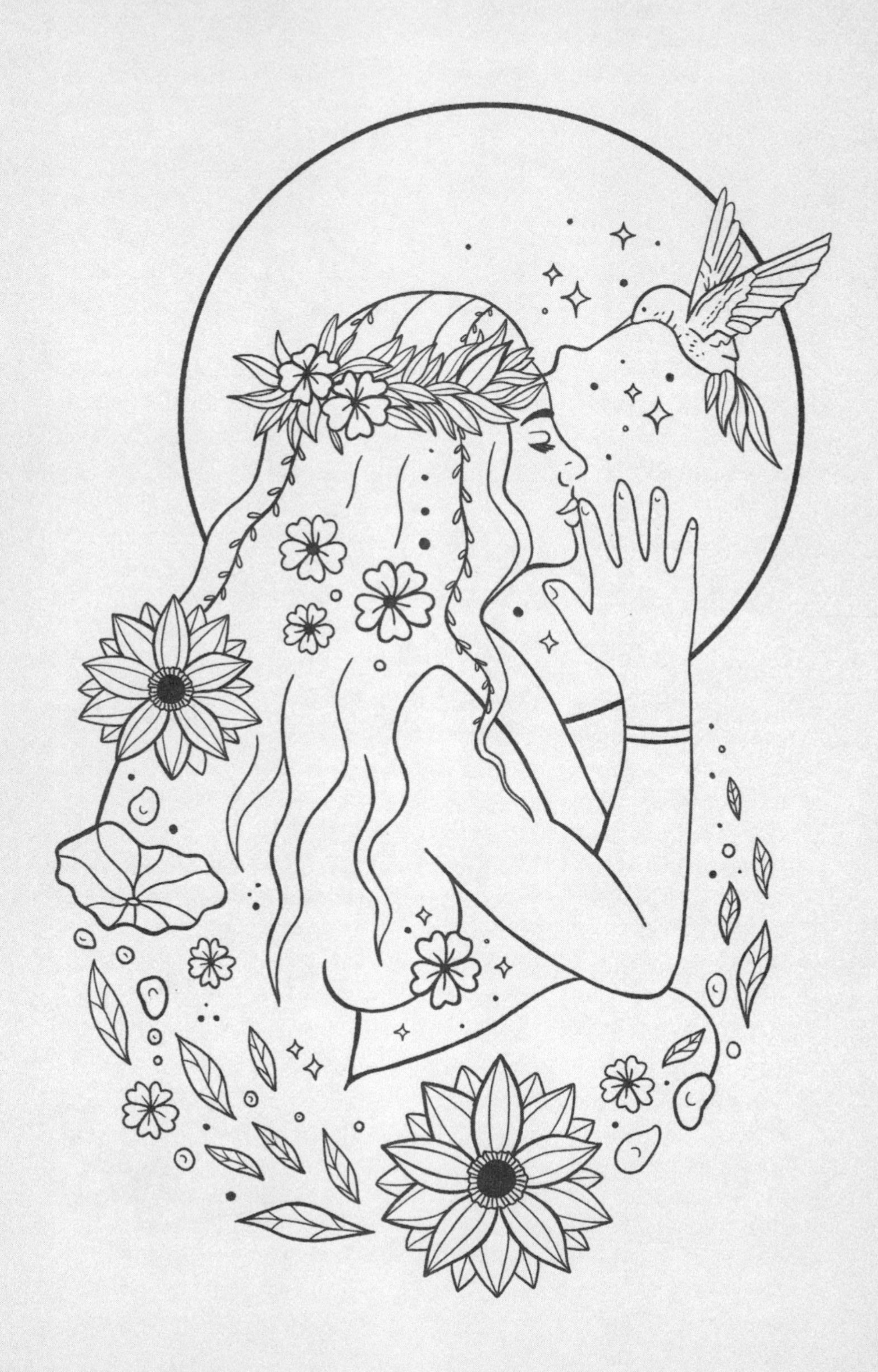

Foundations of Ayurveda

· 1 ·

The state of ill health is a moment-to-moment happening. Healing is moment-to-moment balance, bringing awareness to your thoughts, feelings, and emotions and how you respond.

—Dr. Vasant Lad, author and founder of the Ayurvedic Institute

Ayurveda is a five-thousand-year-old system of natural healing rooted in the ancient culture of India. More than a mere system of treating illness, Ayurveda is a science of life (*ayur* = life, *veda* = science or knowledge) that will guide you not only toward vibrant physical and mental health but also toward a deeper connection to your spiritual nature. It offers a body of wisdom designed to help you stay vital while realizing your full human potential. Providing guidelines on ideal daily and seasonal routines, diet, behavior, and the proper use of your senses, Ayurveda reminds you that health is the balanced and dynamic integration between body, mind, spirit, and environment.

♦

Ayurveda is a science that helps you understand the nature of this world and how the elements the world is made of work together to create harmony or dissonance, health or dis-ease. It guides you toward understanding yourself, your own material makeup, so that you can interact with the world in right relationship. It supports you in navigating life consciously, in making choices that support your health and balance so that you can expand your perspective and seek the deeper, big-picture questions in life: What is my purpose? Who am I? Why am I here?

Ayurveda and yoga are considered to be sister sciences—they are meant to be practiced together. Yoga is the study of spirit, or the soul. It is a science meant to help you understand the nature of your mind and cleanse your heart so that you may awaken to the truth of who you *really* are. Ayurveda is the study of matter, guiding you toward understanding the nature of this world and the elements that it is made of. Practiced together, yoga and Ayurveda guide you toward a way of living in this world-made-of-matter while staying connected to your soul.

PERFECT HEALTH

Real health includes not only a dynamic experience of wellness in the body but also an experience of living a deeply fulfilling life, which includes—but not limited to—mental and emotional well-being, thriving relationships, core alignment with your purpose, and a genuine spiritual connection. Have you ever had the experience of struggling in a relationship and it affecting your state of mind? Or feeling anxious in your mind and the anxiety making your body feel queasy? Any aspect of your life affects every other. Ayurveda teaches that in order to be really healthy, you must take into account the health of your body, your mind, your senses, and your soul. You can be healthy physically, but if you are anxious or depressed, you will not be feeling very well. Or perhaps your body feels great and your mind is steady, but you do not feel a connection to your deepest purpose in life—you do not feel fulfilled. Where many modern medical sciences focus on the health of your body and mind, Ayurveda points to the awakening of the soul—the spark that gives life to all forms—as an inseparable contingent of perfect health.

The word for health in Ayurveda is *svastha. Svastha* literally translates as being situated in the Self, situated within your true Self, beyond the ever-changing body and mind; beyond the senses and their limited perceptions. Discovering the nature of your true Self is the journey and the destination of any authentic spiritual tradition.

THE NATURE OF THE SELF

Because we live in a world and in a body that is made up of matter, we start to identify with it. I think that *I am* my body, *I am* this voice in my head (the mind), and I seek happiness through my senses, in this world made of matter, thinking that it will lead me to lasting joy.

The law of conservation of mass states that matter is neither created nor destroyed, but it is always changing. Everything in this world is made of matter! Anything that can be perceived through your senses, that can be seen, touched, tasted, smelled, or heard, is material. This book you are holding, the ground beneath you, a yoga mat, a cup, even the air all around you is matter. And this body you are in? It is made of the same elements! However, there is something about this lump of matter, your body, that is different from a yoga mat or a cup. Ayurveda and yoga teach us that it is the presence of the soul that gives consciousness, or life, to form—and that is who you *really* are.

Six symptoms of life (or the presence of the soul) are manifest in all sentient beings: birth, growth, the potential to procreate when healthy, maintenance for a while, dwindling or disease, and eventually death. Wherever you see matter cycling through these six symptoms (not only in a human body but also in the body of a plant, a grasshopper, a cat, or a tree) you know that there is the presence of a soul.

If you are driving a 1986 Ford pickup truck, you drive a certain way. You will likely drive slowly, chugging along on the interstate. Another day, you might be driving a brand-new Porsche Carrera, which drives really fast and zooms in and out of the lanes. Depending on the vehicle (or body) that the soul is residing in, it has different abilities and limitations. A grasshopper can do certain things that a plant cannot. A plant can do certain things that a human cannot! But regardless of the vehicle, the quality of the indwelling soul is the same.

The Vedas, the ancient sacred texts of India, use the Sanskrit term *sat-chit-ananda* to describe the soul. *Sat* means that the soul is eternal. The soul is unborn and never dies; it simply moves from body to body at the time of death. *Chit* conveys that the soul is fully conscious and fully aware; the soul is seeing through your eyes, hearing through your ears, feeling through your skin, and so on. And *ananda* signifies that the soul is eternally blissful, with the potential to experience the highest happiness that comes from the love shared between the individual soul and God.

The Vedic literature compares God to the sun and our eternal nature to the sun's rays. The celestial body we call the sun is the source of all light and all heat, and nothing can live without it. The sun's rays are not different from the sun, in quality; they give off heat, they give off light, and they are of the same substance. And every sun ray is coming from the same source; so they are all related, they are all united. But quantitatively, there is a difference between a sun ray and the sun itself: the sun is not coming from the sun ray, rather the sun ray is coming from the larger body of the sun. Similarly, the Upanishads explain *nityo nityanaam cetanas cetananam*: that is, there is one Supreme Truth—God—who is like the sun—from whom everything emanates, and there are limitless, eternal, unique, and individual souls—like the sun rays. Wherever there is life, there is part of God. So in the Bhakti tradition, we are all like those sun rays. We are *sat-chit-ananda;* just like God, we are eternal, full of knowledge, full of bliss.

THE CAUSE OF DISEASE

Ayurveda teaches that disease begins with *raga* and *dvesha*, attachment and aversion, which come from identifying with matter and forgetting who you *really* are. Raga and dvesha cloud your connection to your true essence, as you become caught up in choosing what you want and what you do not want; what you like and what you do not like; what you move toward and what you move away from, based on your previous experiences in life. You make your decisions based on the limited scope of your past, moving toward what you *think* will bring pleasure and away from what you *think* will bring pain, measured and weighed by what brought pleasure or pain before. You have conditioned responses, habits if you will, of action and reaction based on what you have already experienced in life.

You may go for that third bowl of ice cream because you *want* it, even though you *know* that you will not feel good afterward. You avoid deep, loving relationships because twelve years ago your best friend moved away and deep relationship, unconsciously, equals pain. You drink coffee each morning because it is what you are used to doing, even though you experience dryness, irritation, and anxiety (things that coffee will exacerbate!). You seek pleasure in people, places, or things that remind you of past pleasurable experiences, even if choosing those things is not best. You avoid people, places, and situations that remind you of past painful experiences—even if they would ultimately be good. Because you filter all your choices through raga and dvesha, attachment and aversion, based on your past experiences, these govern your entire experience of life and are the cause of all imbalance.

Like and dislike take away your ability to be centered and to perceive things clearly. If you were centered—connected to your self—you would make choices that ultimately serve, rather than being pulled or pushed by what you want or don't want right now. If your baby will not stop crying, rather than being present with them and seeing how you can support them, your mind may say, "I don't like this." It will continue by trying to validate itself and find a solution: you might think, "This is not acceptable," and decide the baby deserves to be hit, or ignored, or yelled at.

Parents will oftentimes respond to their children based on how their own parents responded to them. By observing and experiencing your parents' likes and dislikes and their corresponding reactions, you were programmed to like and not like certain things, and you learned how to respond. So much of your spiritual life, or your attempt to live consciously, is in the practice of noticing what programs run your life and your impulse to respond based on them. The Vedas teach that out of millions of species of life on this planet, the main thing that distinguishes the human form of life from any other species is our ability to *choose*, and to thus consciously evolve and realize the essence of our spiritual existence. All other animals on this planet (including most humans!) are making decisions based on their previous experiences; choosing things that they think will bring happiness and avoiding things that they think will bring pain, based on how they have been programmed by their past.

Once you become aware of this phenomenon, rather than responding to the world based on your personal programmed preferences, you can instead choose to show up in a way that actually serves. Rather than continuing the cycles of dysfunction and dis-ease, you begin to more clearly see and understand the most beneficial way to *be* in each situation. Awareness creates a gap between stimulus and response, and that gap is a crucial skill on the journey of parenthood. When you act from a place of deeper awareness, your actions will be helpful and bring about an experience of balance and ease.

In every circumstance there is right action. Not right as opposed to wrong, but "right" in the sense of what actually serves. Because of raga and dvesha, attachment and aversion, you become unable to make this distinction. By contrast, when you are able to feel steady within any situation you can make a "right" decision based on what is real, rather than a decision founded in your hopes, past fears, and fantasies. When you are present, rather than being pushed and pulled by personal preference and how you think things *should* be, you can choose how to respond based on your values, whether the situation involves what food to eat, whether to stay in a relationship, or how to parent your child. When reacting from a mental or an emotional place, you will often say or do things that do not serve the highest good but instead only serve to temporarily pacify your state of stress, fear, anxiety, unhappiness, or desire.

The mind and emotions are always changing, so being governed by them will never lead you to lasting happiness or a life of true meaning. If your desires are not stemming from a deeper place than your mind and emotions—that is, stemming from a sense of who you really are—acting with those desires as your compass is the cause of all imbalances.

When you have forgotten who you really are, you seek lasting happiness in a temporary world, when what you are actually seeking is *anandamayo bhyasat*—the happiness that is inherent within the nature of your soul. It is said that this inherent happiness is *anandam buddhi vardhanam*—like an ever-expanding ocean of happiness that is not caused by anything! It is not *because* I got the raise, or *because* he looked at me a certain way, or *because* life is unfolding the way that I *want* it to. Anandamayo bhyasat is a happiness that is beyond circumstance, which means that it will not be interrupted as the circumstances inevitably change. This is unconditional happiness, as it is not dependent on conditions or circumstances.

This happiness is what you experience when you awaken to your true Self.

♦

The happiness that you experience in life is often linked to something external being the way that you want it to be. You feel "happy" thinking, "I got the job," "It is sunny outside," "He complimented me." Your happiness, then, is completely dictated by an external experience or circumstance that you have absolutely no control over. This is conditional happiness: happiness based on the conditions of your environment. The other side of that coin is that as soon as things outside of you are *not* the way that you want them to be—or *are* the way that you do *not* want them to be—you become sad, distressed, disappointed, or angry. If your happiness is linked to something outside of you being a certain way, you are going to suffer because it is not going to stay that way.

The Three Causes of Disease

Because you have forgotten who you really are, you might experience the following.

***Prajnaaparadha*, knowing what is best but choosing something different.** Eating something that you know makes you sick just because it tastes good or watching a scary movie even though you know you will have nightmares. Acting from ignorance, you ignore your own wisdom, trying to satisfy particular needs, though in a temporary and unsatisfactory way.

***Asatmendriyartha samyoga*, misusing your senses.** Eating too much or not enough; eating foods out of season or not supportive to your health; watching too many movies; indulging in too much screen time; listening to music too loud; and so on.

***Parinama*, living out of rhythm.** When you ignore opportunities to align with nature's rhythm, the natural rhythmic process of decay over time can pick up speed. You have many opportunities to align your biorhythms through circadian, seasonal, and time-of-life rhythms.

Allopathic medicine can be useful in helping to treat suffering, while Ayurveda guides us toward an end to all suffering by treating its root cause. Even when your body is in a state of dis-ease, when your senses are not working as well as they once did, when conditions in your life are not what you would hope or imagine, or even the day that you are on your deathbed, you can still be svastha—situated so deeply within your Self that you will not be swayed by any of it. This is the real goal of Ayurveda: aligning with the nature of your true self and living your life from that deepest place.

Ayurveda is a practical science; it has to be applied in order for it to be experienced. The practice starts with simple dietary and lifestyle recommendations that will help you feel healthier in your body and more content within your mind. Your diet and lifestyle dictate how you experience your life. When you are aligned with a way of living that supports you in feeling vital, energized, and empowered, you are living a life in alignment with nature—and the nature of your Self. More than two thousand years ago, Hippocrates—the father of modern medicine—suggested that all diseases begin in the gut. In fact, about 70 percent of the immune system is housed in the gut, so making sure that your digestive system is functioning properly can be key to addressing many of your bodily woes.* Indeed, most imbalances can be cured through diet and lifestyle alone. So, however simple, apply these principles that I lay out in the next chapters and experience the profound effects of Ayurveda.

Through purifying your body, mind, and life you begin to live as a higher version of your self. From there, you make decisions that serve to uplift your life and the life of this little soul that you are inviting (or have already invited!) in. You strive to not just provide a healthy body and environment for your baby to develop in, but also the ability to offer them an opportunity to remember who they *really* are so that they can experience true happiness and fulfillment in this life.

This, Ayurveda teaches, is the perfection of parenthood.

* https://www.ncbi.nlm.nih.gov/pmc/articles/PMC2515351/.

ELEMENTS AND DOSHAS: SEEKING BALANCE

In Ayurveda, the five elements found in all things—ether, air, fire, water, and earth—are the building blocks of life. While this foundation unites all beings, the manifestation of these elements also gives rise to the ways in which we are all different. How the five elements appear, and in what proportion, makes each of us physiologically unique.

From the perspective of Ayurveda, there are three universal, holistic, fundamental forces, or *doshas*, that pervade all of material nature: *vata*, *pitta*, and *kapha*. Vata is a combination of the elements space and air (as well as the qualities born of those elements); pitta, of fire and water; kapha, of water and earth. These fundamental forces work in every individual and all of nature and govern all physical, mental, and emotional processes.

All matter manifests from a combination of ether, air, fire, water, and earth in different proportions, meaning that your constitution is made up of a unique combination of all five of those elements—and thus a unique combination of all three doshas—making Ayurveda a personalized science. This particular combination is determined at the moment of conception and becomes your own personal blueprint, or *prakruti*—your perfect amount of each element for ideal health. Your prakruti is fixed and will not change throughout your life—and this fundamental psycho-physical nature can be used as a compass to guide you back to wellness. Based on your mother's diet and lifestyle during pregnancy, however, as well as your own diet and lifestyle throughout life, you may move into a state of *vikruti*, or imbalance—meaning that the proportions of the elements have changed from their original, balanced state.

As you move through life, the three doshas constantly fluctuate—creating vikruti—according to your environment, your diet, the seasons, the climate, your age, and many other factors. Because of this, balance is not something that is ever attained, rather a dynamic state that you constantly move toward as you make micro-adjustments to harmonize with your external circumstances. As they move into and out of balance, the doshas can affect your health, energy level, and general mood.

The goal of Ayurveda is to bring you toward your prakruti; to support you in making the moment-to-moment micro-adjustments that will help you adapt to the time of day, the time of year, and the time of life, as well as help correct any imbalance that you are experiencing. In this way, you can experience vibrant health and your intrinsic connection to Source.

Balance is a dynamic state. You never actually "get there." You are constantly working with your environment to adapt as the circumstances keep changing. The word *dosha* literally translates to "at fault," and that conveys how these forces work within your body. The doshas are constantly affected by whatever comes in through your senses. They are affected by what you see, smell, taste, touch, and hear, as well as by the climate, the season, and the time of day. For example, you might feel very balanced, but then the sun hits the highest point in the sky (around noon time), you take a hot yoga class, and follow that up by going out for a lunch of spicy Mexican food. The time of day and your activities during that time create an increase of the fire energy in your body, thus throwing you out of balance. You might start to notice excess heat in your body, manifesting as irritability, acid reflux, or a skin rash. If you lack awareness, you might opt for picking up a cup of hot coffee as a routine pick-me-up on your way home. However, that will throw you even more out of balance with its heating and drying qualities. With awareness, by contrast, once you notice that you are out of balance, you have an opportunity to make choices that will bring you back. Every choice has the ability to move you toward balance or away from it, depending on where, when, how, and why you make the choice.

Ayurveda uses an understanding of the doshas to guide you toward an awareness of what you actually need (rather than just what you want), helping you to cultivate balance and adjust to your environment, to maintain vibrant and steady health. The doshas are the organizing energies in your body; they each carry with them a bundle of specific qualities, which is the easiest way to define them. For example, you know something is primarily composed of air and ether elements (or primarily vata dosha) when you see the qualities of cold, light, dry, rough, mobile, irregular, and changeable. So, as you will learn later in this chapter, if you have an excess of these qualities—if your skin is very dry, if you're frequently cold, if you experience constipation or bloating from dryness in your colon, if you have no rhythm and things seem to be constantly changing in your life leading you to feel ungrounded or anxious—you would simply bring in the opposite qualities (hot, heavy, moist, smooth, stable, and predictable, respectively) with your diet and lifestyle activities to balance vata.

Knowing your prakruti (your personalized doshic blueprint) is valuable, as it shows you the ways that you are most likely to move out of balance and helps you be aware of activities that should generally be favored or avoided. (The best way to determine your doshic blueprint is to see an experienced Ayurveda practitioner, who can use *ashatvidha-pariksha*, or the eight methods of diagnosis, to identify your prakruti.) In this book, rather than placing emphasis on discovering your prakruti, we will focus on the many ways that you can know if you have an imbalance in any of the doshas, and we'll talk about the tools that will support you in coming back to your ideal state of health.

Although vata is the main dosha to be concerned with during pregnancy and postpartum, it is also possible for pitta and kapha to go out of balance, especially if you already have a lot of pitta or kapha in your constitution. Generally during pregnancy, pitta is concerned with metabolism, hormones, and increased heat in the body, where kapha plays its role with the extra fluids and increased bulk. Let's look at each of these doshas in turn.

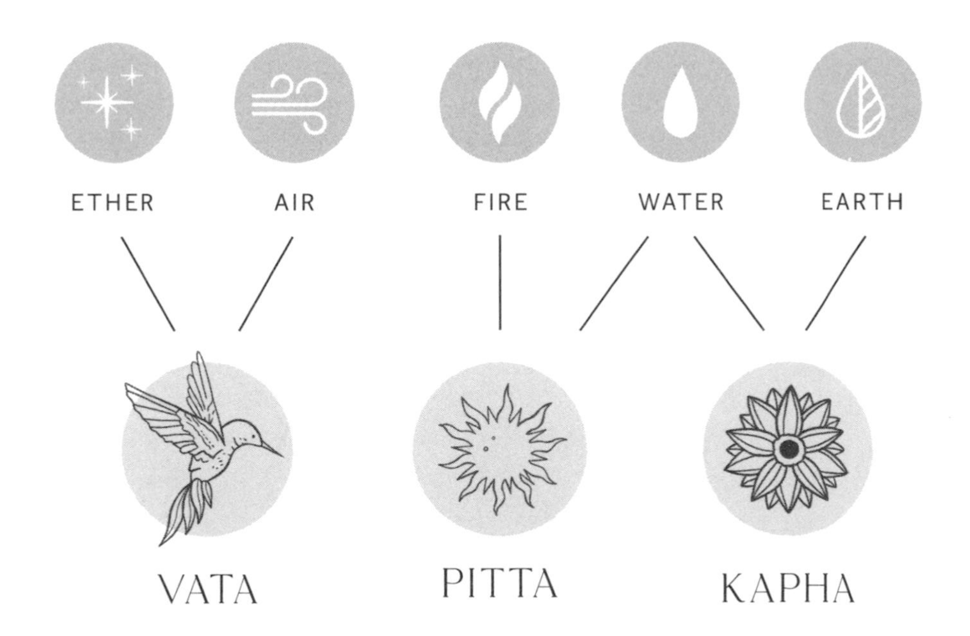

Like Increases Like, Opposites Balance: Twenty Gunas

Ayurveda uses a simple equation to guide you toward a state of equilibrium: "Like increases like, opposites balance." "Like increases like" advises, for instance, that if you feel cold and you drink something cold, you will feel colder. "Opposites balance" directs that if you feel cold and you drink a hot beverage, you will move toward a state of more internal symmetry. If you're feeling heavy in your body and mind, what can you do to bring in the quality of lightness? If you're feeling dry, what foods can you eat or what self-care practices can you do that will support you in counteracting that arid sensation? Ayurveda's equation encourages you to step out of established habits and become aware of your current experience of balance or dis-ease, in order to make the moment-to-moment choices that invite you to thrive.

In chapter 3 we'll talk more deeply about three major qualities of nature, called the *maha gunas* in the Vedic literature. Within those major gunas, Ayurveda recognizes twenty minor gunas—ten qualities and their opposites, which balance each other out—that exist everywhere in our environment: in our bodies, our minds, our activities, our food and drink, and anything else in material existence. The following list of paired qualities is a foundational Ayurvedic tool, and as you embark on your journey as an Ayurveda mama, it can be useful to review the twenty gunas each morning to notice what qualities you are feeling in your body and mind—then invite the opposite quality through your dietary and lifestyle choices to create a state of ease and connection.

Heavy ♦ Light

Dull ♦ Sharp

Cold ♦ Hot

Oily ♦ Dry

Smooth ♦ Rough

Solid ♦ Liquid

Soft ♦ Hard

Static ♦ Mobile

Big/Gross ♦ Subtle

Cloudy ♦ Clear

VATA DOSHA: AIR + ETHER

Vata is the energy of air and ether. When you think of the air and ether elements, do you think hot or cold? Heavy or light? Moist or dry? It is quite intuitive, actually! Vata is cold, light, dry, mobile, subtle, and irregular. Vata is responsible for your energy and movement as well as for nerve impulses, breath, speech, circulation, and many aspects of digestion.

When vata is balanced it brings with it creativity, spontaneity, and enthusiasm. From an excess of these qualities—for example, too much cold food, a cold and dry climate or environment, too much light food, excess talking, too much fast-paced exercise or travel—an imbalance of vata is born. This imbalance breeds fear, anxiety, and nervousness as well as physical symptoms such as bloating, gas, constipation, nausea, and fatigue.

The late fall and early winter months are governed by vata dosha. When you observe nature during that time, you can see that the leaves are starting to dry up; there is more coolness, and more wind in the atmosphere. Because there is more vata in the environment, you will also be affected by the predominance of the air and ether elements and the qualities that come from them. Thus, take extra precautions during the fall and winter months to balance vata dosha.

In an article for *Yoga Journal* titled "Intro to Ayurveda: Understanding the Three Doshas," Scott Blossom, a traditional Chinese medical practitioner and Ayurvedic consultant, offers this overview of vata dosha:

> Vata types tend to be thin and lanky. They are very mentally and physically active and enjoy creative endeavors, meeting new people, and traveling to new places. When they are balanced, vatas are flexible, have lively imaginations, and are original thinkers. When imbalanced they can get anxious, ungrounded, and can seem "flaky" about fulfilling commitments, sticking to a routine, and completing projects. They tend to run cold and dry and enjoy warm, humid weather.
>
> It's common for vata types to experience cold hands and feet, constipation, dry skin, and cracking joints. The influence of the air element in their constitution causes their energy, mood, and appetite to fluctuate dramatically. For this reason, vata types often fail to eat and sleep regularly, swinging from eating heavy foods to ground and sedate themselves, or ingesting stimulants like coffee and sugar to sustain intense physical or mental activity. Insomnia and low immunity are very common problems for the sensitive vata person.*

---

* Scott Blossom, "Intro to Ayurveda: Understanding the Three Doshas," *Yoga Journal*, January 21, 2021, https://www.yogajournal.com/lifestyle/health/intro-ayurveda/.

Whether or not you are generally a vata type, vata is the most important dosha to observe during pregnancy and postpartum. (You should also pay close attention to vata when you are preparing for pregnancy, as preconception is a time where you want to feel nourished, stable, deeply trusting, and supported—all things that you will experience when vata is balanced.) Vata especially governs the first trimester, where there is rapid cell separation and growth, though it is also responsible for the expansion and intense transformation happening inside the mother's body throughout pregnancy. During this time of constant internal movement and change, vata tends to go out of balance quite easily. Excess vata dosha—too much of dry, light, mobile, cool, or clear qualities—may lead to a pregnant mama experiencing constipation, dry skin, nervousness or anxiety, absentmindedness, or difficulty sleeping. An imbalance of vata is also one of the potential causes of disruption in the embryo, early miscarriage, ectopic pregnancy, hemorrhage, eclampsia, and a long, difficult labor. To balance vata, try to bring in the opposite qualities—warm, heavy, moist, stable, and regulated—when planning your meals, your self-care, your workouts, and your daily rhythm.

Watch for the following cues that your vata is out of balance:

PHYSICAL SIGNS

Dry, cracking skin and joints

Dry nails and hair

Gas and bloating (often from dryness in colon)

Constipation

Low back pain, nerve pain, twitches

Fatigue, exhaustion, depletion

MENTAL AND EMOTIONAL SIGNS

Insomnia, restlessness

Inability to focus, scattered thinking

Rapid speech, lost train of thought

Fear, anxiety, nervousness

Feelings of ungroundedness

Feelings of loneliness, isolation

CAUSES OF VATA IMBALANCE

Excess vata dosha can be traced to specific qualities in diet and lifestyle. For instance, vata may go out of balance if a pregnant mama is eating foods that are overly dry, light, cold, rough, or "mobile" (such as raw food, crackers, rice cakes, caffeine, cooling foods such as coconut or cucumber). Having irregular meal times, skipping meals, or eating without full attention on food can also cause excess vata. Living in a cold or dry climate or being in the dryness of the fall or the chill of winter months, traveling too frequently, engaging in excessive movement and talking (or excessive, fast, intense exercise), or being overstimulated by the sensory environment (with lights that are too bright, sounds that are too loud, an overload of screen time, and so on) can likewise send vata into imbalance.

BRINGING VATA INTO BALANCE

The key words to keep in mind for bringing vata into balance are *nourishment*, *warmth*, and *rhythm*. In your diet, these qualities can be achieved in the following ways:

Favor sweet, sour, and salty flavors.

Eat in a peaceful environment.

Eat mindfully; dine quietly or silently.

Avoid caffeine.

Avoid dry, raw, cooling, and cold foods.

Have most of your meals be warm, cooked, and grounding, made from oily and nourishing foods that are easy to digest.

Only eat when you're actually hungry at regular times throughout the day, without snacking (if you do need a snack, opt for a juicy fruit, a few soaked nuts, or a blended soup with digestive spices like black pepper, ginger, cumin, and fennel).

You can also increase your experience of nourishment, warmth, and rhythm by paying attention to self-care and exercise. When you notice signs of excess vata dosha, slow your life down! And try the following activities and lifestyle adaptations to bring vata back into balance:

Reduce sensory stimulation (lower lights, reduce volume, minimize screen time).

Create a quiet environment before bedtime.

Find routine and rhythm with regular waking, eating, and sleeping times.

Do exercises such as belly breathing; long exhalations/sighs (to activate the parasympathetic nervous system, allowing for relaxation), or alternate-nostril breathing (see page 22).

Perform *abhyanga* (self-massage with sesame oil) in the mornings, twenty minutes before your shower (see page 66).

Take baths.

Do slow, rhythmic, stabilizing, and grounding exercises, such as hatha yoga, swimming, tai chi, or walking (especially in nature).

Alternate-Nostril Breathing (*Nadi Shodhana*)

Alternate-nostril breathing (*nadi shodhana*) is a stabilizing breathing technique (*pranayama*) with the following benefits:

Improves ability to focus the mind

Supports lungs and respiratory functions

Restores balance in the left and right hemispheres of the brain

Clears the energetic channels

Rejuvenates the nervous system

Balances the hormones

Removes toxins

Settles stress

1. Take a comfortable and tall seat, making sure that your spine is straight and your heart is open.
2. Relax your left palm comfortably into your lap and bring your right hand just in front of your face. (Reverse "right" and "left" in these instructions if your dominant hand is your left hand.)
3. With your right hand, bring your pointer finger and middle finger to rest between your eyebrows, lightly using them as an anchor. The fingers you will be actively using are the thumb and ring finger.
4. Close your eyes and take a deep breath in and out through your nose.
5. Close your right nostril with your right thumb. Inhale through the left nostril slowly and steadily.
6. Close your left nostril with your ring finger, open your right nostril, and release the breath slowly through the right side.
8. Inhale through the right side slowly.
9. Close your right nostril and open your left nostril. Release the breath slowly through the left side.
10. Repeat for five to ten cycles, allowing your mind to follow your inhales and exhales.

Steps 5 through 9 represent one complete cycle of alternate-nostril breathing. If you're moving through the sequence slowly, one cycle should take you about thirty or forty seconds. Move through five to ten cycles when you're feeling stressed, anxious, or in need of a reset button.

Tip: Consistency is helpful; try to match the length of your inhales and exhales. For example, you can start to inhale for a count of five and exhale for five. You can slowly increase your count as you refine your practice.

PITTA DOSHA: FIRE + WATER

You can recognize pitta when you see the qualities of oily, penetrating or sharp, hot, light, malodorous, spreading, and liquid. According to Ayurveda, this is the dosha responsible for all transformation. Pitta is the force behind your ability to digest, learn, and grow from your life experiences as well as the ability to digest your food.

> Because pitta is a combination of fire and water, especially in the summer months, be mindful of the excess fire energy that is already in the environment.

Healthy pitta is responsible for clarity of perception and focus in the mind. It governs intelligence and the ability to understand. Someone with a lot of pitta in their prakruti will be disciplined, courageous, passionate, and inspiring when balanced.

Scott Blossom describes the pitta dosha constitution in this way:

> Pitta types are dominated by the fire element, which makes them innately strong, intense, and irritable. They tend to have a medium build and endurance with powerful musculature. They often have freckled skin that easily reddens in the sun, during exercise, massage, and when blushing.
>
> They are strong willed and good at doing what they think is right. They approach work and play with the same intensity and

competitiveness. They are natural leaders and quick learners whose ability to easily comprehend and master new skills and concepts can make them judgmental or impatient toward people they feel are slower or less focused than themselves.

They have strong digestion and intense appetites, both for food and challenges. If they miss a meal they are likely to become grumpy and may take a "bite" out of somebody instead. It is common for them to suffer from health conditions such as inflammation, rashes, acne, and loose stool. For balance, pittas need to manage their "fiery" tendencies, channeling them in productive ways and learning to recognize their destructive power.*

During your second trimester you may experience more of the qualities that come with an excess of pitta dosha, though a pitta imbalance can show up any time during pregnancy. The changes in metabolism and increased bodily heat due to pitta (hot, sharp, light, penetrating, or oily qualities) may also lead to irritability, anemia, morning sickness, nausea, heartburn, indigestion, bleeding tendencies, or trouble falling asleep.

Watch for the following cues that your pitta is out of balance:

PHYSICAL SIGNS

Inflammation (any "-itis")

Skin rashes, hives, acne, sunburn, poison ivy that spreads, bug bites that become inflamed

Heartburn, sour burps, acid indigestion

Loose stools

Ulcers

Hemorrhoids

Burning, irritated, itchy, bloodshot eyes

MENTAL AND EMOTIONAL SIGNS

Anger, frustration, irritation, agitation, impatience

Overcompetitiveness

Tendency to be overly critical, judgmental

Propensity toward being manipulative and controlling of others

* **Blossom, "Intro to Ayurveda."**

CAUSES OF PITTA IMBALANCE

Excess pitta can result from a diet that includes eating excessively oily, spicy, and penetrating foods; eating while angry; or drinking coffee, black tea, or alcohol. Lifestyle-associated reasons for pitta imbalance include living in a hot climate or being in the heat of summer months; being in the active middle years of adulthood; being overscheduled (in professional or personal life); having exposure to loud, aggressive sensory input (like violence on TV); or engaging in highly intense interactions including arguing, gossiping, manipulating, or debating. The pitta dosha also goes out of balance because of exercising in a way that is intense, aggressive, or overly competitive; practicing fitness activities in hot, humid environments; or exercising during the hottest time of day.

BRINGING PITTA INTO BALANCE

The key words to keep in mind for bringing pitta into balance are *cooling*, *calming*, and *content*. In your diet, these qualities can be achieved in the following way:

Favor nourishing, cooling, simple yet filling foods (summer harvest foods or foods that are sweet, bitter, or astringent).

Avoid caffeine, alcohol, spicy foods, fried foods.

Eat in a peaceful environment.

You can also try the following activities and lifestyle adaptations to bring pitta back into balance:

Volunteer or perform acts of generosity (this helps you get out of self-centeredness).

Meditate daily.

Avoid overbooking your social or professional schedule.

Listen to calming music.

Take time to rest every day.

Laugh and smile more.

Find ways to cool down: do self-massage with coconut oil; enjoy a cool foot bath; take a cool shower; walk on the cool grass.

Do intermediate or gentle yoga (during the cooler time of day).

Do exercises such as belly breathing, long exhalations, alternate-nostril breathing (see page 22), or the cooling breath (see below).

Go swimming, spend time in nature, relax in the shade.

Cooling Breath (*Sitali*)

"Cooling breath" (Sanskrit: *sitali*) is a pranayama that can be practiced on an empty stomach while in a comfortable seated position. Stick your tongue out and roll the lateral edges upward to form a tube. Inhale through the curled tongue, and exhale normally through the mouth.

KAPHA DOSHA: EARTH + WATER

Earth and water are the elements with the most density. When you think of these elements, you may think of the qualities of heavy, slow, cool, oily, dull, smooth, cloudy, soft, and stable. The common translation of *kapha* is "that which binds things" or "that which holds things together." Kapha is the lubricating factor in the body, which brings the necessary moisture to the brain, gastrointestinal tract, sense organs, joints, and skin. It is associated with the mucosal lining, or the myelin sheath, that protects the nervous system and is responsible for carrying hormones throughout the body. It is responsible for all nourishment in general.

When kapha is balanced according to your prakruti, you will experience contentment, thoughtfulness, and generosity as well as the feeling of being nourished, stable in your body and mind, and safe. Kapha dosha supports memory, emotional calm, mental and physical endurance, and it allows you to feel deeply, to empathize, and to be patient and compassionate.

Scott Blossom summarizes the kapha constitution this way:

> Kapha types have strong frames and are naturally athletic as long as they are exercising regularly to manage their tendency to gain weight. The influence of the earth and water elements makes them innately stable, compassionate, and loyal. They appreciate doing

things in a methodical, step-by-step manner, and prefer a regular routine in their personal and professional lives.

When imbalanced they can become unmotivated, stubborn, and complacent even when change is necessary. Their metabolism tends to be slow and their appetite for both food and stimulation is less intense than vata or pitta types. They benefit from exposing themselves to new environments, people, and occasionally fasting.*

During pregnancy, a pregnant mama's increase in bulk—especially later in pregnancy—is due to (and can lead to) excess kapha: slow, heavy, dull, sluggish, cloudy, cool, and oily qualities. This may contribute to excess weight gain, fluid retention, excess congestion, yeast infections, or excess sleep. Kapha imbalance is most noticeable during the third trimester, when baby is accumulating their fatty tissues and you, mama, may start to feel like a little whale yourself! It is not uncommon to feel more cloudy, tired, and inwardly focused in the last few weeks of a pregnancy.

Watch for the following cues that kapha is out of balance:

PHYSICAL SIGNS

Cold, cough, congestion; excess mucus and phlegm

Springtime seasonal allergies

A heavy feeling in the stomach, sluggish digestion, lack of appetite

Obesity and weight gain

Water retention, swelling, puffiness

Excessive sleeping

Yeast conditions

Lymphatic disorders

MENTAL AND EMOTIONAL SIGNS

Lethargy, depression, lack of motivation (feeling stuck, hopeless, or having heavy emotions)

Feelings of attachment or greed, hoarding

Stubbornness

Having a hard time saying no; being overly passive

* **Blossom, "Intro to Ayurveda."**

CAUSES OF KAPHA IMBALANCE

Excess kapha can be traced to a diet of heavy, dense, thick, oily, sticky, or cold foods; to overeating; or to a habit of eating to offset emotions (like indulging in sweets when depressed). Kapha also becomes imbalanced by living in cool and wet climates and during the cool and damp of spring months. A person's kapha time of life is considered to be the early or childhood years. Excess kapha also results from a lifestyle that is sedentary, lacks variety, or does not have enough physical or mental stimulation. Along the same lines, too little exercise and movement, exercise that is too slow, and exercise that does not have enough heat and circulation can contribute to an imbalance of kapha.

BRINGING KAPHA INTO BALANCE

The key words to keep in mind for bringing kapha into balance are *drying*, *stimulating*, and *expressing*. In your diet, these qualities can be achieved in the following way:

Favor light, simple, cooked foods (spring harvest foods; foods that are bitter, astringent, or pungent; steamed or grilled veggies; dry grains such as millet, barley, and quinoa; and spices such as black pepper, ginger, and cayenne).

Eat in a loving environment.

Include some caffeine in your diet if you wish (black tea, black coffee).

Avoid heavy foods including meat, wheat, sugar, and dairy.

Eat at regular mealtimes without snacking.

You can also increase the qualities of drying, stimulating, and expressing in your life through adjustments to daily behavior including self-care and exercise. Try the following activities and lifestyle adaptations to bring kapha into balance:

Go to bed early and get up before sunrise; don't take daytime naps.

Add variety! Seek out mental and physical stimulation.

Focus on nonattachment in daily life.

Listen to enlivening music.

Do intermediate to vigorous yoga (incorporating movement that is heating and circulating; *vinyasa*, twists, arm balances).

Engage in warming activities such as walking, hiking, dancing, or jogging.

Treat yourself to dry, brisk, exfoliating massage.

Take cold showers.

Receive fast and deep massage with sesame oil.

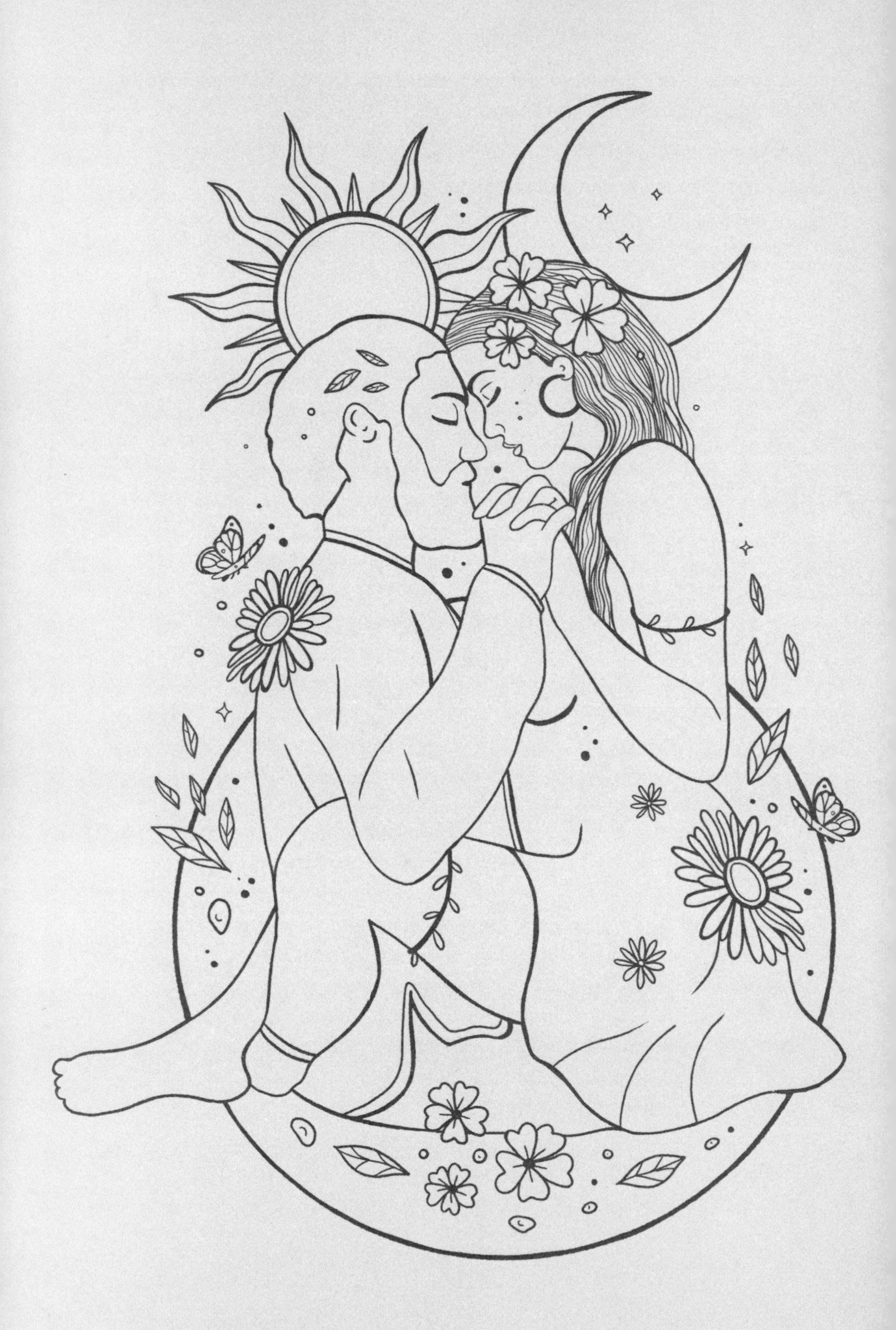

Conscious Conception

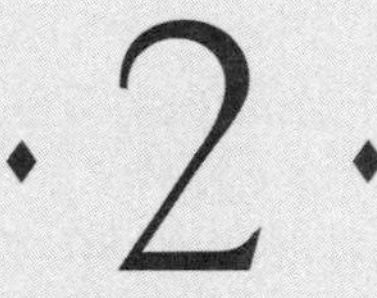

The Ayurvedic ideal goes far beyond merely conceiving. Instead, the emphasis is on creating a child who is mentally, physically, emotionally, and spiritually healthy—a wise and well-rounded child who will contribute to society and become an enlightened citizen.

—Maharishi Ayurveda

Ayurveda teaches that the presence of life is what allows the embryo to grow and transform into a fetus, and then a child. Without life, matter is in a state of dormancy. When consciousness enters matter, you can see all the symptoms of life: birth, growth, maintenance, the ability to procreate, disease (or dwindling), and eventually death. Ayurveda teaches that at the moment of conception the soul enters into mama's womb, and that the physical, mental, and emotional body of the baby begins to form. Thus, Ayurveda emphasizes the value of preparation before conception, as well as intention during conception to call in a soul who will bring more light and goodness into the world by welcoming them with that same energy.

The physical strength of the parents three or four months before and at the moment of conception determines a large part of the foundation of health or dis-ease for the baby. The parents' mental state is a foundation for the baby's overall state of mind. And the parents' spiritual connection (or disconnection) determines the soul who will come in, depending on where the soul is on their own spiritual journey.

From an Ayurvedic standpoint, the process of a woman bringing a life into the world with intention is one of treating herself like a plant in a garden, with four aspects to consider in preparation for conception: the field, the seed, the season, and the water.

Ayurveda teaches that a woman is the channel through which the soul of a new life arrives. Women carry within them the "field" of the uterus, which lives in the larger field of their body, mind, and emotions. The space that a woman lives in, her relationship with her partner, her work, her community, and the planet all make up the greater context of the field that she needs to cultivate with deeper intention. The health of all of these aspects of her life influence the field of her uterus, and therefore, they are all important when considering conception.

Attention to the "seed" is attention to the health of the egg and the sperm. We know that the menstrual cycle, and therefore fertility, is negatively affected by stress, hormonal imbalance, poor diet, environmental toxicity, low body fat, and more. Ayurveda looks at how all these different components of a woman's life might affect her eggs and reproductive organs as well as how the lifestyle of a baby's father affects the quality and quantity of sperm. Stress causes us to clench, which hinders the free flow of *prana* (vitality, life force) and causes stagnation in the body, leading to dis-ease. Part of preparing for conception involves addressing any disorders of the reproductive system such as irregular periods (often because of stagnation or not enough nourishment), ovarian cysts, uterine fibroids, and so on through proper diet, lifestyle practices, and herbal support, which will vary from person to person. Ayurveda thus suggests a cleansing period followed by a rebuilding (or nourishing) period prior to conceiving.

The "season" refers to assessing a time for conception based on the parents' time of life, determining the proper time in the menstrual cycle, and following guidance for living and eating in accordance with the time of year so that the doshas stay balanced. Ayurveda also assesses the season, the phase of the moon, the environment (literally, the room!) that this soul will be called into, as well as the state of consciousness of the parents at the moment of conception.

Last, the "water" is the Ayurvedic approach to the ways in which a woman nourishes herself. The modern love affair with intensity, stress, activity, drive, and ambition oftentimes gets in the way of a woman's ability to receive, and thus to conceive. A woman who has too many stress hormones and not enough nourishment may need to slow down, relax, and really focus on self-care practices that allow her to feel softer, grounded, and cared for.

♦

Through the ancient yet practical lifestyle science of Ayurveda, you learn how to engage with life consciously: how to step into every experience with clarity, wisdom, and intention. This is a dynamic integration of doing everything you can to prepare an ideal environment to welcome a child into but also softening just enough so you do not become rigid within the timing and the rituals. The goal is to trust that, ultimately, there is Divine timing and a bigger plan than your own.

The guidelines in this chapter offer ways to cultivate the field of your body, your consciousness, and different aspects of your life in preparation for conception. Along with dietary disciplines that can assist you in cultivating a strong seed and information to guide you in choosing the right timing for inviting a child into your life, the chapter presents different rituals from the ancient science of Ayurveda that you can use to invoke intention and auspiciousness for the process of procreation. These guidelines are not only for preconception and conception; throughout pregnancy this same energy can be put into the cultivation of your body and your baby's life as you nurture the little soul that is growing in the womb.

PREPARING YOUR CONSCIOUSNESS

Your consciousness can be compared to a mirror. It reflects the impressions that have come in through your senses and the desires that stem from them. If you see a red convertible and really like it, it creates an impression in your mind, and then a desire to have it. Your activities then become motivated by your desire. Ideally, however, rather than your consciousness reflecting the world outside of you, through spiritual practices, your consciousness begins to reflect the pure nature of your soul. When your consciousness reflects your soul, rather than being moved by what you want or don't want, like or don't like (raga and dvesha), your only motive is the desire to serve. Your will becomes aligned with Divine will, and all your activities reflect that connection.

The great teacher of Bhakti yoga Srila Prabhupada gives the metaphor of a mirror that is covered by dust. When you look into that mirror, rather than seeing yourself, all you see is the dust! The dust is compared to the layers and layers of false identifications that have covered your *real* identity: the roles that you play, the job that you have, the heartbreaks and the joys, the pleasures and the pain, the past experiences that have shaped and molded you. These create a "personality" that you now identify with, as well as an endless stream of desires that you actively pursue. You have forgotten who you really are.

Yoga and Ayurveda teach that *you* are not what has happened to you. *You* are not your mind; *you* are not the temporary roles that you play; *your* value is not defined by your status or position; *you* are not the color of your skin or even the body that you are in. Your culture or ancestry may bring deep meaning into your life, though *who you really are* isn't actually touched by any of it. *You* are the one that is seeing through your eyes, hearing through your ears, and smelling through your nose. *You* are the spark of life that gives consciousness to form. The actualization of material desires (desires satisfied by matter) will not ultimately satisfy your soul. You are a pure spirit with the potential of becoming an instrument of the greatest love possible. How can you clear the dust so that you can see who you really are?

It's you and me forever, little one.
And the tears started flowing
just as the rain falls outside of my window
from my heart,
down my cheeks,
onto my belly.

Nothing lasts forever in this world.

I already love you so much.
And I'm already preparing for the little goodbyes
that come with a love so deep.

And it is heartbreaking and beautiful
all at once.

I pray that you know who you really are,
little one.
Beyond the body and mind,
beyond the circumstances and past experiences.
I pray you know who you are
so you do not have to grieve the pain of loss
in the ways that I do.

I pray you know who you really are
so that the love that you give
and the love you receive
is without conditions.

I remember sitting on a rock on the Ganges River this past January
as two of my dear friends offered the ashes of their brother
into the river.

The final destination
for all of us—
whether it is returning to the river
or returning to the earth
or the soul making its way back home.

When will I take this spiritual life seriously?
When will I understand that life is so fleeting
and every moment is so precious and best utilized
in the service
and remembrance
of God?

I flashed forward to the day that my ashes will be
delivered into the current of mother Ganges.

And I saw you, little soul, putting them in.

The cycles and rhythms of life.

It is heartbreaking
And so beautiful
All at once.

YAMAS AND NIYAMAS

In the Yoga Sutras, Patanjali outlines an eight-limbed, step-by-step path for purifying the body and the mind, leading to self-realization and lasting fulfillment. The first two steps of this path are guidelines—restraints and observances—called the *yamas* and the *niyamas*, which outline how to act in the world and what practices to do to purify the mind so that we may experience real happiness. The lifestyle aspect of the five yamas and five niyamas are a great way to cultivate a supportive consciousness for the journey of motherhood. They are guardrails to help keep us living in right relationship with ourselves, with others, and with the world as we move toward the awakening of our spiritual nature.

Many people may think that boundaries or parameters will cheat you out of freedom. When you become aware of what the parameters are protecting you from, you realize that they actually enhance your freedom! For example, you may have boundaries around what you eat so that you do not get sick. You don't eat foods that you're allergic to, which ultimately enhances your experience of health.

You begin to recognize that the journey toward real inner freedom takes a commitment to identifying with the part of you that is steady beyond your mind and body; you are otherwise bound by desires that control you. Inner peace comes from a lifestyle dedicated to the process of self-realization. Vedic traditions had parameters that were built into the culture; the Vedic texts recommend certain values as ideals to hold on to because they keep your train on the track, so to speak, and your consciousness fixed in the right place.

By living a life devoted to these higher values, your mind becomes situated in *sattva*—that is, purity, goodness. You begin to live with more clarity, from a place deeper than the ever-changing mind and emotions.

The yamas and niyamas help in managing your life energy, balancing your outer life and your inner development. They help you to see yourself with compassion and awareness and guide you toward leading a conscious, spiritual life. They clean up your life, in a way, so that you are not full of guilt, shame, and toxins—and you can start to gain some momentum on this very, very deep path. The yamas and niyamas are about living in integrity with your true Self. Living according to these principles is about living your life in a better way, and thus becoming an example for your little one.

THE FIVE YAMAS

The yamas lay out guidelines about how to live and interact in relationship to other beings and the world.

AHIMSA

The first yama, *ahimsa*, calls for noninjury, or nonharming; it requires the awareness and practice of nonviolence in thought, speech, and action. Ahimsa advocates the practices of compassion, love, understanding, patience, self-care, and worthiness on the deepest level.

Ahimsa is the fundamental acknowledgment of the soul within all beings—the understanding that wherever there is life, there is a soul, whether in the body of a human, a grasshopper, a tree, or a blade of grass. The different bodies in which the soul can reside are many. Each body has certain abilities and certain limitations. The quality of the indwelling soul, however, is the same for all of us.

But recall that out of the millions of species of life on this planet, the thing that separates humans from all other animals is the ability to choose. Rather than being pushed by your past or pulled by your self-satisfying desires, you can establish your identity as a pure spirit soul and move through life making decisions from that deepest place, where we are all united. Rather than making choices that may satisfy your own senses but bring harm to another, you can choose to live with a broader perspective and allow all your actions to be an expression of compassion. When established in the Self, all your choices are ahimsa—not just nonviolent, but compassionate. You understand that all beings are pure spirit, deserving of love, compassion, and life, regardless of the body that they are temporarily inhabiting or the conditions and circumstances that have shaped them to act in certain ways.

How can you live with more compassion? How can you be more compassionate toward yourself? What might you start or stop doing, buying, or eating if you were living in alignment with ahimsa?

SATYA

Satya means truthfulness or living an honest life. Are there little white lies? Exaggerations? Excuses? Satya is taking responsibility, or accountability, for your life and living a life of integrity.

Sat means eternal, which means that in order for something to be Truth, it must have been true in the past, is true in the present, and will be true for all of time to come. In my late teens, I started seeking Truth: the big, capital-letter-T Truth. I saw that so many people and so many spiritual traditions had *their* truth, which too often negated the truth of another. I felt that real Truth had to be so big, so great, so vast that it could hold within it all truths, without making any one wrong.

There is an underlying Truth that pervades all of reality. This Truth is the essence of all spiritual traditions, and what all real religion points us toward.

Yes, satya means not telling lies. But more important, it means living in alignment with Truth. You practice satya when your thoughts, words, and actions stem from that deepest place of *being*; situated in that which is sat, that which is eternal (the soul), without attachment to results or aversion to circumstance. Satya calls for living from a deeper place than thinking, being, or doing from your temporary likes and dislikes. It is living deeper than seeking lasting happiness in a temporary world. It is establishing values based on a Truth that is beyond convenience and preference.

Think of ways that you are living out of alignment with your values. It can be something as simple as "I don't recycle and I'd like to," "I eat meat, though I don't believe it is kind," "I don't meditate each day, though I know I'd feel better if I did." Examine those misalignments and then act: start recycling, stop eating meat, meditate. Live from a deeper place than your likes or dislikes. Live bigger than convenience. You will feel empowered when you start living from a place of integrity; when how you act is aligned with how you feel, which stems from a more enlightened place of thinking, born from a deeper way of being.

Surround yourself with people who are servants of Truth, living a life of integrity, and you will learn how to be as they are.

ASTEYA

Asteya refers to the virtue of "nonstealing": everything has been given to you by nature; nothing is really yours. How can you utilize everything that you have, including your thoughts, your time, and your body, in service to the Source of all that is?

If you knew that you would be given everything that you need, where would be the need to take more? Mother Nature provides enough for everyone's needs, though not for everyone's greed. If you trusted that you would always be provided for, you would take only what you needed. You wouldn't buy things just because they were on sale or take something just because it was free. If you knew that you were always taken care of, you would be able to discern what is rightfully yours, and what should be left for someone else, or passed on.

Asteya means not taking what is not yours, or what is not freely offered. Stealing can manifest in obvious ways but also in more subtle ways, as in taking people's time and energy. You can steal unwittingly when you are not grounded, when you are not seated in your Self. This can show up as demanding energy from the same person over and over again, rambling, complaining, or asking too many questions. Make sure that you are not asking for too much or giving too much. This is where healthy boundaries come in. Every interaction should be balanced—treated as a co-creation.

You can apply asteya by honoring your teachers and recognizing that everything you are and everything you know has been given to you by someone else. You learned it from a relationship or an experience, or you heard it from a teacher. When you acknowledge this, you remain humble, and humility is the soil in which gratitude grows. Everything that you have is a gift.

BRAHMACHARYA

Brahmacharya translates as "that which brings you back to Source"; it refers to energy management and the practice of controlling your senses so that your senses do not control you.

All of us can be dragged about by desires, by wanting to feel something (taste, smell, see, hear something). We are pulled toward an experience because we think it will bring us the pleasure we are seeking, when what we actually seek is the pleasure that is inherent within the Truth of who we are.

When you are disconnected from yourself, your attempts toward happiness are attempts to fill a bottomless void that you are experiencing within your own heart. If you are caught up in your thoughts or distracted doing too many things at once (whether it be a situation as difficult as trying to work at multiple jobs and still have time to parent or something as simple as eating while watching TV), then you miss out on the actual *experience* of your life, and thus feel empty and dissatisfied no matter what you do. When you are engaging in activities to satisfy your senses from a disconnected place within yourself, you will likely choose things that only bring momentary happiness and lead you to feeling even more disconnected than before.

You'll overeat because you aren't allowing yourself to *fully* taste what you're eating. In the same way, you'll oversleep if you aren't being rejuvenated from your sleep. If you don't allow yourself to be nourished by what you allow into your senses then your senses are constantly craving more (more sex, more TV, more food, more sound, sight, taste, touch, smell). You then overindulge, which dulls your senses, meaning that you need *more* in order to satiate. Though in that disconnected state, you will never, ever be satisfied.

As always, it's an inner shift that is necessary—the movement from a distracted way of existing to a more connected way of *being* in your life.

When you are connected to yourself, you make choices that nourish rather than deplete you, and you are present enough to actually allow yourself to be nourished by whatever it is that you choose. You become present enough to not only touch, but *feel*; not only eat, but *taste*; not only listen, but *hear*; not only smell, but *savor*; not only look, but *see*. When you become present to what you are experiencing in the moment—chewing each bite, tasting it fully—you become present enough to *know* when you've had enough. In that way, you are able to maintain balance, and thus an ideal experience of health.

Brahmacharya acknowledges that if the senses are not regulated, they drive your life, your decisions, your relationships, your everything. They end up controlling you. Without trying to starve the senses, yoga guides you toward a lifestyle where you reestablish your Self as the driver, choosing sensory impressions that serve to uplift your experience of life, bringing you closer to your true nature.

Sensory impressions (things that you see, hear, touch, taste, smell) serve if they reconnect and remind you of who you really are. They distract when they bind you into the maelstrom of false identification with the body, mind, and emotions. What are you allowing in? It takes willpower and discipline to choose what serves, rather than what would feel (taste, touch, sound, smell) good right now.

The yoga scriptures say that, of all sensory pleasures, sexual desire is the hardest to regulate. You can see that sex has the incredible ability to create families, though if not regulated—you controlling it, rather than it controlling you—it can also destroy them. Because the sexual act is so powerful—do you know of any other activity in the world that holds the power to create life?!—Ayurveda encourages you to regulate it. Then, rather than being an impulse that needs to be tended to whenever the desire comes, it is something that you enter into with more consciousness and intention.

Yoga guides you toward sense control (or regulation) so that you can stay balanced. If you have already eaten to your full satisfaction when the dessert comes out, you know it would be best for you to not eat any. But the tongue might say otherwise! You might eat the dessert anyway and end up feeling sick. In the same way, overindulgence in any sensual activity will lead to disharmony and depletion. Through regulation, however, you gain the ability to discern what actually serves you in the long run from what would serve your senses immediately.

APARIGRAHA

Aparigraha is nonattachment, nonpossessiveness or nongrasping: loving completely with the willingness to let go, because all things (material) must pass.

Aparigraha is not an attitude of cold-heartedness. Nor is it detachment, and thus disengagement. It is not “this is temporary, so why be attached?” Rather, it is the understanding that matter is always changing; form is always changing. It’s the realization that the body we have is temporary, but while it is here, we should take care of it. It’s awareness that the forms our relationships take are temporary and seeing that as a reason to love that much more deeply while we can.

Rather than making you detached or aloof, being aware of the reality of impermanence helps you to engage more deeply with life and to love more fully in relationships; it invites you to generate gratitude for the multitude of blessings that are here, now. You stop getting caught up or burdened by "what ifs?" "should haves," and "might bes." You instead show up in love. You do your best, without focusing on results. You love and live from a deeper place, not swayed by circumstance (the highs and the lows) because all of it keeps changing. What stays the same?

The soul.

You.

Simple Practices to Uplift

Become conscious of the impressions that you are allowing in through your senses, and as much as possible, allow them to be light and uplifting. What type of music are you listening to? What movies are you watching? What type of food are you eating? All these things have a huge effect on your consciousness, so choose things that bring joy and clarity.

Meditate daily. Mantra meditation is powerful; it is one of the fastest and easiest ways to uplift the mind. (See page 83.)

Start a gentle yoga and pranayama practice to settle your thoughts and become grounded in your body.

Think about the qualities you would like this little soul to embody. Make a list! Be as detailed as possible. How can you embody these qualities more? You will begin to attract this soul into your life.

> The universal character of anyone on any religious or spiritual path—if they are really doing it right, in a deep meaningful way—is that they are going to have common characters and values that are universal: compassion, honesty, self-control, generosity, wisdom, insight. Whether one is a Christian or a Muslim or a Jew or a Hindu or whatever, these are the common values we find in the scriptures and in the lives of the saints. The realized people—a saint could be a mother with three children, or a monk who is traveling around and preaching.
>
> —Radhanath Swami, author, spiritual teacher, and activist

THE FIVE NIYAMAS

The niyamas are about self-regulation—they are positive duties that help you maintain a conducive environment in which to grow. Their practice harnesses the energy generated from the cultivation of the yamas.

SAUCHAM

Saucham is cleanliness and purity. It is said that how a person keeps their home reveals the inner workings of their mind. A clean and clear mind cannot live in a cluttered or dirty home. A cluttered and busy mind is not likely to live in a tidy and clean home! Cleanliness in your mind, body, and surroundings creates the most conducive environment for conscious living and Self-realization.

Purify. Meditate to clear the mental clutter that has accumulated for years and years (and lifetimes) of preference, of false conditionings and identifications, of memories (generally the extremes of what you loved and what you wish never happened). Purify the mind and, naturally, your life will start to clean itself up. Your relationships, your closet, your perceptions will all become clearer.

If your mind is too messy for meditating, then first clean your drawers, then your house, then your car, then start to clean up your diet. Assure that you are showering at least every morning. Upgrade your lifestyle choices. Prioritize self-care. It is amazing how more space in your closet creates more space in your mind, which creates more space in your life.

Then, meditate. Not just to meditate, but to change the way you live, the way you love, the way you consume, the way you eat, and what you listen to. You will notice that it all affects the state of your mind, which in turn creates your entire experience of life. Again, purify. Then you can experience things as they are rather than through the dusty lens created by your past.

SANTOSHA

Santosha means contentment or satisfaction. Your mind tells you that you'll be happy when the world outside of you is the way that you want it to be, and that you'll be sad when the world outside of you is *not* the way that you want it to be. In this way, your happiness is completely controlled by something outside of you—something that you have absolutely no control over—and your other emotions follow suit.

You swing back and forth and up and down on the mental and emotional seesaw, because you are so caught up with this identification with your mind. Thoughts like "I'll be happy if . . ." or "I'll be happy when . . ." can come up in your mind; happiness stays elusive, always one step ahead of where you are now, and you never feel satisfied. You set yourself up so that you can only have peace when the circumstances are just right. But then the circumstances keep on changing.

No peace will ever last when the quest is outside.

There is a deeper way to live.

Your true Self is not swayed by circumstance, only your mind and emotions are. When you identify your Self as deeper than your mind and emotions, you will be satisfied, content, okay—regardless of what is happening outside of you.

Rather than spending your precious moments trying to contort and control the world outside of you or trying to "fix" or change people so they will not trigger your emotional wounds, work on your Self. Work on developing that indwelling connection so that you can be deeply satisfied, and then move through the world from *that* place: beyond the fickleness of the mind, beyond conditioned desire, beyond the ever-changing stream of emotion.

What if you practiced believing that you already have everything you need? What if you practiced feeling that you are enough—that what you know is enough, what you have is enough, and who you are is enough? What if you let yourself be satisfied—as it is, and as you are—right now? What if you accepted rather than resisted reality and then showed up in every situation in a way that uplifts and actually serves? When you are already satisfied, your actions stem from a place of wanting to give rather than wanting to get, and it is truly in giving that you will receive. Let each moment become better because you were there.

TAPAS

Tapas is discipline or austerity. It is the fire between what you want *now* and what you want *most*, between an old habit and a new one. The moment when you crave your first cigarette after deciding to quit or pass by that first coffee shop after giving up caffeine. Every single part of you is wired to reach for the cigarette or to get a cup of coffee. In that moment there is a fire that will transform you . . . if you let it.

Tapas is choosing something different. It is the ability to wait. It is the willingness to sit in the heat, to tolerate the discomfort that arises, not because you want it, but because you know that you need it. It is acknowledging the neuroplasticity of your brain and your ability to rewire old habits in order to build pathways to freedom.

SVADHYAYA

Svadhyaya is Self-study: know who *you* are. Know the highest vision—the highest version—of yourself for this lifetime, and also know who you will be beyond this life. The moment *you* entered into your mother's womb, cells divided and multiplied—and will keep dividing and multiplying, transforming and changing, until, one day, *you* will depart.

Know who you are, beyond your body and mind, your roles and positions. Hear Truth every day. Read, meditate, and learn from Self-realized teachers. Seek shelter in those who know. Knowing your Self is the greatest treasure you will offer the world. By living from that place, you will inspire and remind many others to do the same. When you know who you are, kindness, compassion, truthfulness, sense control, and understanding the temporary nature of this world all come with it. When you know who you really are, you see the soul within all beings, regardless of the body they are inhabiting. You'll show up every moment of your life in a way that ultimately serves.

ISHVARAPRANIDHANA

Ishvarapranidhana is "surrender to the Divine": offering everything that you have and everything that you do to God—because where does it all come from, anyway? Humility is vital on the path: ishvarapranidhana calls for surrendering the idea that you are the controller, the maintainer, and the owner of it all; it calls for letting go of the notion that you know best or know everything and requires opening to the possibility that there is a scope much larger than your own.

Just because you have not seen something does not mean that it is not real.

Would the fish in the tank believe you if you told them of the ocean? Humility is the ability to say, "I don't know, could be!" rather than shutting out a larger perspective than what your limited experience has shown you. When you are humble you are able to recognize someone who has a larger scope than your own, someone who has touched Truth, and you'll have the desire to learn.

When you trust, you can begin to love. When you love, it is natural to put your self-centered desires aside and show up in a way that truly serves. To fully serve means that you have surrendered your own personal will to a much larger one—realizing that you are a part of something greater.

"Thy will, not mine" becomes your life's mantra.

NURTURING YOUR RELATIONSHIP

Whether you are going through the journey of pregnancy with a partner or on your own, having the support of people in your life is invaluable. The field of your relationships serve as a sacred container in which your little one will grow. Before inviting this soul into your life, it is important to cultivate a sense of deep trust, nourishment, and genuine care in your primary relationships, as these are the energies that will nourish your babe.

If you are in a committed partnership, part of the preparation for pregnancy will be to give yourself completely and fully to that other person. The level and depth of commitment required to enter into the parenthood phase of a relationship is profound. To invite a soul into the field of your and your partner's love is a powerful step to take as a couple. When inviting a child into your relationship, the relationship is no longer just about the two of you, but about serving something greater. It is a bonding at a very deep level that requires a container of profound trust, conscious communication, and commitment.

DEALING WITH CONFLICT

Whatever the dynamic (whether it be a mother and daughter, a romantic partnership, or something else), a great relationship does not mean that there are never disagreements. It means that when they do come up, both parties have tools, skills, and the ability to listen, reflect, and grow from whatever arises. A strong parenting relationship will involve a mutual commitment to growth. This will be especially important once your little one arrives, as you are the model for the relationships that they will seek in the future.

It may sound like a lot of pressure, but try to see it as an opportunity to strengthen your commitment; to refine your communication skills; to redefine your need to be "right"; and to cultivate qualities such as patience, forgiveness, steadiness, and gratitude, which you will pass on to your little one through your example. If you are able to practice these things before your baby comes, you will be much better prepared during pregnancy and once baby is here to meet any challenges that will arise in your relationships.

Ayurveda teaches that during pregnancy the mother should always feel happy, and that the partner's only job is to assure her happiness. Remember that the baby experiences everything that mama experiences, so, as much as possible, bathe yourself in uplifting environments, conversations, tastes, sights, and sounds.

I remember during month three of my pregnancy I was feeling really frustrated in one of my primary relationships, and at the same time I was feeling heavy guilt knowing that my baby was experiencing the emotions that I was feeling. I called one of my girlfriends and shared my experience with her, and she offered me the following gem of wisdom:

> It is not about not feeling the other emotions. Your baby needs to know that it is okay to feel what they feel and that they do not have to be happy all the time. How do you move through it? How do you process it? How do you grow from it? What is important is that you teach them, through your example, how to move through emotions as they arise in a healthy way.

She assured me that conflict is nothing to fear and that we should raise our children to know that. Then, rather than avoiding conflict or being afraid when it comes up, they witness and learn how conflict (if dealt with consciously) can be fertile soil for growth and connection.

After the first time my husband and I got into a disagreement in front of our six-week-old baby, we had the discussion about what boundaries to have around that happening again. Is it okay to argue in front of him? We decided that it is okay, as long as we are communicating effectively (which includes listening and reflecting), and as long as we are committed to coming out the other side with more clarity and connection. In this way, we model *real* relationship: there will be bumps and challenging times, but it is nothing to fear. Conflict does not mean that someone is going to get hurt, or shamed, or worse, leave. Conflict is not something to run away from, but rather something to move toward with the intention to understand and move closer together.

Many of us fear conflict because we have seen our own families torn apart by it. We are afraid of arguments, because we fear that it is the end of something: "Dad is going to walk out." "Mom is going to break something." We fear it is going to lead to horrible outcomes because that may have been what we experienced as children. We fear that our children will carry the burden of our disagreements, because we took responsibility for our own parents' separation. We feel that it is not safe to argue, because we never felt safe when our parents argued.

Begin to create guidelines. Build safety around conflict so that your children will know that disagreement does not need to be feared. Learn how to communicate your needs, boundaries, and desires effectively so that your children will learn the same. Raise children who know that with any disagreement there is an end, a solution, and a deepening of love.

BUILDING TRUST

Building trust is the necessary groundwork for a relationship to thrive. Trust is the fertile soil that allows for the seed of commitment to grow deep roots. With every new layer of established trust, you enable a deeper level of commitment.

The foundation of trust is built on the knowing that your partner respects you and genuinely wants what is best for you. Perhaps it is easy for you to trust, or maybe you have a hard time trusting because of past relationship scars, childhood trauma, or in the ongoing experience of a relationship where your partner says something and then does something different. To build or rebuild trust is a process.

Whether trust is at a low point or high point in your relationship, if both of you believe that the character of the other is intrinsically good, trust can be built. You show you are committed to building trust by following through with what you promise to yourself and in your relationship. If you tell your partner that you will be home by a certain time, show up on time.

If you promise quality time, make sure you show up with your full presence. If you tell your partner that you will not talk to your ex, then do not talk to your ex. Follow through on your words.

Trust is practical. Reliability may start with small things, but over time you give energy and life to your relationship with each commitment that you follow through with. More and more trust builds upon the foundation of your previous commitments. When you see someone consistently following through with their commitments, it speaks for itself.

If you have somehow broken the trust in your relationship, you need to be patient. You cannot build anything of value unless there is integrity in the foundation. Would you enter into a building if you did not trust the foundation holding it up? Know that trust is built gradually over time, and the pain caused by breaking it can be devastating.

Whether your breach of trust was something small or something severe, these next steps will help assure, if your partner is willing to forgive you, that you are doing the work necessary in order to reestablish a stable foundation for your relationship.

First, accept responsibility.

Oftentimes when we have broken trust, we give excuses, reverse blame, or even lie about it, which further breaks down trust. Accept responsibility for what you did by stating what your agreement was and how you broke the agreement.

"I told you I would be home by 6 p.m. and I am forty-five minutes late."

Next, acknowledge.

What you did may have caused pain to the person you love. Get into a space of reflecting on how they might feel, whether you agree with them or not. Acknowledge how you can see why your actions may have hurt them.

"I can imagine it being so frustrating waiting for me, especially because you had dinner ready, the table set, and you were looking forward to a really nice evening together."

Then, account.

While still fully accepting responsibility, honestly share what happened. If the breach of trust was that you showed up late, maybe your boss demanded you finish the report before leaving the office, or traffic was horrible and caused you to be late. Maybe something unforeseen came up that you could not avoid, or perhaps you just lost track of time. Accounting is not making excuses, but is simply sharing what happened.

"I was on a call at the office and totally lost track of time."

Now, apologize.

Genuinely apologize for your actions, recognizing how they caused a breakdown in trust.

"I am sorry for coming home late and not acting in alignment with our agreement. I acknowledge how that has the potential to break down your trust in my word."

Finally, amend.

Let them know how you plan to act in the future when something like this comes up, and ask them what they would need to see from you in order to rebuild trust. Do everything in your power to follow through with whatever shared agreements you come to.

"In the future, when we have a date planned, I will be more conscious of the time. Is there anything else that you need from me in order to reinstill that trust?"

When you follow through with shared agreements, you build and rebuild trust in your relationship. Over time, the challenging moments are looked at in hindsight as catalysts for growth and deeper connection, built off shared love and trust.

What if the other person has been responsible for breaking your trust? Broken trust can be crippling for a relationship; it is one of the main reasons relationships come to an end. When you have had your trust broken, you first need to search your heart and take guidance from reliable friends to determine whether you feel confident that you can rebuild trust with this person. If the answer is yes, then move forward with the following steps.

If they have genuinely taken responsibility for their actions and understand their damaging effects, you take the first step toward reestablishing trust. If you are confident that they are sincerely sorry for what they have done, you build confidence in their moral compass: that they know what serves your relationship and what damages it.

The next step is often the most challenging and may take some time, so do not rush it. If you want to move forward, you must be willing to genuinely and fully forgive them and to let go of the past. This often takes a power greater than yours, a higher power that can heal your heart so that it can open again.

If they are not willing to be patient and give you the time that you need to fully forgive them, this can be a warning sign that they may not understand the magnitude of their actions and might break your trust in the future. If they are patient with you, while they work on themselves, and you are able to genuinely forgive them, you can continue the relationship with simple shared agreements and commitments. When they see these commitments as opportunities to gain your trust and you see them following through with them, the process has begun.

Gradually, if you see steady follow-through with commitments, you will be able to trust them with bigger agreements and more vulnerable aspects of yourself. As you trust their character and commitment more and more, you might then be able to envision a long-term committed relationship with them. However, it is not always possible to reestablish trust with someone. Depending on their character and the pain that has been caused, it may not even be healthy to push for it. Rebuilding trust takes sincerity on their end, and the ability to forgive on yours.

WORKING ON CONSCIOUS COMMUNICATION

When you get triggered, how do you process and communicate it so that there is growth? Communication is a skill. It is not something that we are all raised knowing how to do, but it is something that we can learn.

Creating a conscious relationship requires communicating consciously—that is, in a way that invites both parties to take responsibility for their emotions and their actions and allows for both people to feel understood. When you feel understood, you can let down your armor, meet the other person where they are, and grow together. In the same way, when you reflect back to the other person what they have expressed to assure that you've genuinely understood their perspective and then respond in a way that serves to uplift your relationship, it allows your connection to deepen.

To learn skills and techniques for building trust and communicating consciously, I highly recommend reading *Relationships That Work: The Power of Conscious Living* by David B. Wolf and *Nonviolent Communication* by Marshall Rosenberg, listed in the references section at the back of this book.

DEEPENING COMMITMENT

What are you committed to? Knowing what you and your partner are committed to together will create a solid ground for you both to come back to as the inevitable waves wash in. A lasting relationship must be built atop a foundation that lasts.

What assures you that the commitment of your relationship will last, beyond the temporary experience of "I love them because of how they make me feel"? Anyone in a long-term relationship knows that their commitment to each other is not simply based on a feeling. Feelings change. The nature of the mind is that sometimes you like each other and sometimes you don't. Sometimes you are happy, sometimes you are not. Today you might "love" them, and tomorrow you might feel different, yet you stay. Real love lives deeper than the circumstantial feelings. When everything is always changing, what can you depend on? Where is there stability? Commitment invites both you and your partner to connect to the parts of yourselves that are steady even as feelings change.

Ayurveda recognizes that your spiritual connection is the one thing that is steady, as everything else in your life and in the world inevitably shifts, and the Ayurvedic approach emphasizes building a relationship that serves to connect you back to *that* reality. A spiritual relationship is one in which the deepest values are aligned, and in which the deepest commitment is to helping each other awaken to the reality of your soul—the only part of you that is consistent, as everything else changes. To build a love that lasts—because its foundation is built upon the only part of you that is lasting—here are suggestions for deeper commitments you may choose to make in your relationship:

Help each other awaken to the part of you that is unchanging (beyond the body, mind, emotions, and situation).

Learn how to love from that deepest place.

Practice loving, even when it is hard.

Hold space for each other when you forget who you really are and how to act.

Take responsibility for your actions and communicate effectively so that you grow together.

Be honest and transparent because you respect each other.

Acknowledge the parts of yourselves that have been broken by circumstance, and come back the part of you that is (and has always been) whole.

Help each other learn how to love God, acknowledging that the most profound experience of relationship is when you are instruments of that love and that compassion in the world.

Make each other happy, knowing that ultimately your happiness is not the other's responsibility, though real joy is experienced in loving exchanges (both in giving and receiving love).

Live a life of service, knowing that that is where real happiness comes from.

Questions to Explore as a Couple

Before your little one comes, it is invaluable to sit down and discuss your vision for becoming parents, sharing ideas about what that might look like. This assures that you and your partner are both on the same page about building this next part of your life.

What is your intention for inviting this little soul into your lives?

How do you envision yourself as a mother/father?

Practically speaking, what will your day-to-day life look like? Will one of you take primary responsibility for your child as the other one works? Will it be a 50/50 split? Will there be anyone else supporting with childcare?

How do you see yourselves raising this little one? What values (spirituality, purpose, nature, health, family, discipline) are important?

Are there any habits that you would like to rid yourself of before baby comes?

Are there any mental or emotional patterns that you would like to work on, so as not to pass them on?

Are there any dynamics or past experiences in your relationship that need to be healed?

How might your relationship change?

When and how do you feel most supported by the other?

What fears do you have around becoming a mother/father?

What are you excited about?

PREPARING YOUR BODY

By human adolescence, each female ovary holds 250,000 eggs. Over the course of a woman's lifetime, about four hundred of those eggs will be released.* Each month, in preparation for pregnancy, one egg is released. This "chosen egg" is being prepared for three or four months and slowly making its way through all other eggs toward the top of the ovary.

* https://courses.lumenlearning.com/atd-fscj-childpsychology/chapter/unit-4-foundations-of-child-and-adolescent-psychology.

Ayurvedic medicine is attentive to an understanding that the health (or dis-ease) of the egg, and thus the long-term health (or dis-ease) of the child, is largely established in those three or four months before it is released, based on the mother's diet and lifestyle.

Similarly, Ayurveda emphasizes the importance of a father's dietary and lifestyle choices. It takes about three months for sperm to get from where they are produced to where they are ejaculated—almost exactly the same as the egg maturation period! Consequently, a man's ability to procreate and the health of his sperm, and thus the health of his child, are affected by his diet and the way that he lives.

Ayurveda teaches that there are six bodily tissues—plasma, blood, muscle, fat, bone, and nerve tissue—on which the health of the reproductive tissues—the seventh tissue—are dependent. To the degree that plasma is nourished, blood will be nourished. To the degree that blood is nourished, muscles will be nourished, and so on. The final tissues to be nourished are the reproductive organs.

The health of all of the tissues are dependent on having good digestion, referred to in Ayurveda as *agni*, which controls how well food is assimilated into the body (see more on agni in chapter 8, starting at page 270). Your tissues are literally composed of what you are able to digest and assimilate. The first step in producing healthy sperm and eggs is to ensure digestion is working optimally—a goal achieved through deep internal cleansing to balance the doshas and remove toxins. If it suits your unique circumstance, both parents should begin the following cleanse starting six months before trying to conceive:

Six months before conception: gentle cleansing. Eat an easy-to-digest, whole-food diet that is well cooked. Any of the recipes in chapter 8 will be appropriate for this time. Eliminate—or at least avoid as much as possible—processed foods, dairy, vegetable oils, meat, caffeine, and alcohol. Eating at the same times each day without snacking between meals will support the body's regulation, metabolism, and ability to digest accumulated waste. Regarding digestion, Ayurveda says that how you eat is just as important as what you eat. Take this time to work on being present while eating and chew your food thoroughly so that it is easier to digest.

Five months before conception: more intense cleansing. If a *panchakarma* center is accessible to you, undergo panchakarma for at least two weeks. Panchakarma is an Ayurvedic regimen that includes oil massages, herbal steam baths, and detoxifying Ayurvedic processes and herbs to move any toxicity from the deeper tissues of the body to the gastrointestinal tract, where they will then be eliminated. If panchakarma is not possible, follow a home cleanse routine for two weeks to a month, eating a mono-diet of *kitchari* (see page 294 for the recipe) with well-cooked seasonal veggies and sipping on warm lemon water, ginger tea, or cumin, coriander, and fennel (CCF) tea (see the recipe for CCF tea on page 288) throughout the day. Perform daily oil massages, take baths, and sweat every day.

Four months before conception: gentle cleansing. Ease back into the routine of a gentler cleanse, as in the first month. Minimize or abstain from intercourse. This time of cleansing requires extra energy and reserves. Abstinence is a yogic practice used to conserve physical energy, mental energy, and *ojas* so that a more introspective and clearer mindset is maintained. *Note:* In the practice of Ayurveda, *ojas*, meaning "vigor," is thought to be responsible for strength, health, longevity, immunity, and mental and emotional wellness.

Ashoka Bath

When preparing for conception, Ayurveda recommends bathing in water infused with the herb ashoka. *Ashoka,* which means "remover of sorrow," heals physical and psychological pain associated with your reproductive tract and supports female fertility by promoting healthy ovarian and endometrial tissues. Enjoy an ashoka bath one to three times weekly in the months before trying to conceive. Boil the herbs and draw the bath with intention.

Boil ½ cup of ashoka powder in 5 cups of water, reducing until 3 cups of water remain.

Add to a hot bath and soak in it for at least twenty minutes.

While in the bath, try to suck in the perineum to draw the herbal water and its effects close to the uterus.

Ojas Milk

Ojas is the final product of the digestion of food after it goes through all seven layers of tissue. During the months before conception, milk brewed with ojas-building ingredients is an incredibly nourishing drink for your reproductive organ. Also, once you start trying to conceive, you can bathe, and then drink a glass of this warm milk after intercourse. Saffron is particularly nourishing to the reproductive tract and good for ojas-building.

- 1 cup of milk
- pinch of cardamom
- pinch of saffron
- pinch of ginger powder
- pinch of ground almond powder

Warm the milk on the stove and add the spices and almond powder. Bring to a light simmer (watch that the milk does not foam over the edges of the pot!) for three minutes.

Let cool and add sweetener if you desire. Enjoy warm after your bath.

After a cleanse, the three months prior to conception are focused on rebuilding and deep nourishment. Both parents should aim to follow a diet of organic, fresh, and whole foods rich in prana (vitality, life force) for the remaining three months prior to conception. The following foods and spices are deemed to nourish reproductive tissues, increase ojas, and support fertility (provided that they are digested well):

Spices: saffron, cloves, cardamom, nutmeg, cinnamon, ginger, cumin, ajowan, turmeric

Dairy: ghee (clarified butter), raw butter, cream-top milk, yogurt, paneer (fresh cheese)

Sweeteners: dates, honey, maple syrup, sucanat (unrefined whole cane sugar), jaggery (unrefined brown sugar)

Nuts and seeds: black sesame seeds, pumpkin seeds, soaked almonds, soaked walnuts

Grains and beans: urad dal (black gram dal), mung dal, whole grains

Produce: fresh, local organic juicy fruits and vegetables

In the months prior to conception, avoid consuming substances that diminish ojas: for instance, foods that are highly starchy, antibiotic- and hormone-laden meat and milk, nonfat or low-fat milk, canned foods, foods containing preservatives and other chemicals, artificial sweeteners, MSG, artificial flavoring and coloring, alcohol, caffeine, tobacco, soda, nicotine, trans fats, and refined carbohydrates. You can also reduce your estrogen load by avoiding commercial beauty and oral care products.

Build the plasma and blood. These are the life-giving and nutrient-giving tissues of your body, to the extent that the blood volume increases by almost 50 percent during pregnancy.* Ensure you're staying well-hydrated in a healthy way by consuming juicy fruits, cream-top milk, herbal teas, mineral water, and electrolytes. Eat organic and local foods rich in nutrients. Most women are underfed, undernourished, and overworked. Not eating enough will create hormonal imbalances, increase stress hormones, and down-regulate the thyroid. You can supplement your diet with calcium, iron, vitamin B_{12}, and folate as needed. An organic food-based multivitamin is the easiest source.

Prioritize mineral intake. Minerals are what make your cells run and are the foundation in which your body works. They are the catalyst for your hormones, and without them thousands of enzymatic reactions are compromised. When you don't have adequate levels of certain minerals, specific physiological responses become compromised (like hormone regulation, thyroid function, and digestion). Prioritize your major minerals: magnesium, potassium, sodium, and calcium.

A vata-pacifying diet and lifestyle (as described on pages 21–22 in chapter 1) should be honored preconception to ensure that you will feel nourished, grounded, and ready to receive this new life. (Within the first days of pregnancy, when rapid internal movement begins to take place, a vata-pacifying diet and lifestyle preconception will assure stability in the midst of so much change.)

For women, it is always important to take care of yourself during menstruation and particularly during the preconception months. Follow the Ayurvedic guidelines for that time: avoid traveling; avoid skipping meals; eat foods that are warm, nourishing, and easy to digest; and take real rest as needed during your menstrual cycle.

The following herbs can help offset the effects of stress in the busy lifestyles of today, as well as nourish the deeper tissues of your body:

Ashwagandha. Ashwagandha is a highly rejuvenating herb that both promotes semen production and strengthens the uterus. Its name refers to the strength of a horse, and it acts as a natural aphrodisiac.

---

* https://pubmed.ncbi.nlm.nih.gov/4075604/.

Brahmi. In Ayurveda, *brahmi* is considered the feminine essence of Universal Consciousness. This herb, also known as water hyssop, promotes fertility and supports implantation. It balances all three doshas and all seven tissues in the body, but it is especially known for supporting brain functions and helping to pacify anxiety. Brahmi is beneficial in preconception and pregnancy because it brings the quality of sattva (purity) into your mind and body and relieves symptoms that may be coming from excess pitta. During the postpartum period, it helps in clearing brain fog, otherwise known as "mama mind/ milk mind."

Chyavanprash. *Chyavanprash* is a delicious traditional Indian nutritional jam made from around forty different herbs, ghee, and honey. The main ingredient is *amalaki* (Indian gooseberry, also known as amla), a powerful antioxidant. It has been used in India to promote immunity, strength, and fertility.

Shatavari. *Shatavari* (*Asparagus racemosus*, a type of asparagus root with many uses in Ayurveda) is a powerful fertility-enhancing herb whose name means "she who has a hundred husbands." It can be taken to strengthen the uterus without altering the estrogen balance. *Note:* shatavari is contraindicated for any woman who has a history of any estrogen imbalances, such as cysts, fibroids, or reproductive cancers. In such cases, *guduchi* (*Tinospora cordifolia*, or heart-leaved moonseed) can be used.

Shilajit. *Shilatjit* is rich in fulvic acid which helps to improve your ability to absorb essential nutrients and minerals from food. It also improves digestion, boosts immunity, reduces inflammation, and increases energy levels in your body. Apart from this, shilajit also contains essential minerals (such as iron, selenium, zinc, and calcium).

Triphala. *Triphala* is a blend of three fruits: amalaki, *bibhitaki* (*Terminalia berecilla*), and *haritaki* (*Chebulic Myrobalan*). Along with being a powerful immune enhancer, triphala is considered a *rasayana*—that is, it is a rejuvenator that nourishes all the tissues in the body. Triphala is also used as a detoxifier, as it cleans out the gastrointestinal tract and promotes healthy digestion and elimination, so vital for good health.

See the resources section on page 325 for more information on where to find these herbs.

TIMING OF CONCEPTION AND SEASONAL ADJUSTMENTS

The mental condition of a child depends upon the mental status of his parents at the time he is conceived. According to the Vedic system, therefore, the garbhādhāna-saṁskāra, or the ceremony for conceiving a child, is observed. Before begetting a child, one has to sanctify his perplexed mind. When the parents engage their minds [in connection to their higher power] and in such a state the child is born, naturally good, conscious children come. When the society is full of such good population, there is no trouble from [dysfunctional] mentalities.

—Srimad Bhagavatam Canto 3, chapter 20, verse 28

An Ayurvedic approach to conception emphasizes the importance of appropriate timing. Ayurveda offers an optimal daily rhythm to prepare for pregnancy and also takes into account the ideal time of your life, the time of the month, and the necessity of adapting your lifestyle based on the time of year in order to maintain your best health.

When Ayurveda considers the appropriate time of life for conception, it considers the age of the parents and other factors. Is it a good time in your relationship to have a child, where there is harmony, respect, and love? Is it a good time in your career, where you will have enough time and energy to nourish your little one? Ayurveda suggests that the best biological time of life for conception and pregnancy is between the ages of eighteen and thirty for women and ages twenty-one to forty for men. The traditional understanding is that this is the period when the reproductive tissue, *shukra dhatu*, is fully matured. Although it might be physically easier to conceive during those windows of life, that does not mean that it will necessarily be hard to have a baby later on in life (or easier to raise a baby earlier in life). The guidelines and ideas about daily, monthly, and seasonal rhythms described in this chapter are Ayurvedic approaches to having fertile tissues and the ability to bring a healthy and happy baby into the world even after what would traditionally be considered “peak” biological time.

The Ayurvedic principle of living your life according to the flow of the seasons is called *ritucharya*. *Ritu* means "season" and *charya* means "regimen." An Ayurvedic adage states, "as is the macrocosm, so is the microcosm." In order to maintain balance in your body and mind, your habits, routines, and dietary choices (the microcosm) should have a seasonal rhythm (following the macrocosm)—that is, ebbing and flowing with the time of year. While this idea may at first seem daunting, many people find that the recommended seasonal adjustments come quite naturally and that a few simple changes can dramatically improve your health and sense of well-being while you are trying to conceive.

Using the equation "like increases like" and "opposites create balance," Ayurveda offers ways to stay balanced and precautions to take throughout the seasons. The following pages describe the qualities of each season and explain how to invite the opposites to maintain balance throughout the year. (Of course, because the seasons vary widely from one place to another, as do the qualities that they engender, you may need to make your own location-specific adjustments to this Ayurvedic template.)

LATE WINTER INTO SPRING: KAPHA SEASON

Late winter into spring is kapha season: a time of year characterized by still cool weather and a sense of heaviness from increased moisture in the air. As the sun gets warmer it melts the lingering snow. In the same way, the warmth begins to liquefy accumulated kapha in your body so that it can be eliminated with ease. This process can either be a revitalizing event or can trigger congestion, colds, hay fever, and allergies, depending on your diet and lifestyle during this time.

Toward the end of winter and into spring, you'll want to invite extra lightness, sharpness, dryness, and heat so that you can support your physiology in its natural process of springtime renewal and revitalization. As well as following kapha-pacifying lifestyle habits from chapter 1 (see pages 28–29), favor pungent, bitter, and astringent tastes and eat warm, light foods that are relatively easy to digest. These habits help to balance mucus production, regulate moisture levels, and open the channels of elimination that are critical for purification.

SUMMER: PITTA SEASON

The weather of summer, considered pitta season, is characterized by the hot, light, and sharp qualities. To balance the excess qualities of pitta season, focus on staying cool, mellowing intensity, deepening relaxation, and grounding your energy. During the summer, your body naturally craves light foods and small meals that are easy to digest because the digestive fire—a strong source of internal heat—disperses in order to help keep you cool.

As well as following pitta-pacifying lifestyle habits from chapter 1 (see pages 25–26), summer is a time to favor the sweet, bitter, and astringent tastes and to relish cool and cooling foods. Most unrefined sweeteners except for honey and molasses are cooling and can be enjoyed in moderation during the summer months.

FALL AND EARLY WINTER: VATA SEASON

Fall and early winter is a time of year where the environment gets cooler, the wind picks up, and the leaves dry and fall from the trees. Vata season is a time of transition. It harbors a certain emptiness that can leave you feeling exposed and a little raw, but it is also filled with possibility—it's a time when you, too, can strip down to a quiet essence of *being* and savor the simplicity.

To pacify the vata qualities (cool, dry, light, and mobile) during this season, you want to fill your life with warmth, oiliness, deep nourishment, loving relationships, and a sense of stability, routine, and groundedness. Favor the sweet, sour, and salty tastes and eat mushy, warm, and oily foods.

♦

Because like increases like and opposites balance, if your constitution tends to be more vata, it may be better to conceive during kapha season, and vice versa. If you tend to be more pitta, it might be best not to conceive during the hottest time of year. Considering postpartum is already a time to be mindful of stabilizing vata; it may be a bit more challenging if you are going through your postpartum window during the vata time of year. All of that being said, these are ways to stay balanced and precautions to take no matter what time of year it is. You can consult with an Ayurvedic practitioner or an Ayurdoula to guide you in this process.

YOUR MONTHLY RHYTHM

Monthly rhythm is another important element of Ayurveda's emphasis on timing. Ayurveda encourages women to understand their particular menstrual rhythm and to become aware of any imbalances, in order to come back into a vital state of health before becoming pregnant. Women should honor every phase of their monthly cycle, which is intimately tied to the lunar cycle of approximately 29.5 days—coinciding with the average length of the menstrual cycle for most ovulating women. According to Ayurveda, the healthiest flow—one that is most in tune with the lunar phases—will start on a new moon, with ovulation occurring around the time of the full moon. When the moon is full, it is at its peak energy, pulling the egg from its home in the ovary.

You can treat many menstrual disorders using tips from chapter 1 and keeping in mind the guideline "like increases like, opposites bring balance." Here are some general things to watch for:

Vata imbalances. Pain in the lower abdomen or back, stiffness, anxiety, fear, nervousness, dark red blood, scanty blood

Pitta imbalances. Increase in body temperature, headache, acne, nausea, diarrhea, swelling, anger, irritability, heavy flow, foul-smelling blood

Kapha imbalances. Water retention, yeast infections, bloating, increased sleep time, depression, emotional eating, heavy and long flow

Understanding your monthly rhythm also allows for tracking your cycle to know the best time for conception. Three things are valuable to look for:

1. Check and track your basal body temperature each morning.
Basal body temperature is your temperature at rest as soon as you wake up in the morning. Right before ovulation, basal body temperature usually drops, before rising slightly right after ovulation occurs. By recording this temperature daily for several months you will be able to predict your most fertile days. Usually a woman's basal body temperature rises by only 0.4 to 0.8 degrees Fahrenheit, so to detect this tiny change, you must use a basal body thermometer, which is more sensitive and precise.

Basal body temperature differs slightly from person to person. Anywhere from 96 to 98 degrees orally is average before ovulation. After ovulation most women have an oral temperature between 97 and 99 degrees. The rise in temperature can be a sudden jump or a gradual climb over a few days. Record your temperature daily so that you can determine a pattern over the months.

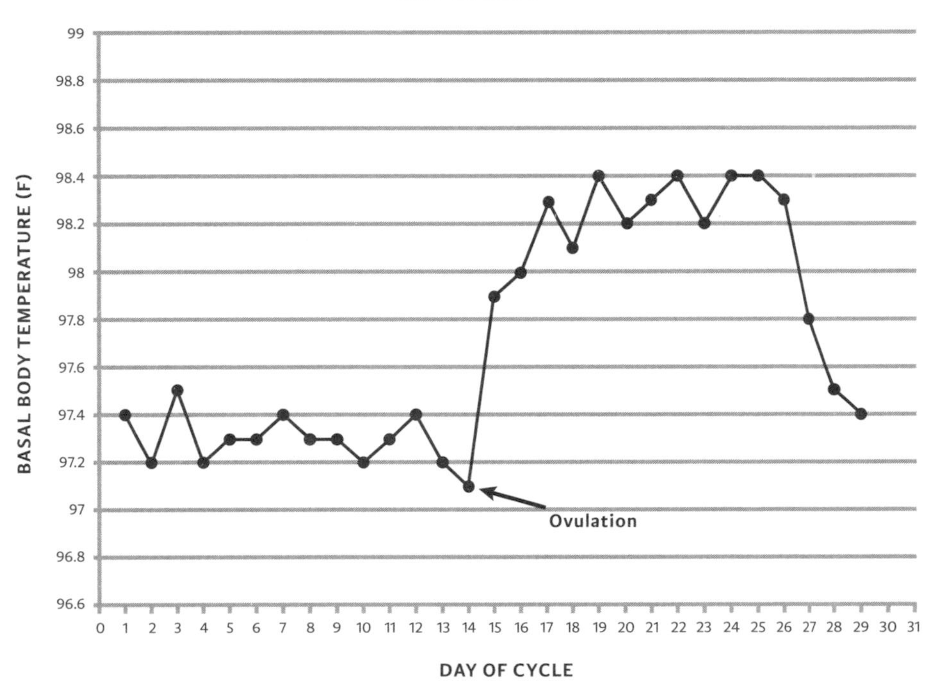

After ovulation, your body temperature stays at the higher level until your period starts. You are most fertile and most likely to get pregnant two to three days before your temperature rises (ovulation), and twelve to twenty-four hours after ovulation. A man's sperm can live for up to five days in a woman's body. The sperm can fertilize an egg at any point during that time. If you try to conceive two or three days before ovulation there is a better chance of becoming pregnant.

2. Become aware of your vaginal discharge.

The hormones that control your menstrual cycle also change the type and amount of mucus you have before and during ovulation. Right after your period, there are usually a few "dry days," when there is no mucus present. As the egg starts to mature, mucus increases in the vagina, appears at the vaginal opening, and is white or off-white in color and cloudy, wet or shiny in consistency. The greatest amount of mucus appears just before ovulation. During these "wet days" vaginal mucus becomes clear in color and slippery in consistency, like raw egg whites. It's generally tacky or can be stretched apart between your fingers. This indicates that you are at your most fertile window; it is the best time to conceive.

About four days after the wet days begin, the mucus changes again. There will be much less and it becomes cloudy, and then you might have a few more dry days before your period returns.

3. Feel for the position and texture of your cervix.
During ovulation your cervix rises to a position high in your vaginal cavity and also becomes more soft, wet, and open. This is the best time to try for conception. After ovulation, your cervix becomes lower in the vagina and becomes more firm, dry, and closed. The majority of women have not touched their cervix; hence, when they touch it, they cannot make out how firm is "firm" and how soft is "soft." The best way to get familiar with your cervix texture and position is to simply check it throughout your cycle to feel the difference.

YOUR DAILY RHYTHM

The tradition of *dinacharya*, or adopting a daily routine, is one of the most powerful Ayurvedic tools for improving overall health and well-being and one of the most important practices to stabilize vata dosha. Nature moves in cycles (day to night, winter to spring), and all the animals and plants follow suit with their own daily and seasonal routines. As humans living in a fast-paced world, we can easily grow out of touch with our natural, circadian rhythms.

Adopting an appropriate daily routine is one of the most grounding and nourishing things you can do for yourself. The following are Ayurveda's recommended daily practices for starting the morning:

Wake up before the sun. The early part of the day, before the sun rises, is governed by vata dosha. If you wake up during this time you will feel lighter and more energized upon waking and throughout the day.

Meditate. Meditation is essential for creating space between your mind (the voice in your head that is always saying something about everything) and your Self (the one who is steadily witnessing, beyond the mind and emotions). The more you can identify with your true Self rather than your mind, the more steady, content, and happy you will be in your life.

Do an oil pull. Put 1 or 2 teaspoons of coconut oil or sesame oil into your mouth and swish it around for ten or twenty minutes. Then spit it out and rinse. Oil pulling promotes oral hygiene; strengthens teeth, gums, and jaw; draws fat-soluble toxins out of the body; reduces inflammation; boosts immunity; whitens teeth; and more!

Scrape your tongue and brush your teeth. Gently scrape your tongue with a tongue scraper or a spoon, from back to front eight to fifteen times, removing the coating that has accumulated overnight. This stimulates the internal organs, helps digestion, improves taste, and removes dead bacteria. Then brush your teeth using a bitter or astringent toothpaste rather than sweet.

Do self-massage. Abhyanga, or self-massage, is one of the most nourishing practices you can do! (See page 66.)

Drink warm water with lime. Warm water first thing in the morning gently awakens your gastrointestinal tract, stimulating peristalsis, encouraging elimination, and therefore supporting digestive health. Limes are high in minerals and vitamins and help loosen *ama*, or toxins, in the digestive tract.

As you go through your day, the Ayurvedic approach calls for attention to some more general principles:

Engage in movement. In the morning, support the waking of your body in a way that you enjoy, whether it be taking a brisk walk around your neighborhood, dancing around your house, going to the gym, or dedicating time to your yoga practice. The afternoon is a prime time to get the blood flowing. After your largest meal of the day is consumed (Ayurvedic tradition says this should be midday) give yourself at least ten or fifteen minutes for a walk to promote blood flow. Evening calls for gentler movement, such as a gentle yoga practice, so that you can wind the body down in preparation for a good night of sleep.

Nourish properly. Ayurvedic tradition encourages eating your meals at the same time each day without snacking in between. Breakfast can be a light yet nourishing meal that awakens your body's digestive fire and gives you enough energy until lunchtime. Lunch should be your biggest meal of the day, followed by a light dinner eaten at least two hours before bedtime. The Ayurvedic approach is to avoid having snacks between meals, so rather than your body digesting food all day it has an opportunity to burn fat as fuel—the most sustainable and efficient form of energy for your body and mind. (A "snack" is considered anything that you eat when your body is not actually hungry.)

Get to bed early. Ayurvedic teachings encourage us to wind down with the sun and to be asleep no later than 10 p.m. This likely means that you begin winding down from your day no later than 8 p.m.—turning off electronics, dimming lights, taking a bath or shower, and brushing your teeth. At 10 p.m., pitta energy fills the atmosphere, often giving you a "second wind" if you are still awake. Ideally, the body is able to use that pitta energy while you are sleeping to break down and metabolize any toxicity or undigested food that has accumulated throughout the day, so that you wake up in the morning feeling bright-eyed and bushy-tailed!

Abhyanga: Self-Massage

The Sanskrit word *sneha* can be translated as both "oil" and "love." Ayurvedic tradition suggests that the benefits of abhyanga, or self-massage with oil, are similar to those received when one is saturated with love.

Because abhyanga gives a deep experience of stability, nourishment, and warmth, it is one of the greatest practices for balancing vata dosha. After self-massage, you will feel more steady in your mind, more balanced, and more energized throughout the day. You will feel more joy, even in the body itself, and more ease in your entire nervous system. Feelings of agitation, depression, sorrow, fear, and anxiety will dissolve.

By soothing the nervous system, abhyanga creates a protective shield between yourself and the world so that you will feel less affected by aggressive or unwanted stimuli. Your energy will seem soft and more contained. You will feel nourished, so you will respond to the world from a nourished, centered place. Abhyanga stimulates the lymphatic system, increases immunity and circulation, lubricates joints, tones muscles, heightens mental alertness, improves sleep, and helps excretion of impurities from the body.

Your self-massage can be long and luxurious or can be as short as ten minutes—depending on the amount of time you have each day. When performing abhyanga, the loving attention you offer yourself makes all the difference. Be present and really feel the warm oil being applied to your body. Allow your hands to be an expression of your heart, delivering love to every single cell. Your intention and loving attention go a long way in regard to your experience of feeling held, balanced, and deeply nourished.

1. Warm about a half cup of oil for your entire body. You can use sesame in the cooler months or coconut oil in the hot months (or when you feel an excess of pitta).

2. Use long strokes on your long bones, circles around your joints, and clockwise around your belly. Really rub the oil into your tissues so that your body absorbs as much as possible rather than a deep, slow massage.
3. After massage, keep the oil on for fifteen or twenty minutes, allowing it to absorb into your body.
4. Take a warm bath or shower, using soap only where necessary.
5. Pat dry after your shower, rather than rubbing the oil off.

RITUALS FOR THE DAY OF CONCEPTION

Traditionally in Ayurveda, after individuals hoping to conceive have spent some months preparing their bodies (through cleansing and rebuilding), their lives (through the ways they are living and the values they are cultivating), and their consciousness (by nurturing relationship with each other and with their spiritual nature)—while also giving attention to seasonal and monthly rhythms and their daily routine—they would seek guidance from an astrologer to determine the optimal timing for conception. The astrologer would ensure that the time of life was beneficial for both parents and assess whether a particular cycle had the possibility for conception. This process required detailed knowledge of the prospective mama's monthly cycle. If the particular cycle were favorable, the astrologer would then give an auspicious date for conception as well as a specific time of day (in Sanskrit, *muhurta*), for performing the *garbhadhana samskara*: the intentional and spiritual process of planting the seed that then carries the Soul into the mother's womb. Garbhadhana samskara is the science of calling in a spiritual being of pure consciousness. A *samskara* is a rite of passage that marks an important event in one's life. It is an intentional action that leaves a deep impression in the mind in a way that affects all future actions.

Many different rituals are explained in the Vedas with the purpose of making this experience as infused with intention and meaning as possible to guide you in how to engage in the act of lovemaking in a way that creates more positive energy and an ideal environment for conscious conception to take place. Rituals are empty in and of themselves, but if infused with your full awareness and depth of intention, the activity has the potential to be deeply transformative—to be a samskara. In other words, the intention behind the action gives power to that action. By performing the following rituals on the day of conception, you will be stepping into the activity of conception fully aware of the goal of your actions, and thus infusing it with consciousness and intention.

Spend the full day in prayer. Spend hours meditating, praying, chanting, and reading sacred texts. Infuse your consciousness with spiritual vibration so that you can attract a soul with a similar vibration.

Both partners should take showers and anoint their bodies with pure essential oils of rose or sandalwood, both cooling and sattvic (pure) scents.

Prepare the bed with clean, white sheets. Decorate the bedroom with white flowers, banana leaves, candles, and all-natural incense. You and your partner can also dress in all white, representing purity.

Set up an altar with images of great souls whose qualities you would like your child to imbibe.

Before entering into bed, sit in front of your altar with your partner and say prayers, inviting deep intention for the conception of your child. You can recite the following prayer from the central Ayurvedic text *Charaka Samhita* (Ayurveda's oldest text on the science of life) in unison:

> O creator and the cosmic truth, please bless us with a courageous and strong child with a long life and health, with the qualities of Brahma (power to create), Brhaspati (power to alter the future), Vishnu (power to maintain), Soma (power to flourish), Surya (power to be successful), Mitra (power to love), and Varuna (power to nurture).

Allow the act of lovemaking to be more than just physical sensation. Be present to the subtle exchange of energy that is happening between you and your partner and the atmosphere that the energy is creating. Use this time to truly connect with your partner: see how you can satisfy them; synchronize your breathing; be present in the moment; repeat a mantra in your mind or even out loud together. How can you experience the presence of the Divine through this act? Ayurvedic tradition suggests that in lovemaking, the woman should be lying on her back and the man should be on top, to help vata stay stable and balanced. Likewise, tradition advises that lovemaking should not be done during the daytime; at dawn or dusk, during an eclipse, full moon, or new moon; when hungry or thirsty; or within two hours after eating.

At the moment of orgasm, let your attention go toward the Divine—really feeling the sacredness and profundity of the moment. Partners can repeat a mantra together or recite the name(s) of God.

After lovemaking, the woman's belly can be sprayed with cooling rosewater and covered with a cool damp cloth.

Bathe, and then both partners can drink a glass of warm milk boiled with a pinch each of cardamom, saffron, ginger, and ground almond powder. (As noted earlier, saffron is especially nourishing for the reproductive organs and ojas.)

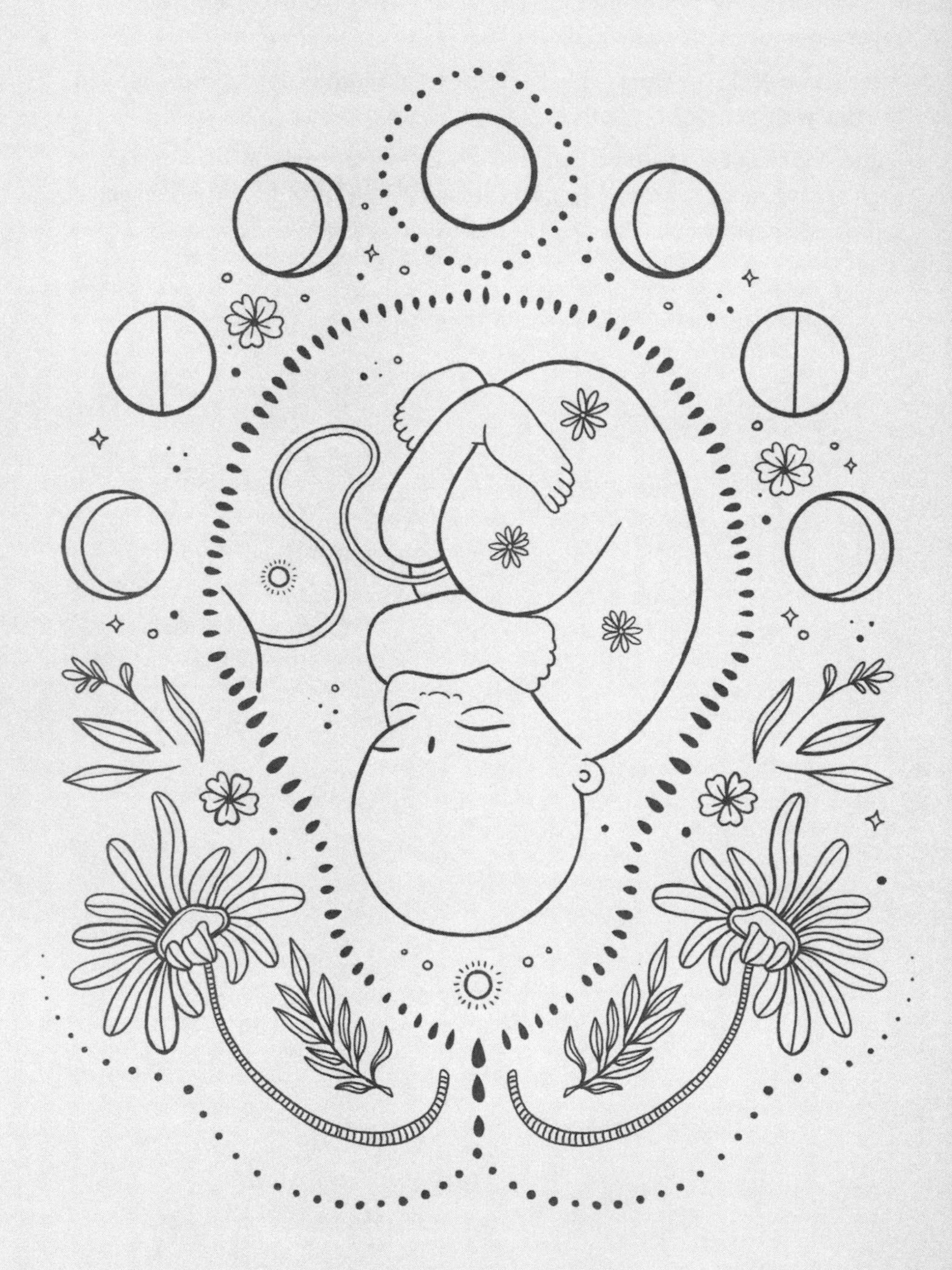

Cultivating the Seed

HOLISTIC HEALTH DURING PREGNANCY

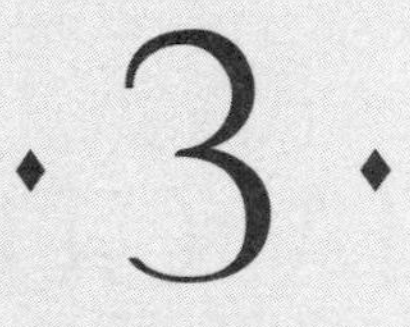

Action that is virtuous, thought through, free from attachment, and without craving for results is considered Sattvic; Action that is driven purely by craving for pleasure, selfishness and much effort is Rajasic; Action that is undertaken because of delusion, disregarding consequences, without considering loss or injury to others or self, is called Tamasic.

—Bhagavad Gita, chapter 18, verses 23–25

The science of Ayurveda takes a holistic approach to caring for this little soul as its body is growing inside of you. Whereas Western medicine places emphasis more narrowly on a mother's diet, Ayurveda acknowledges that you receive nourishment not only from the food that you eat but also from everything coming in through all your senses. The sounds you hear, the scents you smell, everything you see, touch, and taste all shape this little being's body, mind, and consciousness.

According to Ayurvedic thought, the constitution of your baby, as well as any imbalances that they are born with, are formed by several factors, including the genetic makeup of both parents, the parents' balances and imbalances, their psychology and consciousness at the moment of conception, the mama's diet and emotions during pregnancy, environmental influences during pregnancy, and the samskaras (subtle impressions from past actions) from previous lives. In Ayurvedic teaching, however, the most important thing in pregnancy is that mama is happy and feels positive emotions. A mama's emotions affect a baby more than any other factor, so it's crucial to focus on sattva (uplifting sensory impression) during pregnancy.

This chapter will explore how sensory impressions either serve to support the health and happiness of your babe or bring more discomfort, discontent, and dis-ease to the little one developing in your womb. This chapter also explores the growth of your baby, month by month, according to the teachings of Ayurveda on a physical and energetic level, and it will talk about how to support the health of your little one throughout each phase.

MAHA GUNAS

We are what we associate with.

Every person has an energy that vibrates in and around them. Your energy is a combination of all the energy you pick up from the people you spend time with, the places you go, the foods you eat, and everything that comes in through your senses. Wherever you go you carry this vibration, as you simultaneously pick up the energies of the people, places, and things that you interact with. When you spend time with another person, you pick up not only their energy but also the energy they have picked up from their other associations. When you go to certain places, you pick up the energies of the people that have been there.

The great teacher A. C. Bhaktivedanta Swami Prabhupada used to give the following example about the power of association: If you place an iron rod in fire, in a bit of time it begins to take on all the qualities of fire; if you touch it, it will have the same effect as fire does! That same iron rod, if you place it in ice, after some time it begins to take on the qualities of ice. Every interaction that takes place changes you. The teachings of yoga and Ayurveda urge you to become conscious of the ways that you are affected by what you associate with, and to choose associations that uplift you.

During pregnancy your senses are the gateways between your own inner and outer world, and they also are serving as a filter for your growing baby—so everything a pregnant mama tastes, sees, touches, hears, and smells should be nourishing to both the mother and the child. Whatever comes in through your senses shapes not only the body but also the mind of your little one.

In Ayurvedic teaching, the sensory impressions you bring in through your eyes, ears, mouth, nose, and skin are described in terms of three primordial qualities called the *maha gunas*, which weave through the subtle nature of all matter. If your sensory impressions are proper and balanced, you feel happy, clear, and uplifted; this quality of experience is described as sattvic, as it stems from the association with *sattva* guna. If your sensory impressions are in excess, deficient, or imbalanced, you feel disturbed and agitated; these experiences are rajasic or tamasic in nature, and they arise from exposure to raja or tama gunas. These three gunas are like the three threads that make up the fabric of the material world or like the three primary colors that mix to create every other color that exists.

Qualities and Characteristics of the Three Gunas

Sattva. balancing, pure, luminous, serene, good, light, ease, harmony, order; signifies knowledge

Rajas. stimulation, movement, passion, restlessness; responsible for motion and activity

Tamas. inert, impure, dull, dark, degenerating, ignorant or sloth and torpor (lethargy)

You are constantly engaged in energy transfers. You pick up different energies simply by walking into another house or environment. Upon entering some places—perhaps a temple, your yoga studio, a clean and orderly house, or even a library!—you might suddenly feel uplifted, clearer, and more connected to your Self. Certain people that you spend time with might also bring you that feeling of connection and clarity, as might some of the foods that you eat, music that you listen to, and scents that you smell. These grounding energetic sensations that bring ease, harmony, and clarity to your mind are *sattvic* impressions, coming from people, places, and things that carry a vibration of goodness.

In the same way, certain places—the New York City stock exchange, a disco club, or any place during rush hour—might make you suddenly feel intensely energized! In the company of certain people, you might find yourself planning for the future, setting goals, perhaps feeling anxious, competitive, critical, or a bit angry. Some of the foods you eat, music or sounds you hear, or scents you smell might make your mind more active—make you feel more unsettled, future-oriented, and overstimulated. These rajasic impressions come from association with people, places, or things in the mode of passion.

Then there are places you might find yourself in that have a dulling effect on the mind: places that are dark and dirty; someone's home where the shades are closed, the sink is full of dirty dishes, and you cannot even see the countertop because of the mess; a night club at 2 a.m. when everyone is intoxicated. In the company of some people you might suddenly feel your consciousness being pulled down: you find yourself resenting past experiences, feeling hopeless and depressed. Certain foods you eat, music or sounds you hear, and things you smell might color your mind with more inertia, stagnation, and heaviness. These are all tamasic impressions, or energy that is imprinted upon the mind from the lower vibrations of ignorance or inertia.

The natural state of the mind is sattvic, though depending on what comes in through your senses, the mind may be colored by rajas or tamas. Ayurvedic tradition views rajasic and tamasic impressions as the cause of all dis-ease because they distort your perception and hence your ability to make decisions from a clear and centered place. You begin to choose what you want *now* rather than what you want most—a choice often based on short-term sensory stimulation that fails to lead you toward the real joy and satisfaction that you ultimately seek.

When the mind is distorted by rajas and tamas (by associating with rajasic and tamasic sensory impressions), you fail to see things as they are and instead see things through the lens of your conditioning. It is as if you are looking through red-tinted glasses, so you are always seeing red! You live from a dulled or more reactive state, triggered by life's past experiences, responding to this moment in a distorted way. Influenced by qualities of rajas and tamas, you will constantly seek your sense of self-value, self-worth, and experience of satisfaction in the world outside of you—in people, places, and situations that are always changing. The charts on this and the following pages summarize signs that identify each of the three gunas, along with a list of the sensory experiences that magnify the effect of each.

Sattva

Some signs of sattva include the following:

Receptivity	Inner quietude	Healthy relationships
Clarity	Clear memory	Healthy habits
Peace	Calm sleep	Nonviolence/compassion
Joy	Compassion	Truthfulness
Healthy detachment	Selflessness	Cleanliness

The following types of sensory input increase sattva:

Smell: scents that uplift the mood and invoke clarity, such as the natural scents of rose, jasmine, lavender, and sandalwood

Taste: mindful eating and a diet of organic, freshly prepared vegetarian foods, including fresh fruits and vegetables; nuts, seeds, grains, and legumes; ethically and freshly produced milk, ghee, and paneer; and natural sweeteners

Sight: clean and uncluttered spaces and uplifting sights such as the sky, sacred spaces, and natural environments

Feeling: good company, uplifting and peaceful environments, the effects of meditation and pranayama, gentle and nourishing movement and self-care practices

Hearing: *kirtan* (to call, recite, praise, or glorify some form of Divinity through song), uplifting conversations, spiritual discussions, ambient or classical music

Rajas

Some signs of rajas include the following:

Aggression
Overcompetitiveness
Frustration
Agitation/impatience
Anxiety/worry
Insomnia/disturbed sleep
Restlessness/klutziness
Overstimulation
Discontent
Turbulence in relationships
Self-criticalness
Judgmentalness
Self-righteousness
Narrow-mindedness
Ambition
Arrogance
Powerful sensory desires
Greediness
Jealousy

The following types of sensory input increase rajas:

Smell: scents that activate the mind, including rosemary, peppermint, coffee, citrus, and cinnamon

Taste: caffeine, alcohol, overly sour and spicy foods, onion and garlic, foods with a strong flavor, distracted eating or multitasking while eating

Sight: competitive sports, action movies, too much activity, fast movement

Feeling: overstimulating and busy environments; excessive movement, working, or talking; exercising too intensely; competitive or future-oriented company; impulsive behavior

Hearing: gossip, loud noise, music with a strong beat, uncontrolled thoughts

Tamas

Some signs of tamas include the following:

Sluggishness and lethargy
Stubbornness
Lack of motivation
Depression
Dull mind; foggy thinking; feeling "blah"
Lack of sensitivity
Deep-seated emotional blockages
Being stuck in the past

- Needing excessive sleep
- Dishonesty
- Lack of intelligence
- Lack of self-control
- Being easily influenced
- Taking drugs
- Having a negative idea of self
- Dirtiness
- Dependence
- Being identified with body
- Addiction

The following types of sensory input increase tamas:

Smell: putrid, rotten smelling things, scents that activate trauma and memory

Taste: processed, packaged, canned, microwaved, leftover, stale, and fast foods; food that has been produced using cruelty and that has caused suffering; overeating

Sight: sex- and violence-based media; violence; not having time in nature; not having access to fresh air, sunlight, and moonlight; too much social media or TV time (or other ways of visually "numbing" oneself)

Feeling: sedentary lifestyle, not enough movement, being indoors too much, darkness, fearful situations, too much sleep, drugs, passivity

Hearing: music with violent and degrading lyrics, music that numbs emotions and makes one depressed, hearing about violence

During pregnancy especially, you want to lean into a more sattvic lifestyle and sattvic dietary habits to promote more clarity and inner connection. When you are eating sattvic foods, immersing yourself in sattvic environments, spending time with sattvic people, listening to more sattvic sounds, and seeing sattvic sensory impressions, your mind will become lighter, clearer, and more luminous. You will naturally begin to feel an inner satisfaction that is not swayed by the external circumstances, and you will make decisions that serve to bring you back into a state of balance.

You can choose the sensory impressions that you allow in based on what leads you to feeling peaceful or agitated, connected or disconnected. While you do not have control over every sight, smell, and sound you encounter, there are still an infinite number of other choices to be made. Choosing your sensory input wisely is the easiest way to alter your mind and uplift your consciousness, as well as uplift the mind, body, and consciousness of your little one.

The gunas categorize material nature by revealing how all matter has a certain frequency and specific energy that it exudes. Even sattva, however, has the potential of binding you into the cycles of material identification; although it is the preferred guna, sattva is still material energy—so it is often mixed with the energies of the other gunas, and therefore generally brings with it a bit of rajas and tamas.

Although the gunas affect your mind and your body, they can never color the soul. From a sattvic consciousness, you can choose to enter into the realm of spirit. Spiritual energy transcends matter (the gunas) and directly reaches the soul. Spiritual discourses, sacred literature, and spiritual sound vibration in the form of kirtan—the calling or glorifying a form of Divinity through song—and mantra meditation are powerful ways to introduce spiritual energy to your little one. These are the frequencies that you want to bathe in the most, as they will directly touch the essence of your babe and allow them to remember the Truth of who they really are.

SPIRITUAL PERCEPTION

Everything in its essence is spiritual, as everything comes from the same Source, even matter. So how do you begin to see matter as spiritual rather than material? By seeing it connected to its Source! Everything can be experienced as spiritual, depending on how it is perceived and how it is utilized. "Spiritual" or "material," then, are simply our state of consciousness.

A microphone, if used to amplify your ego, serves to bind you more deeply into identifying with your false ego (the temporary roles that you play and the conditions that you have based on your circumstances and past experiences). That same microphone, however, if used to amplify spiritual knowledge, or kirtan, becomes spiritual. When you utilize matter to serve spirit, it becomes spiritual. When you acknowledge that everything is a gift from the Divine, you can utilize everything in this world in a way that ultimately serves.

With that spiritual awareness, you are no longer bound by the gunas (which you cycle in and out of and are constantly affected by) and instead you enter into the spiritual realm. The following are ways that you can enter into that consciousness, and thus surround your growing baby with spiritual vibrations.

Feeling this little angel kicking has been one of the most special things.
I've always known it was a miracle,
to grow a baby inside of you,
though I've never really felt it in the way I do now.

The perfect design.

A little person,
a little soul,
is growing their body
in my body.

I got back to New York in the beginning of April,
and it's honestly been magic since then.
I generally feel like I have more energy than I've ever had in my life.
I feel grateful.
Humbled.
So blessed.
And purpose-filled in a way I've never felt.
I'm not looking for
or planning my
"next big thing."
I'm not looking for a purpose outside of this one.
Because I know this will be my most meaningful offering to the world:
raising this little being with love, focus, and intention
. . . starting now.

In the evenings, papa rubs my belly with belly balm and says the most beautiful, heartfelt prayers.
It's his main time of connecting with little one . . .
and it's oh so sweet.
I'm doing yoga about four days per week and walking miles each day.
I'm receiving *marma* sessions (Ayurvedic pressure points) each week and doing massages each morning.
I don't notice a huge shift in my hunger and haven't had any cravings or aversions.

I feel healthy and happy
and like I'm part of a miracle unfolding —
and it's so, so special.

Little babe listens to the Brahma Samhita each morning and Bhagavad Gita *shlokas* daily.
As one of my mentors has said, "She or he will learn the Gita and become intelligent, as Sanskrit is the most intelligent language."
At this stage, the baby absorbs their environment
and that is what creates and develops their sense of self.
"I am my environment."
So we are infusing the environment with as much love and spiritual sound vibrations as possible.
Letting little soul know how how much they're cared for and wanted
and what a special little being they are.

PRASADA: THE POWER OF SPIRITUAL FOOD

You eat food with the purpose to nourish your body. How can that same food nourish your soul? Yoga and Ayurveda teach us that the energy and the mood of the chef, as well as the atmosphere that the food is prepared in, is cooked into the elements (the matter) of the food. When you eat food, the elements that the food is made up of feed the elemental components of your body, whereas the consciousness and environment that the food was made in feeds your mind and conscience.

You therefore want to be mindful of not only *what* you are eating but also of who prepared it and what their consciousness was during that time. If you eat a healthy meal prepared by someone who is frustrated, the healthy food nourishes your tissues, but the frustration colors your consciousness, making you feel frustrated. In the same way, you may eat some greasy comfort food that was made with a lot of love and feel satisfied, nourished, and uplifted from it.

Food becomes spiritual when it is prepared as a meditation, in the mood of loving service, to satisfy and please the Divine. In India, millions of people keep altars in their homes. They cook with the thought that they are preparing food for the Supreme as an act of love.

Everything in this world comes from the Divine. When you prepare your food in gratitude, as an offering to the Divine, that mood and intention infuses the food with spiritual energy. The prayerful offering, accepted by the Beloved, transforms food into *prasadam*, or spiritual food, that not only nourishes the five elements that make up your material form, but also serves to awaken the soul. In *The Journey Within*, Radhanath Swami writes,

> Of course the Supreme Beloved does not need our food. Mothers and fathers provide for their children. If the children take the ingredients provided by the parents and cook a meal for the parents, it's natural that the parents will be pleased. Similarly, the Supreme is pleased by our devotion when we cook and make our heartfelt offerings.

Prasadam is made with sattvic foods that heal and energize your body so that your body becomes an ideal home for the soul to reside in. Lord Krishna in the Bhagavad Gita advises that the foods that best help to develop your consciousness are juicy, wholesome, and pleasing to the heart. This type of food purifies your existence and gives strength, health, happiness, and satisfaction. In this way, preparing, cooking, and eating food becomes a meditation and a spiritual practice that will connect you deeply to yourself, to all of nature, and to the Source of all that is.

To Make Prasadam

First, take a shower and put on clean clothes. Assure that the kitchen you are using is scrupulously clean. When your body and environment are purified, your mind naturally becomes more clear.

Play a recording of kirtan or a spiritual lecture that attunes your mind toward Truth. This assures that your mind is absorbed in hearing spiritual sound vibration rather than wandering into the past or future.

Say a prayer that your preparations become infused with Divine love.

While cooking, make sure not to snack or sample a dish before it is finished and offered. Remember, this meal is a loving gift that you first want to offer to the Divine before enjoying it yourself. This also maintains a standard of cleanliness.

Once preparation of the food is complete, make a small plate and place it on your altar or personal sacred space. (Traditionally, you would use a plate that was only meant for this purpose.) Close your eyes, take a few deep breaths, and offer the meal with love and gratitude to whatever form of Divinity you connect with. The Divine accepts the love, devotion, sincerity, and intention behind the offering. After the offering, take the prasadam off the altar and transfer it to another plate.

Share it with others and enjoy!

ASSOCIATION WITH SACRED SPACES

Sacred places are infused with spiritual energy, energy that brings you back to your spiritual nature. When you enter into a spiritual environment, the stresses of your days may fall away as you remember what is really of value in life.

You may feel supercharged after visiting holy places of pilgrimage, perhaps feeling the difference in yourself for days. Holy places are infused with the energy of the people who have frequented them and the mood those people have brought to the spaces. They carry the energy of great saints, great knowers, and great seekers of Truth. They are steeped in the power of prayer and thus the presence of Divinity. Whether or not you believe that the dent in that rock was made by Buddha or that God really appeared in the burning bush, it is hard to ignore the profound way that others experience the sacredness of these sites. The presence of faith elevates these spiritual places, making them more than the sites of a mere stone or tree.

ASSOCIATION WITH SPIRITUAL PEOPLE

When you spend time with holy people, people who are dedicated to living a life in alignment with Truth, their vibration affects you in a deep way. Their energy, lived knowledge, and depth of realization affects the atmosphere by bringing cleansing, connection, and clarification. Just being in their presence begins to shift your inner experience through an energy transfer that takes place beyond anything that they say or do. By associating with spiritual people, whether in person, by listening to lectures, or through reading books or biographies, you will begin to take on qualities of those people. By serving these great seers of Truth, Truth awakens within your own heart and the heart of the little one in your womb.

SPIRITUAL SOUND VIBRATION

Technology allows spiritual sound vibration to be easily accessible anywhere, at any time. Listening to Truth from sacred literature is a good way to refocus your priorities, purify your heart, and attract Divine grace. The purer and more realized the source of the knowledge, the more powerful the effect.

Another form of receiving spiritual sound is the practice of mantra meditation or kirtan. Mantra is spiritual energy encased in sound structure. In Sanskrit, *man* means "mind" and *tra* means "to free." Mantra meditation is a practice known for its ability to free the mind from the fear and anxiety that stems from forgetfulness of your true Self. Chanting has a profound effect on the body, mind, and spirit, and there are many different mantras that each have their own potency, carrying with them many different effects.

The following mantra, the maha mantra, was first mentioned in the Kali-Santarana Upanishad and is said to carry within it the power of all other mantras. It uses only three words, repeated to express a mantra that consists of sixteen words in total: *Hare* (pronounced ha-ray), *Krishna* (pronounced krish-na), and *Rama* (rhymes with "mama"). *Hare* invokes the presence of the Divine feminine, and with that, all of Her qualities, such as compassion, divine grace, and pure love. *Krishna* is one of many names for the One (or God) meaning "attractive to everyone," and *Rama* means "one who gives pleasure"—that is, who awakens you to the pleasure inherent within your own heart.

This mantra is a prayer and a meditation. As a prayer, its intention is to serve—to awaken you to the Truth of who you really are and help you remember your loving relationship with the Divine. As a meditation, its practice is to focus your attention completely on the sound of the mantra, whether you say it silently or aloud, and to really allow yourself to bathe in the vibrations and be nourished by them. Whenever the mind wanders (usually to the past or to the future), invite it back—simply focusing your attention on hearing the sound. When the mind wanders again, bring it back again. Then it will wander again. Bring it back. The mantra becomes a place for your mind to rest.

This mantra is said to permeate through all layers of matter and directly touch the soul. It revives your original, pure consciousness. It helps you to awaken to the deepest reality and allows you to become an instrument of God's grace, love, and compassion in the world. (For more details on mantra meditation, I suggest reading *The Living Name* by Sacinandana Swami.)

Maha Mantra Meditation

Repeat this mantra over and over again, out loud or in your mind, focusing your attention completely on the sound vibration for a minimum of five minutes per day, working up to twenty minutes in the morning and twenty minutes each evening.

Hare Krishna Hare Krishna
Krishna Krishna Hare Hare
Hare Rama Hare Rama
Rama Rama Hare Hare

PREGNANCY MONTH BY MONTH: THE AYURVEDIC APPROACH

FIRST TRIMESTER

Upon conception all three doshas begin to increase in your body. During the first trimester of pregnancy, you are likely to notice an increase of vata, pitta, or kapha appearing in different ways. Immediately after the egg is fertilized, it takes time (and needs stability!) in order to be implanted into the uterine wall. During the following weeks, inner activity increases as the "details" of your little one's newly forming body develop. Cell differentiation takes place, the baby's senses and motor organs are formed, the genitals develop, and cartilage turns into bones. Ayurvedic practice strongly recommends against traveling during this trimester to promote stability in the uterus, and it favors gentle exercise (rather than fast-paced and intense), such as walking and yoga.

First month: Immediately, from the moment of conception, the sperm and egg unite to form a soft mass of cells called *kalala*, "the first expression of creation." Immediately there is consciousness in the embryo, and everything you consume through your five senses will leave an impression on your little one. In Ayurveda, nutrition starts even before conception. All seven *dhatus*, or tissues, begin to form from this soft mass, and by the end of the first month, the *rasa dhatu* (plasma and lymph) has matured. Ayurvedic tradition recommends eating butter, ghee, and hot milk regularly in the first month of pregnancy and taking special care not to overheat. (See page 287 for a recipe for making ghee.)

Second month: In the second month the three doshas—vata, pitta, and kapha—are formed in the baby's body from the five elements. *Rakta dhatu* (blood) matures by the end of this month. Hot milk, lightly spiced with sweet spices, is a beneficial drink during this time.

Third month: Mamsa dhatu (muscle tissue) matures in the third month. Warm milk with half a teaspoon of honey and 1 teaspoon of ghee is good for mama and baby throughout this month. A gentle yoga practice can also be beneficial, especially hip openers and postures that increase the mobility of pelvic joints, as well as balancing *asanas* (yoga poses) to build strength in your legs and increase circulation and stability. Good asanas to practice include tadasana (mountain pose), virabhadrasana (warrior pose), prasarita padottanasana (expanded leg stretch), parshva konasana (side angle pose), adho mukha svanasana (downward-facing dog pose), janu shirshasana (head-to-knee pose), and savasana (corpse pose).

SECOND TRIMESTER

In the second trimester of pregnancy some mamas start noticing cravings. If that happens, Ayurveda strongly recommends that you honor these cravings if they are not harmful to your health or the health of your babe. During this time, the emotions you feel and the desires you have may actually be coming from your baby, as your hearts are so connected. The *Sushruta Samhita*, a classical Ayurvedic text, notes that during the fourth month the fetus is endowed with awareness, especially as it pertains to the energetic heart (considered the seat of consciousness). Tradition suggests that during this trimester, the baby still remembers its past lives, and through prayer, mantra, kirtan, spiritual association, and scriptural study, the baby's samskaras (past conditioning) can be washed away. Ayurveda considers this the stable period; if you were wanting to go on a "baby-moon," this is a good time to do it!

Fourth month: By the end of the third month of pregnancy, the baby's heart is formed. Ayurveda teaches that a woman has two hearts during pregnancy, and because of this—she feels so much! A mother experiences her baby's feelings and emotions as well as her own. Any experience that is harmful to her emotions will affect the physical and emotional heart of her baby at this point. Therefore, the relationship between the mother and her partner should be kept happy and peaceful.

The desires of the baby are being reflected as cravings. These cravings should be satisfied in order to support the health of your baby. Around the fourth month, *meda dhatu* (adipose tissue/fat) also matures. You can have warm milk blended with two and a half teaspoons of butter. For exercise, continue practicing the yoga asana sequence from month three.

Fifth month: During the fifth month the brain forms, and your baby's mind begins to register subtle impressions. If you have not already focused on surrounding yourself with sattvic impressions, the fifth month is a good time to start. When your navel begins to protrude, your ability to sense the environment and those around you increases dramatically, thanks to the 72,000 nerve endings that unite underneath the navel that are now exposed to outer vibrations. Your sensitivity to your surroundings should be respected, as it protects both you and your baby. *Asthi dhatu* (bones and cartilage) matures in the fifth month. 1 or 2 teaspoons of ghee daily is recommended. Prenatal yoga can continue with the addition of the squatting pose.

Sixth month: During the sixth month the fetus begins to experience some emotions, and more sensitive mothers might be able to read feelings of pain or pleasure coming from the baby in the womb. *Majja dhatu* (marrow, nerve tissue, connective tissue) reaches maturity. Ghee with demulcent herbs can be taken as needed to reduce inflammation. During prenatal yoga, add in restorative postures such as balasana (child pose), upavishta konasana (wide angle pose), supta baddha konasana (reclining bound angle pose), and savasana (corpse pose).

THIRD TRIMESTER

The third trimester of pregnancy is the time to start slowing down. It is a great time to introduce a meditative grounding practice if you have not already started. This period is when you really want to focus on building kapha and stabilizing vata dosha so that your body can be nourished and prepared for a more ease-filled delivery and postpartum window. During the eighth month, you may have wavering feelings of joy and sorrow because of the unsteadiness of ojas. Ayurvedic thought suggests that during this time, ojas goes back and forth from mama to baby, baby to mama. That is why it is especially important to rest during this time so that you and baby can be stable when the ojas is not.

Seventh month: The final tissues to mature are the *shukra dhatu* (male reproductive tissue) or *artava dhatu* (female reproductive tissue). By the end of the seventh month all the tissues in your baby's body are fully formed. Ghee infused with medicinal sweet herbs like shatavari and cardamom is suggested. The yoga asana practice can include more chest openers to relieve any tension in your back and neck. A beneficial asana sequence for the seventh month would be as follows: tadasana, virabhadrasana, squatting pose, trikonasana (triangle pose), prasarita padottanasana, virasana with arm movements (hero pose), and savasana.

Eighth month: In the eighth month ojas begins to spread and give stability to your entire body. Ayurveda recommends eating thin rice gruel prepared with milk and ghee (see the recipe at page 277). Around this time you can begin the traditional Ayurvedic treatment called *yoni picchu* (see the discussion on page 126), a practice of vaginal oleation that prepares the body for delivery and prevents tearing. Balancing poses such as vrikshasana (tree pose), utthita hasta padangushthasana (extended side-hand-to-big-toe pose) can be added to the asana sequence.

Ninth month: During the ninth month, try to stay well rested and relaxed but also keep your body strong and active. Walking every day is beneficial for strength and endurance. Ayurveda recommends a sitz bath at least several times a week for the six weeks prior to birth, as a way to soften the perineum. (A sitz bath is a basin that fits perfectly into your toilet seat and lets you get a soothing soak of the important parts without having to immerse in a tub. See page 126 for two sitz bath recipes.) For diet, healthy fats are important during the end of pregnancy to lubricate deeper tissues. Freshly prepared foods that are creamy, soft, warm, and sweet will be beneficial. Add ghee to everything you eat, and prepare a thick rice gruel cooked with milk, cardamom, and ghee when desired (see page 277). The following sequence of asanas is recommended for the end of pregnancy: tadasana, virabhadrasana, squatting pose, trikonasana, chakravakasana, adho mukha svanasana, balasana, and savasana. (Previous sequences/poses can also be practiced, if they feel comfortable.)

AYURVEDIC FESTIVALS FOR EACH OF THE FIVE SENSES

According to Ayurveda, the baby's five senses develop one month at a time over five consecutive months of pregnancy. Traditionally, Ayurveda calls for a celebration during each one of these months, in which the focus of the party is to bring extra attention to nourishing the specific sense that is developing. As mama's senses are engaged, baby develops a keen sense and the ability to perceive through it clearly.

THIRD MONTH: SENSE OF SIGHT

In the third month, the baby's sense of sight is developing. During a celebration of this new sense, we want everything mama sees to be aesthetically pleasing and beautiful! To this end, you can decorate for the celebration using lots of color, or perhaps host the celebration in a beautiful garden. Have extravagant floral arrangements and lots of candles. For activities, do art projects such as painting watercolor images for baby's room, tie-dyeing onesies, or painting squares to put together as a quilt.

FOURTH MONTH: SENSE OF TASTE

In the fourth month, the baby's sense of taste is developing. During this celebration, we want to have foods that are pleasing to mama's palate. Perhaps have mama create a list of her favorite foods and host a potluck, with each guest bringing one dish. Make sure all six tastes are available in the potluck (sweet, sour, salty, pungent, bitter, and astringent). Have different tables with different types of items so that the presentation feels super abundant! You might have one table with cut-up fruits and fruit drinks, another table with all the desserts, another table with savories, and so on! This could also be a good time to start talking about plans for a postpartum meal train—where people deliver home-cooked meals to mama and family after the baby is born—and educating guests about what will be needed postpartum for mama (and start a sign-up list!).

FIFTH MONTH: SENSE OF SMELL

In the fifth month, the baby's sense of smell is developing, and the celebration will be one that indulges mama's sense of smell! One possibility is to have a warm fresh meal prepared so that the aroma fills the house. Light aromatic candles and have multiple diffusers on with mama's favorite essential oil blends. Make beautiful teas, have aromatic flowers all around, and bring mama gifts of all-natural and aromatic soaps, teas, and oils.

SIXTH MONTH: SENSE OF HEARING

In the sixth month, the baby's sense of hearing is developing. In the celebration for this month, we want to infuse the atmosphere with uplifting and supportive sound vibrations. This is a perfect month to host a kirtan at your home! If you do not play instruments, you can play your favorite songs and sing along, as well as dance together. A sharing circle can also be a part of the celebration, with each guest sharing blessings for the new baby and family.

SEVENTH MONTH: SENSE OF TOUCH

In the seventh month, the baby's sense of touch is developing. During this celebration, we want mama to *feel* amazing. One way to do this is to hold a gathering that includes some gentle massage for mama with many hands all at once. Belly painting is also a beautiful idea! Those gathered could engage in hair brushing or ceremonial hair braiding while mama receives a rosewater foot bath. This is also a great time to let your girlfriends know that you would like gentle, soothing, oily (Ayurvedic style) massages after your birth experience to facilitate your recovery and mothering strength.

FOUR IMPORTANT SELF-CARE PRACTICES DURING PREGNANCY

Along with the various recommendations discussed so far as ways of nurturing mind, body, and soul in the months between conception and birth, Ayurveda specifies four main self-care practices for nourishing yourself and your little babe throughout pregnancy, as follows.

ABHYANGA: SELF-MASSAGE

If you have been practicing abhyanga massages steadily for at least three months prior to conception (details and instructions on page 66), it is safe to continue massages throughout pregnancy. Otherwise, Ayurveda advises waiting to begin your massages until the second trimester, when your pregnancy is more stable. During pregnancy, abhyanga should be done slowly, lightly, and with your loving attention, really honoring your body as a sacred vessel that is growing your little one. Abhyanga is one of the most powerful ways to stabilize vata dosha and to assure that mama and babe are nourished, happy, and at ease.

LONG WALKS

Walking is a low-impact exercise that gives many benefits to the pregnant mama. Taking long walks boosts mood and energy levels, eases back pain and other aches, helps you sleep better, relieves constipation, supports overall cardiovascular health, aids in a more ease-filled labor and delivery, and much more.

Ideally, walk barefoot in nature! You'll have the perfect all-around self-care practice for maintaining mind-body wellness. Connection with the natural world soothes and heals the nervous system and invites us to connect with something larger than ourselves. Researchers have observed that spending time being present in nature lowers blood pressure, brings down heart rate, and reduces levels of harmful hormones circulating in the bloodstream—including cortisol, which your body produces when it's stressed.* Walking in nature can help put you (and babe!) in a more calm and relaxed state. If you live in a city, even spending time in an urban park can have a positive impact on your sense of well-being.

HERBAL BATHS

Baths are known to soothe tired or achy muscles, reduce stress, support digestion, boost immunity, promote relaxation, and more. When you add herbs, salts, clays, flower essences, and essential oils to your bath, the additions bring qualities that increase the bath's ability to support you in many ways. Cultures throughout history have recognized the importance of bathing, not only for personal hygiene, but also to open pathways to the soul's inner guidance.

There's nothing quite like an herbal bath. It's like soaking in a large cup of tea! Because the skin is the largest organ in the body, it draws in the medicinal compounds of the herbs that are added to the bath and delivers them to your entire system in a holistic way. Bathing in botanical baths gives you the opportunity to reconnect with the natural world and to reset your body toward ideal health and vitality.

Water is healing, soothing, and regenerative. It has a profound ability to bring clarity to the mind, supports you in *feeling* your emotions, and helps you to release what no longer serves. It has a "holding" ability: it literally will hold you and carry anything that feels too heavy or burdensome so that it can be released through the drain when your bath is finished.

Water also holds intention, so if you draw your bath with intention—perhaps the intention to bring more beauty, ease, or joy into your life—the water will deliver that energy into your body. You can increase the intention by simply adding more attention to what you are infusing into the bath. Use crystals, oils, herbs, and flowers to invite more healing—and thus a deeper connection to yourself.

To make an herbal bath, use any of the options in the instructions on page 199 and soak for twenty to thirty minutes in a water temperature that feels soothing.

---

* See for example Bum Jin Park et al., "The Physiological Effects of Shinrin-yoku (Taking in the Forest Atmosphere or Forest Bathing): Evidence from Field Experiments in 24 Forests across Japan," *Environmental Health and Preventive Medicine*, May 2009.

Guidelines for an Herbal Bath

Use ½–1 cup of your chosen fresh or dry herbal blend and decoct into a bath tea. If using a powdered herb, 2 tablespoons is plenty. To make a decoction, boil your herbs with 8 cups of water until the water has reduced to 4 cups. Strain before adding to your bath. If using more delicate flowers like rose, lavender, calendula, or chamomile, you can simply add flowers at the end of making your decoction (once the heat is off) or add to a French press and steep for twenty minutes before adding to the bath.

If using essential oils, add 3–10 drops to Epsom salts or honey and then add to the bath.

Clays are grounding and they soothe and heal the skin. You can add ½–1½ cups of clay to your bath.

Salts purify, offer magnesium, ease pain, and relax muscles. You can use ½–1 cup per bath.

Milk nourishes and softens skin. Use ½ cup of full-fat milk or a milk alternative

Colloidal oats soothe dry, itchy skin and are anti-inflammatory. Use ½–1½ cups per bath.

Honey softens, moisturizes, and nourishes the skin. Use ½–1 cup of honey per bath.

Other additions that will add a sense of ritual, beauty, and ceremony to your bathing experience: light candles, add fresh organic flowers to float atop the water, have crystals on hand to invite their specific energies, use sacred smoke to cleanse the area before and after the bath.

MEDITATION AND MINDFULNESS

Taking time each day to settle your mind and connect deeply to yourself is invaluable in the pursuit of living a fulfilling and intentional life. Whether it's practicing mantra meditation (page 83), working with your breath, or some other ritual that calls you deeply into the present moment, making time for meditation and mindfulness will anchor you and your little one into a deeper current of reality so that you may live into your day with more clarity, ease, connection, and intention.

LIFESTYLE ADAPTATIONS DURING PREGNANCY

The following are Ayurveda's recommendations for how to address and adapt sleep, sex, and natural urges as they arise during pregnancy.

SLEEPING POSITIONS

During the first three months of pregnancy you can lie down to sleep in any position, as your little one is tiny and tucked into your pelvic cage. After that, however, it is likely that lying on your stomach will feel quite uncomfortable for both you and your little one! After the fifth month, it is generally best to avoid lying on your back for more than twenty to thirty minutes at a time. Ideally you'll sleep on your left side, as your enlarged uterus may put pressure on the aorta, which reduces the amount of blood to your lower body, including your uterus, potentially affecting your baby's blood supply. All that being said, as long as you are comfortable, it is likely that your baby is also just fine. Trust your body. It will tell you if things are not right. Using pillows to get yourself comfortable on your left side during the later months of pregnancy is hugely beneficial for restful sleep. You can put a pillow beneath your tummy and between your knees, and anywhere else that feels supportive so that you can relax completely.

SEX DURING PREGNANCY

Rather than approaching the topic of sex during pregnancy in the mood of "right and wrong" or "good and bad," I will share the Ayurvedic perspective about how it affects the doshas. Because sex is an experience that breeds intimacy, connection, self-expression, and pleasure, please take into consideration the information below and then adapt it in a way that will maintain balance and harmony in your body and your relationship.

Ayurveda recommends abstaining from sex during pregnancy, especially in the first and third trimesters. Because the first trimester is governed by vata dosha, Ayurveda calls for doing everything you can to stabilize vata during that time. If vata is out of balance, it can cause miscarriage, preterm birth, back pain, constipation, anxiety, fear, and overwhelm. While sex in moderation may feel nourishing to your body and to your relationship, sex is light, mobile, and drying, and sex in excess will increase those qualities in your body.

Sex also involves the release of ojas, which takes over a month to produce! Recall that ojas is the final product of the digestion of food after it goes through all seven layers of tissue. It is absolutely necessary for nourishing your embryo and becomes especially important in the later part of pregnancy, when you share it to an even greater degree with your babe.

Abstaining from overindulgence in any sensory pleasures (such as too much food, too much TV, and the like) is beneficial, as you now know that the health (or dis-ease!) of your body and mind has an effect on the body and consciousness of your little one. Overindulgence in anything will affect the state of your mind. If you eat too much, you feel groggy. If you scroll Instagram for too long, you probably feel disconnected from yourself. In the same way, Ayurveda teaches that having too much sex will deplete your bodily tissues and leave you feeling dissatisfied. The discipline of regulating sexual engagement may also instill within your little one the knowledge that the real pleasure they seek is beyond the senses and that real satisfaction comes from within.

That being said, if mama has a strong sexual desire, her desire should not be suppressed; instead it should be regulated so that she stays balanced and vital. In general, those who already have a lot of vata in their constitution will be more affected by this and are advised to have sex only once or twice in a month. Those with a stronger, kapha constitution can have sex more frequently without throwing their doshas out of balance.

Because babies begin to know themselves as their environment, many *vaidyas* (Ayurvedic doctors) would suggest practicing celibacy to conserve that vital energy for internal and spiritual connection. Although celibacy might be a challenge, the benefits could be worthwhile for your little one's development. Deliberately avoiding sex does not mean that something is wrong in your relationship. If entered into consciously as a couple, celibacy can be a great opportunity for you and your partner to explore different ways to express affection, intimacy, and love. Some ideas could be holding hands, massaging each other, cooking and sharing meals together, or sharing loving and affectionate words.

A recommendation to abstain from sex during pregnancy arises if your experience includes any of the following:

- You have unexplained vaginal bleeding.
- You're leaking amniotic fluid.
- Your cervix begins to open prematurely (cervical incompetence).
- Your placenta partly or completely covers your cervical opening (placenta previa).
- You have a history of preterm labor or premature birth.

If you do choose to have sex during pregnancy, be sure to replenish your vital energy by eating ojas-building foods such as soaked almonds, ghee, dates, and hot milk with digestive spices; be consistent with your abhyanga (self-massage); and get plenty of nourishing sleep.

SUPPRESSION OF NATURAL URGES

Ayurveda details fourteen natural urges that should never be suppressed, as suppression of the urges will disrupt the proper movement of vata in the body. Pregnant mamas should especially avoid the following three: resisting flatulence, urination, and defecation.

Holding the urge of flatulence might put pressure on the uterus, as well as cause nausea, burping, and a burning sensation in the chest. Holding in urine increases the chance of developing a urinary tract infection, and the filled bladder may cramp and put pressure on the uterus. Resisting the urge to defecate will create a more toxic environment in your body and may also make you feel more "full" or bloated, and thus less hungry, so you are more likely to miss meals. These three urges are also governed by apana vata (the downward flow of vata), which is the direction of movement that we want to assure is efficient as mama gets closer to birthing her babe.

YOGA AND EXERCISE DURING PREGNANCY

During pregnancy, the intensity and style of exercise that you choose deserves extra consideration. You will want movement practices that nourish rather than deplete your tissues; Ayurveda suggests yoga and light cardio such as brisk walking, swimming, or the elliptical, which will tone your muscles and circulate your blood without increasing vata dosha.

Traditionally, asanas, or yoga poses, were meant to open the channels in the body to allow for the free flow of energy to take place. Ayurveda talks about many different channels in the body, from gross channels like the gastrointestinal tract, where your food is digested and assimilated, to smaller channels like the veins and arteries, where blood pulsates and oxygenates the entire body. Then there are the more subtle channels, like the channels of the mind and the heart, where thoughts and emotions move, as well as prana—your life-force energy—bringing awareness and thus vitality and vibrancy to the entire organism. The Ayurvedic approach suggests all dis-ease starts with stuck or stagnated energy in one or more of these channels and always originates in the more subtle channels before manifesting in the gross.

Rather than trying to "get a good workout," the focus of exercising during pregnancy is to move energy that has become stuck or stagnated in these channels through deep stretches, joint rotations, and gentle cardiovascular movement. These types of movement will distribute fresh blood and oxygen, as well as awareness, throughout your entire body. When these gross and subtle channels are unobstructed, your body naturally finds its perfect state of balance, whether that means you need to gain weight or lose it, gain muscle mass or soften a bit.

Your breath and your awareness have an intimate connection. As you breathe more deeply into your body, you invite your awareness inside—often our awareness is everywhere but there! Dr. John Douillard, a globally recognized leader in the fields of natural health, Ayurveda, and sports medicine and founder of the Ayurvedic resource LifeSpa, writes that "only when self-awareness is cultivated can the system fully recognize underlying problems or imbalances and elicit appropriate responses to heal them."* As you invite your attention to the space inside of you, you begin to heal. Your attention provides the space for your body, mind, and emotions to rearrange themselves—moving from dis-order to order, dis-ease to health. Your body knows how to heal and knows how it needs to *be* in order to be balanced. Your breath and awareness begin to awaken the innate intelligence that already exists within you by creating the proper environment for healing to happen.

Every emotion has a corresponding breath pattern, and your breath

---

* **John Douillard, LifeSpa website, "Get High on Massage," December 19, 2021, https://lifespa.com/health-topics/stress-management/get-high-massage/.**

pattern alone can stir up an emotion. When you are present, connected, and relaxed, you may notice that your breath is deep and full. When you are feeling anxious or scared, or simply lost in your thoughts, your breath is short and shallow. Even by unconsciously taking short and shallow breaths, you may begin to feel unsettled and anxious. By deepening your breath, you will become more present, connected, and relaxed.

While growing your little one, you want to focus on exercises that allow for you to maintain a steady rhythm of breath. If you notice your breath becoming strained, slow down or back out of the posture, find your steady breath, and then enter back into your exercise from a more ease-filled place.

Vata-stabilizing yoga poses that strengthen your legs and lower back—such as chair pose, the warrior poses, and balancing postures—will be supportive. You can also choose postures that bring circulation to your hips and reproductive organs, such as pigeon pose and bound-angle pose. Joint rotations help to move stuck energy in the body as well as deliver circulation and heat in a gentle way. Again, focus on nourishment and ease in your movement practice and in your life.

COMMON IMBALANCES DURING PREGNANCY

As your body shifts and changes to accommodate your growing babe, many challenges can arise, including certain health difficulties that Ayurveda lists as common in pregnancy: weight loss, nausea, dryness of mouth, vomiting, edema (swelling), fever, anemia, retention of urine, and diarrhea. These things may be hard to avoid, though the wisdom of Ayurveda can support you in your attempt to stay balanced throughout the journey.

Any woman who has been challenged through her pregnancy will tell you how defeating it may feel when health difficulties affect daily life. Some women feel so nauseous during their first trimester that they can barely eat; they become skinny and malnourished, and their digestion is affected. Many women in their third trimester will have a list of complaints: their feet are swollen, they feel heavy and tired, they get heartburn or acid reflux when they eat certain foods, they have to pee all the time, their digestion is affected, their pelvic bones may hurt when they walk or turn over in bed, they may not be sleeping well; the list can go on. Other women feel vibrant, vital, and healthy throughout their entire pregnancy, with no digestive upsets, swelling, or any discomfort at all!

Ayurveda approaches health with a perspective of prevention first. In chapter 2, we discussed the importance of cleansing your body of any imbalances prior to conceiving, and then nourishing and rebuilding with the proper diet and nutrition before conception—this preparation is a means not only to ready your body, mind, and consciousness for the time of conception, but also to best prevent difficulties from arising during your pregnancy. However, you may be living with chronic imbalances that have accumulated over years and years because of environment, lifestyle, and diet. Cleansing for a few weeks or even a few months may not be enough to fully purge these deeper imbalances. Nonetheless, any level of cleansing before conception will help improve your situation for a healthier pregnancy.

I wrote this chapter (and much of this book) with the intention of honoring traditional Ayurvedic wisdom while also providing practical solutions to things that may still arise because of life influences you face. Sometimes the challenges that come up are out of your control, or due to factors that are not easily affected by diet and lifestyle, and you need some tools to move forward with practical and helpful solutions.

ACID REFLUX/HEARTBURN

As the size of the baby increases, the space for mama's intestines and internal organs decreases. For this reason, it is common for a pregnant mama to experience heartburn or acid reflux and digestive problems (constipation, gas, and indigestion) toward the last stage of pregnancy. Acid reflux and heartburn are conditions that arise from pitta dosha. Avoiding pitta-aggravating foods will prevent heartburn. (See chapter 1 to understand the qualities of pitta, and follow the pitta-pacifying lifestyle tips and diet starting at page 25). Here are some tips to alleviate heartburn and other digestive symptoms:

Eat smaller meals, more often (making sure your previous meal is fully digested before eating the next one).

Drink diluted buttermilk with a pinch of cardamom daily.

Remain upright for at least two hours after eating.

Take a gentle walk after meals.

Reduce oil and salt in your diet.

Make a warm tea with equal parts cumin, coriander, and fennel to sip with your meals (see the recipe for CCF tea on page 288).

Sip yogurt lassi.

Drink anise and fennel tea.

Carry soaked, raw almonds with you to chew as a snack when you're feeling symptoms.

Consume amalaki (Indian gooseberry) by mixing 1 teaspoon in 1 cup of warm water to drink as needed.

Consume guduchi by mixing ½ teaspoon in 1 cup of warm water as needed when you experience heartburn.

Consume shatavari by adding 1 teaspoon to your spiced milk before bed.

Use licorice to help with digestive issues by either adding ½ teaspoon of powdered licorice to your spiced milk or making it as a tea by itself.

ANEMIA

Anemia arises when the amount of hemoglobin in your blood dips below normal, which can cause headaches, weakness, fatigue, loss of appetite, and insomnia. The increase in blood volume during pregnancy commonly leads to mild anemia, but anemia may also be the consequence of a diet lacking in the right combination of foods or of living a life so busy that mealtimes are hurried and feature too many processed foods devoid of nutrition. With the high nutritional demands of pregnancy, falling short can especially lead to anemia from folate or iron deficiency.

Here are some ideas for helping to counter mild anemia caused by increased blood volume:

Eat a handful of soaked black raisins daily.

Eat two to six dates with ghee daily.

Eat green veggies and beets. Always add lime, as citrus makes the iron in these foods more bioavailable.

Eat foods or herbs high in vitamin C such as citrus, rosehips, elderberries, blackberries, Schisandra berry, pomegranate, and amalaki fruit.

Take 1 teaspoon of the Ayurvedic herbal jam chyavanprash, twice daily.

Take 2 teaspoons of spirulina or alfalfa powder daily.

Take 1 tablespoon of brahmi-infused ghee in hot milk or water each evening. (See page 287 for a recipe for making ghee.)

Anemia caused by deficiency in folic acid can be countered by eating the following folate-rich herbs and foods:

- Watercress
- Parsley
- Chicory
- Dandelion
- Amaranth
- Whole grains
- Leafy greens

If you are diagnosed with iron anemia, the following iron-rich herbs and foods can help restore healthy red blood cells:

- Yellow dock root and dandelion root (in small amounts)
- Parsley
- Nettles
- Kelp
- Amaranth greens
- Beets

ANXIETY

In Ayurvedic medicine, the *Sushruta Samhita* describes anxiety as a derangement of bodily doshas that affects the nerves and thereby produces a distracted state of mind. Simply put, aggravation of vata dosha in the nervous system and the mind can cause anxiety, insecurity, and fear. And during pregnancy, especially in the first trimester when so much change is happening and there may be too much lightness, coolness, dryness, and mobility in your diet or lifestyle, vata commonly goes out of balance in this way.

To treat acute anxiety, Ayurveda calls for reducing vata dosha. Keeping in mind the principle of like increases like and opposites balance, the treatments for anxiety will be grounding, lubricating, and nourishing and will include oleation and heat, both internally and externally. Use the dietary and lifestyle suggestions in chapter 1 to balance vata dosha (starting on page 21) to reduce anxiety during pregnancy. Herbs such as ashwagandha, chamomile, lavender, oatstraw, and skullcap can also help.

CONGESTION

Runny nose and congestion are common symptoms during pregnancy as a result of excess hormones and blood volume causing the blood vessels in your nose to swell and produce more mucus. To clear your nasal passageways, try the following:

Start your day with a warm, steamy shower.

Drink plenty of hydrating fluids such as mineral water, coconut water, and fresh juices.

Soak a washcloth in hot water and then put a few drops of essential oils such as rosemary, tea tree, or eucalyptus on it. Hold the hot washcloth toward your face and take deep inhales through your nose.

During the day, get mild exercise such as yoga, swimming, or walking.

At night, use a vaporizer or humidifier in your bedroom.

Use a diffuser for essential oils of eucalyptus, tea tree, rosemary, or peppermint.

Sleep with your head slightly elevated.

CONSTIPATION

Many women experience constipation at different stages in their pregnancy. Sometimes constipation is the result of hormonal shifts that cause digestion to slow down, or sometimes it is related to an excess of vata, which causes coolness and dryness in the colon. Later in pregnancy, the growing uterus may be putting pressure on the intestines, constricting the movement of waste through the colon. Ayurveda emphasizes the importance of daily bowel movements for vital health, and going to the bathroom each day remains important during pregnancy. The following tips can help maintain regular elimination:

Drink warm water throughout the day.

Add 2 teaspoons of ghee to your warm water first thing in the morning.

Eat four prunes that have been soaked overnight before breakfast.

Follow a vata-pacifying diet.

Have ojas milk (see recipe on page 56) with 2 tablespoons of ghee at bedtime.

Eat a teaspoon of roasted fennel seed with a glass of warm water at bedtime.

Have 1 tablespoon of amalaki in warm water once per day.

Try to fit in a gentle walk each day to help waste move through your intestines.

EARLY PREGNANCY LOSS

I have been asked by quite a few mamas who have experienced previous miscarriages what to do to protect the little one they are now carrying. Many women experience miscarriages in their first trimester, so although that is never easy, please know that you are not alone. Your individual biology cannot be generalized, so doing everything "right" and still losing a pregnancy is not the fault of your body or necessarily caused by anything that you did or did not do.

Ayurveda is a highly individualized science, but I will attempt to generalize with some Ayurvedic tips to nourish your body and mind before and during pregnancy in ways intended to help prevent miscarriage: The main focus is to strengthen and stabilize an aspect of vata called apana vata, the downward movement of energy (such as evacuation, ejaculation, and menstruation), as well as vata's ability to hold, so you can retain your little babe within your womb—and also so you don't experience incontinence. (This is especially important in your first and third trimesters.) The Ayurvedic approach to strengthening apana vata includes the following:

Maintain a vata-pacifying diet and lifestyle, including regulation with your eating and sleeping times; seek things that are warming, grounding, nourishing, stabilizing.

Focus on grounding yoga poses that strengthen your legs—for instance, chair pose, warrior poses, and squats.

Avoid dry, light, and cooling or cold foods.

Move slowly. Eat slowly. *Be* slowly.

Avoid fast-paced activities and exercise, as well as intense conversations.

Consume ghee, dates, spiced milk, and soaked almonds, which are ojas building and supportive.

Avoid (or greatly reduce) sexual intercourse. Sex disperses the energy of vata throughout the body, moving it from its most stable place in the pelvis.

Start connecting with this little soul; bring your hands to your belly throughout the day and send at least ten deep, intentional breaths to your little angel daily, with as much presence, love, and attention as possible.

Let this little soul know
that they are wanted,
safe,
loved,
and so cared for.
And then, allow.
Whether it is forever or for now.
This little soul is so blessed to have you as its mama.

EDEMA

Edema (swelling) is a fairly common condition in pregnancy and is often a result of the pressure of the uterus pressing on the draining lymphatic fluid from the legs, resulting in swelling. However, if it is associated with any other signs, especially hypertension (high blood pressure), then you should consult your physician. According to Ayurveda, swelling during pregnancy can also be due to lack of exercise, lack of iron, or lack of protein. Try the following approaches to reduce the swelling of mild edema:

Make sure that you are drinking ample water with minerals and electrolytes to help flush the lymphatic system and keep the fluids moving in your body.

Take Epsom salt baths (see "Edema Foot Soak" on page 313).

Practice abhyanga massage (see page 66).

Drink CCF tea (see the recipe on page 288) and ginger tea.

Walk every day for twenty to thirty minutes to improve circulation.

Raise your feet above your heart (to help drain lymphatic fluid).

GESTATIONAL DIABETES

Gestational diabetes is a condition in which women without previously diagnosed diabetes exhibit high blood-glucose levels during pregnancy. Often, diabetes is a kapha disorder that arises when agni, your digestive fire, is impaired. Ayurveda recommends these traditional practices to support agni and reduce the risk of gestational diabetes:

Follow a kapha-pacifying diet, especially avoiding overconsumption of sweets.

Eat more fresh veggies, lightly steamed or baked so that they are easier to digest.

Put 1 cup of water in a copper vessel overnight and drink it in the morning.

Consume turmeric—which is supportive for stabilizing blood sugar—either in capsule form or as a turmeric tea. (Add a pinch of black pepper to tea, to make the medicinal qualities more bioavailable.)

HYPERTENSION (HIGH BLOOD PRESSURE)

Because a woman's blood volume increases dramatically during pregnancy, blood pressure is likely to increase as well during this time. Hypertension is the term for higher-than-normal pressure in the veins and arteries as your blood pumps through them. Ayurvedic medicine typically views high blood pressure as reflecting an imbalance in vata and pitta doshas, but in pregnancy, hypertension often results from an increase of kapha. Vata is responsible for narrowing of the arteries, whereas kapha is responsible for fatty deposits that make their home in the artery walls and increase blood viscosity. To reduce high blood pressure, apply the following Ayurvedic recommendations:

Tame the physical and emotional stress that may increase blood pressure through practices such as *yoga nidra* (a form of guided meditation also known as "yogic sleep") and meditation.

Practice breathing exercises such as nadi shodhana (see page 22) or sitali (see page 26).

Let go of unnecessary responsibilities.

Restrict salty, spicy, sour, fatty, and fried foods.

Drink half a cup of fresh cucumber juice daily.

IRRITABILITY OR MOOD SWINGS

Pregnant women are known for their mood swings! The high levels of hormones in your body may cause your emotions to feel more intense than you are used to. In addition, you are going through a huge shift in your life (physically, mentally, spiritually, relationally), and as you process these shifts, so many feelings can come up.

Although this shift can be challenging, please do not look at your mood swings as a negative symptom of pregnancy. Instead, see your fluctuating emotions, reactions, and triggers as insights into what you most need. Your sensitivity right now is a gift. Your ability to feel everything right now is your strength. You are becoming crystal clear about what works for you and what does not, what serves you and what does not. When you are feeling strong emotions, ask yourself: What needs do I have that are not being met? What is this emotion here to teach me?

It is important to allow yourself to feel, though it is also important that you express your feelings in a way that is effective. Being pregnant is not an excuse to become bossy or unkind or to allow your emotions to run the show. If you are feeling resentful, unsupported, frustrated—how can you express your emotions without making the other person "wrong"? You are not the victim of your experience. Use your superpower of *feeling deeply* to support you in rearranging what needs to be shifted in your life and to upgrade your all-around experience during pregnancy. To be proactive in balancing emotions, consider these tips:

Practice meditation and pranayama exercise.

Use affirmations.

Journal.

Receive counsel from someone you trust, or gather your closest women friends and meet weekly to connect and share your hearts.

If your emotions are affecting your daily life and leading to depression, try the following:

Cut out white sugar and moderate sugary foods (excess sugar—especially when eaten without protein—can lead to blood sugar swings, fatigue, and depression).

Eat high-protein snacks like soaked nuts, yogurt, raw milk, or raw cheese.

Take 5 drops of motherwort tincture in a glass of water (motherwort restores emotional balance).

Drink skullcap tea (to support your nervous system).

According to Ayurveda, the desires of the pregnant mama are the desires of the baby in her womb. You are intrinsically in tune with your child's needs and wishes even before you have met them! Ayurveda teaches that it is important that mama stays happy and feels supported, and that her needs be fulfilled, in order to grow a happy, healthy child who knows that this world will provide them with everything that they need.

MORNING SICKNESS

Nausea, or "morning sickness," during early pregnancy is common. More than half of women experience some degree of nausea or vomiting during their first trimester. For some mamas, nausea will start by the fifth or sixth week of pregnancy and may be the worst toward the beginning of the third month. Morning sickness usually disappears around the start of the second trimester, though for a small percentage of women, the nausea may last longer. For some, it is merely a food aversion—a strong reaction to certain smells or tastes. For others, it is periodic queasiness, often peaking in the morning and dissipating after lunch. For a few, it is an overwhelming feeling that lasts all day.

According to Ayurveda, these symptoms occur mainly due to the aggravation of pitta dosha. The hormones estrogen and progesterone are both essential to the progression of pregnancy, but they are also high in pitta qualities. In order to minimize nausea, the aggravation of pitta needs to be brought back into balance. Morning sickness might also be related to low blood sugar. Ayurveda offers these recommendations to help bring pitta into balance and ease nausea during pregnancy:

Start the day off with a little food.

Eat an energizing snack when you feel nausea coming on to help to raise your blood sugar.

Eat smaller, more frequent meals that are high in protein. (An empty stomach has more acid secretion, which can cause stomach irritation and nausea.)

Roast black cardamom seeds, grind them, and eat small pinches throughout the day.

Sip on ginger tea throughout the day.

Drink a cup of boiled milk each evening to which you've added a few drops of rosewater and a teaspoon of ghee (to prevent nausea in the morning).

Inhale the scent of mint, lemon, or orange essential oil to help alleviate nausea by placing a cotton ball or tissue infused with the oil under your nose (or put these essential oils in a diffuser).

Sip on coconut water with 1 teaspoon of lemon juice

See if exercise helps your symptoms: take an extra walk during the day, go for a swim, or join a prenatal yoga class.

Slow down: clear your schedule and take time to relax.

Practice sitali, also known as cooling breath (page 26), which helps reduce pitta dosha and ease the stomach.

PELVIC PAIN

Toward the end of pregnancy, a hormone called relaxin begins increasing in your body, which loosens the joints, muscles, tendons, and bones in order to make it easier for your body to open up during childbirth. During the third trimester, as the pubic and pelvic bones begin to loosen, you may experience pain in those bones when walking, getting out of bed, turning over in bed, or bending down to put your pants on.

Severe pain of this type is referred to as symphysis pubis dysfunction (SPD). A few things can be done to avoid making the pain worse, but unfortunately it's not always possible to relieve the pain completely. Also unfortunately, this pain may continue after childbirth, so maintaining some level of treatment for stability is important for long-term relief. If you are experiencing SPD, ask your care providers about regular visits to a physical therapist, chiropractor, acupuncturist, or craniosacral therapist. You can also use these tips to get you through your third trimester:

Stabilize your pelvis by using a belly belt, a Mexican rebozo, or a scarf wrapped tightly around your pelvic bones to help hold them in place.

Take a warm Epsom salts bath daily (using 2 cups of Epsom salts) for twenty minutes or longer.

Adapt your daily activities to increase your comfort: sit down while putting on pants, hold your knees together while turning over in bed, lift your legs with your hands when getting in and out of the tub or the car, have someone help you get out of bed in the morning, move slowly, and so on.

Avoid standing or sitting for long periods of time; keep moving.

Get physical therapy to learn exercises that can help create more stability in the pelvis and relieve some of the pain. (Ask your midwife or doctor for a reference to a physical therapist or a pelvic floor therapist who works with pregnant women.)

Find a chiropractor who does adjustments for SPD. (Ask your doctor or midwife to refer you to a chiropractor who is familiar with these specific adjustments.)

Get acupuncture or craniosacral therapy treatments.

Exercise in gentle ways like swimming or walking.

An important note about birth positions and SPD: If you are suffering from SPD, certain birthing positions will make your labor much more difficult and painful, and some positions should be avoided because they bring the risk of permanently damaging your pubic bone. Ask your doctor or midwife about birthing positions safe for SPD, or do some research on your own.

PREECLAMPSIA

Preeclampsia is a specific kind of high blood pressure some women get while pregnant or after giving birth. Also known as metabolic toxemia, preeclampsia is one of the most serious complications during pregnancy. The condition is signaled by edema (swelling), hypertension, and protein in the urine. Other signs and symptoms of preeclampsia may include severe headaches, changes in vision (including temporary loss of vision), blurred vision or light sensitivity, upper abdominal pain (usually under the ribs on the right side), nausea or vomiting, decreased urine output, decreased levels of platelets in the blood (thrombocytopenia), impaired liver function, and shortness of breath. Sudden weight gain and swelling—particularly in the face and hands—may occur with preeclampsia, but these also occur in many normal pregnancies, so they're not considered reliable signs of preeclampsia on their own.

Preeclampsia usually occurs in the third trimester, but it can also arise earlier in pregnancy. Although the medical model of care does not recognize any one cause of preeclampsia, traditional medicine sees a connection to the mother's diet and teaches that it is the result of malnutrition during pregnancy. If you are showing signs of preeclampsia, be sure to manage this condition with your doctor, as it can be serious if not monitored properly. The following is a list of tips for preventing and treating preeclampsia from Susan Weed's *Wise Woman Herbal for the Childbearing Year*.

PREVENTING PREECLAMPSIA

Eat salt! Insufficient salt intake during pregnancy can lead to preeclampsia.

Consume 60–80 grams of protein daily; see recipes in chapter 8 for spiced milk (page 290), kitchari (page 294), dal (page 294).

Eat 2,400 calories per day.

Take 1,000 grams of calcium daily.

Drink raspberry leaf tea, nettle tea, and dandelion tea throughout pregnancy.

Add fresh or cooked dandelion greens to your meals.

TREATING PREECLAMPSIA

Drink mint tea, chicory tea, and dandelion tea for a potassium boost.

Drink 4 ounces of raw beet juice daily to balance sodium and potassium.

Grate raw beet and raw apple together for a daily snack.

Take a supplement of 100 milligrams of vitamin B6 daily.

Take 3 tablespoons of spirulina or chlorella daily.

Eat seaweed daily.

SLEEP

At various times during your pregnancy, you may experience difficulty either falling asleep or staying asleep—perhaps because of an excess of vata dosha leading to restlessness or an active mind, or perhaps because you can't find a position you are comfortable in. You have many traditional approaches to choose from if you're trying to achieve more restful sleep:

Engage your body in healthy activity during the day. Do yoga, take walks, swim.

Avoid taking naps during the day. (According to Ayurveda, this makes for a lazy child!)

Drink plenty of fluids during the day.

Meditate before bed.

Do a head and foot massage before you go to sleep. Your head and your feet have many *marma* points (see "Mama Marma Therapy" at page 211) similar to pressure points or acupuncture points. When oil is applied to your feet and massaged in, your entire nervous system will calm and help prepare your mind and body for sleep.

Drink warm milk with nutmeg before sleep. Nutmeg's sedative effect will help you relax and fall asleep, and having this light snack will help prevent you from waking up hungry in the night.

Sleep on your left side to improve blood flow to your baby.

Use support pillows between your knees, under your belly, and behind your back.

Focus on your breathing as you fall asleep.

If you wake up in the middle of the night, it may be your baby waking you! Try talking to your baby and soothing them back to sleep.

If heartburn is waking you up, avoid eating a couple of hours before sleep and avoid spicy, oily foods.

If you feel active at night or have a sensation of restlessness in your legs at nighttime, try massaging your legs with warm oil or taking a warm bath before going to sleep. Also check to make sure you are not iron or folate deficient.

If your partner tells you that you have been snoring and you are just exhausted throughout the day (more than you would expect), consider getting checked for sleep apnea. Sleeping on your side and propped up can help temporarily.

Get to sleep before 10 p.m.

Avoid stimulation such as movies and social media after sunset.

Take magnesium baths or take a magnesium supplement.

STRETCH MARKS

Stretch marks are a result of the body's fascia, or connective tissue, stretching thin and spreading out. The inner layer of the skin then cracks or splits. Stretch marks occur from the inside out and therefore are prevented from the inside out, starting with nutrition. Ayurveda recommends eating lots of healthy fats—like nonhomogenized milk, raw butter, and ghee—to prevent your skin from cracking. Daily abhyanga massages followed by a warm shower or bath will also help prevent stretch marks as the oil seeps through the pores into the inner layers of your skin. You might find it helpful to treat the dryness or itchiness that comes with a stretched belly by using belly butter, but do make sure that you are using one that is either homemade or has all clean, organic ingredients.

WEIGHT GAIN

There is no "one size fits all" approach to pregnancy weight gain. The amount of weight any particular woman should gain generally depends on how much she weighed before she became pregnant. That said, a vata mama (thinner body frame) is suggested to gain 25–40 pounds over the course of her pregnancy; pitta mamas (average body size) should put on 25–35 pounds; and a kapha mama (larger frame) may only need to gain 15–25 pounds. If you are carrying twins, what is considered healthy weight gain is much more! The most important thing is to keep your weight gain to a safe and healthy level for you and your little one.

Ayurveda suggests that the most important guideline is to maintain a steady weight increase while eating wholesome and healthy foods. If your diet is high quality and you are really listening to your body, you shouldn't have any worries about whether the weight gain is too high or too low. Along these lines, don't worry about "eating for two" during pregnancy. What is important is that you really tune in to your body and recognize when you are hungry or when you are in need of some other form of nourishment (perhaps a bath, an oil massage, or loving touch).

Only some of the weight you gain during pregnancy will be body fat. The other factors causing weight gain will include the extra weight of your baby, the placenta, amniotic fluid (the water surrounding your baby), your growing breasts, increased blood, and natural fluid retention.

The main thing, not surprisingly, is that you want to make sure vata is pacified. Believe it or not, when vata becomes exacerbated, you can actually gain unhealthy weight! Most people associate high vata to weight loss, but let me tell you why some pregnant mamas (and people in general) may gain an unhealthy amount of weight even if they are hardly eating or are eating light foods like salads, working out for hours a day, and staying super busy.

Vata weight may stay on in order to ground a person who is airy and scattered. A high level of mental stress, irregular meal times, skipping meals, unhealthy food choices, or eating too many foods that are dry, cold, light, or raw increases vata dosha in the body and can severely impact your metabolism, causing it to be sluggish and unresponsive.

Because of this, you may accumulate *ama* (toxins) in your body, which leads to clogged channels. When ama blocks the channels of digestion and the channels that circulate nutrients throughout the body, metabolism slows down and weight gain results. When the channels are clogged, nothing can move in or out and you start to hold on to weight. You may then become even more active, trying to lose the excess weight, and thus create an acidic environment in your body. At this point, your body will need to hold on to even more fat to protect the tissues from the acid . . . and so begins a cycle.

I have seen, time and time again, people coming to my gentle yoga classes and saying, “I was going to the gym for two hours per day and couldn’t lose those last ten pounds. But as soon as I started attending restorative yoga classes, the weight just fell off!” When you pacify vata through slow movement, relaxation, routine, and warm, cooked, nourishing meals eaten at regular times throughout the day, the channels in your body relax and open, your digestion regulates, and any excess weight is able to leave the body.

Many of us are acculturated to seeing food as a major source of comfort, because it gives an immediate sense of feeling grounded and satisfied—but too often that tendency leads to overeating or to eating when we are not actually hungry. We may also get caught up in the many “shoulds” around what and when to eat—so caught up that we forget to listen to our own bodies. Ayurveda suggests that you are not actually what you eat, but rather what you digest. And in order to digest anything, there has to be real hunger.

Try to stay tuned in to your real hunger before eating, and then to eat to your satisfaction. Let yourself be nourished by what you’re eating by staying present with your food, chewing and really tasting each bite, and actually enjoying it. Believe it or not, this will have a drastic effect on your ability to digest, absorb, and assimilate food efficiently! Aim for regular mealtimes, as vata thrives with routine (and so does your digestive system). Eat foods that are easy to digest yet nourishing. Sip on warm water and hydrating teas throughout the day, which will open the channels in your body and gently stoke the digestive fire. Warm food and digestive spices will nourish vata and also help pacify excess kapha in your system.

Since pregnancy is already a time when vata dosha is increased, use this time to invite more grounding, nourishing, and stabilizing routines into your life. Rather than doing high-intensity fitness classes or a lot of cardio, opt for yoga classes, long (perhaps brisk) walks, and conscious relaxation. When the channels in your body are open, and when you are truly nourished, your body knows what it needs or does not need and can find its optimal state of well-being.

A LATE-PREGNANCY BLESSING

Traditionally in the last months of pregnancy there would be the following ceremony to honor the pregnant mama and to bless her with the necessary strength, surrender, and confidence to enter this next season of her life.

Simantonnayana: Parting of the Hair Ceremony

Simantonnayana is a traditional ceremony held in the third trimester of pregnancy meant to invoke blessings and auspiciousness for the final stages of gestation and the upcoming moment of birth. The mantras are said to release lifetimes of past trauma from the baby so that the new child can enter the world with a deeper connection to themselves.

During this ceremony, the expectant partners gather together with friends and family. The father offers mama his affectionate attention as he parts her hair down the center line three times, each time with different objects (traditionally, darbha grass, a porcupine quill, and a stick of viratara wood). Each time, he recites different mantras.

He offers flowers to her and feeds her sweet and nourishing fruits, to symbolize her nourishment and happiness and to honor her for carrying their child during this sacred time in their lives. Other mantras are recited to give mama confidence and mental strength. Mama and baby then receive individual blessings from each mother who is present for the ceremony.

After the *simantonnayana* ritual and until the birth, the woman is expected to not overexert herself and her partner is expected to be near her and to not travel to distant lands.

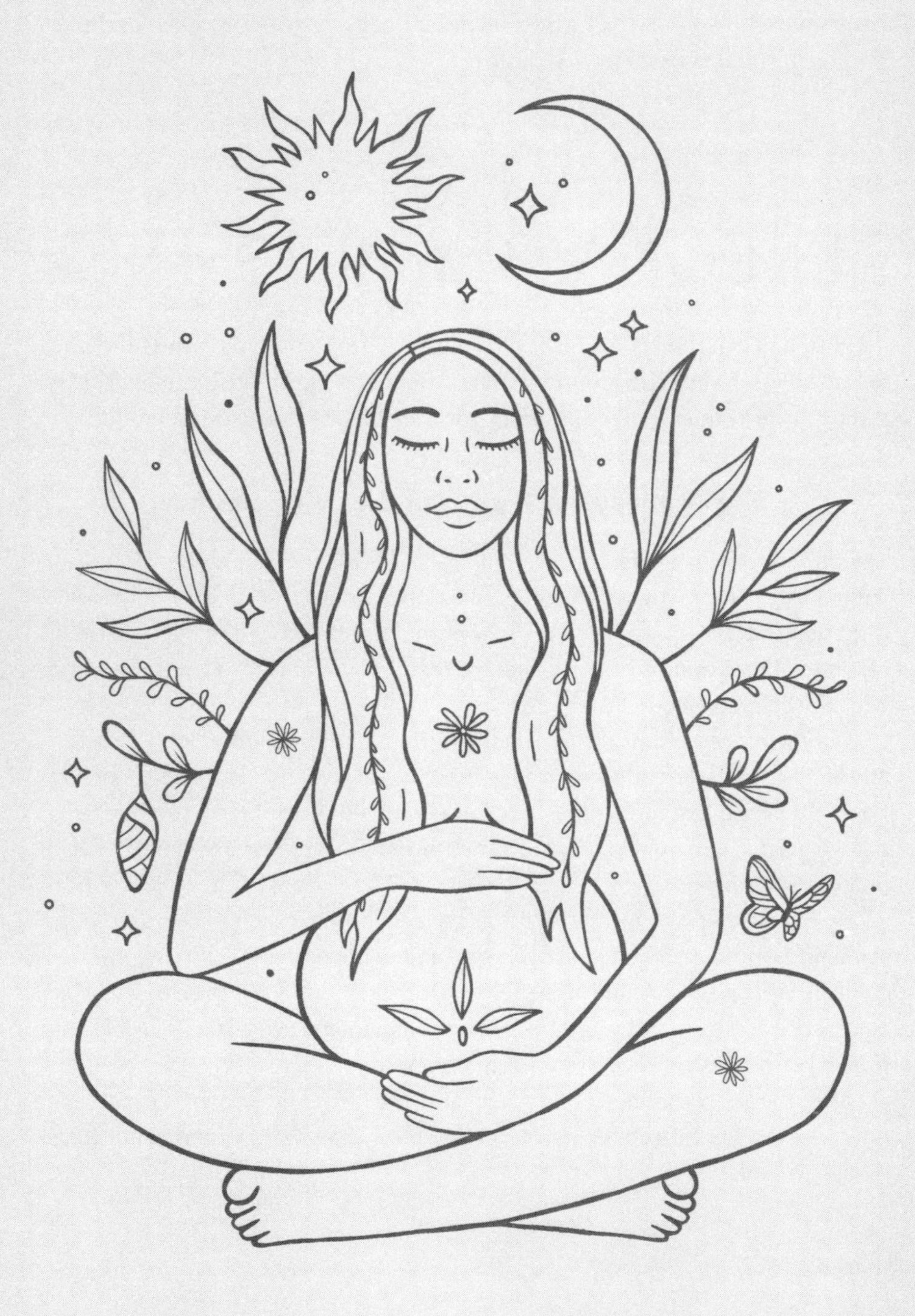

Preparing for Birth

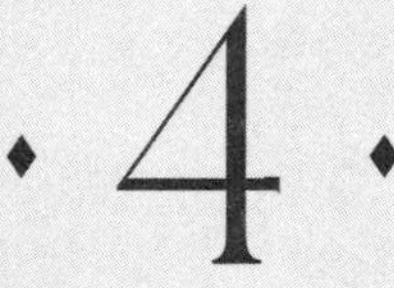

For far too many, pregnancy and birth is still something that happens to them rather than something they set out consciously and joyfully to do themselves.

—Sheila Kitzinger, *The Experience of Childbirth*

Doing everything that you can to prepare for your labor and birth allows you to show up fully for your own unique, empowered birth experience and to surrender completely to the process as it unfolds—from a place of deep trust and confidence. Where do you plan to give birth? How do you want to give birth? Who will be there? How will you prepare? Is it possible to feel prepared?! A million questions may be buzzing in your mind as you consider the many options of how you will birth your little one. How you choose to give birth takes consideration, thought, and research, whether you prefer a free birth at home with just you and your partner; a home birth with attending midwives, doulas, and family; a vaginal birth at the hospital; or a plan to schedule an induction or C-section.

How and where you give birth matters. The people present; the energy in the space; mama feeling empowered or subservient, trusting or fearful; who receives baby; what happens immediately following birth—it all matters. The environment that your babe is born into is their first impression of the world outside of the womb. Before deciding on your birth plan, reflect on the beliefs that you have around birthing. Do you believe that it is powerful and beautiful? Do you think it will be unbearably painful? Do you trust that it is a natural process, designed to go well? Do you feel that things often go wrong? Perhaps you have heard stories of your family and friends giving birth, and you think that your experience will be similar. Maybe you have seen a woman in labor on TV or in movies and think that your water will break, then you will be rushed to the hospital and scream the whole way through. If the beliefs that you have surrounding your birth cause fear or anxiety, you may want to take some time to reframe your thoughts and open up to other possibilities. Every single birth is completely and utterly profound. Your birth story will not be like any other birth story you have ever heard.

Every woman should have the opportunity for a healthy, safe, and empowered birth. Giving birth can be a deeply positive and transformative experience. In an oft-cited quote from her book *A Bun in the Oven: How the Food and Birth Movements Resist Industrialization*, the sociologist Barbara Katz Rothman emphasizes: "Birth is not only about making babies. Birth is about making mothers—strong, competent, capable mothers who trust themselves and know their inner strength." I suggest reading stories of positive birth experiences and researching facts and statistics on different methods of birth and birth interventions. From there, make an informed decision from an empowered place rather than a fearful one. *Ina May's Guide to Childbirth*, by the renowned professional midwife Ina May Gaskin, is perhaps one of the most valuable books a pregnant mother can read before making her birth plan.

In this chapter, I share information that will support you in preparing your birth plan, home, body, mind, and life to welcome your little one into the world. I share my personal plan for my home birth along with my hospital transfer plan, which includes my own personal choices in the case that I needed to be transferred to the hospital during labor. I hope that sharing my choices will inspire you and give you some practical direction while thinking of what to research when creating your own birth vision. I share this information solely from my personal experience and not to give any medical advice.

This little cabin,
the little window,
that little table surrounded by the biggest trees
and the biggest love I know.

We left from San Francisco airport this morning:
him on United Airlines: a plane to New York City.
Me on Alaska airlines: flying back to Florida.
On the way to our terminals
little tears were rolling down my cheeks,
and once I got off at my terminal,
leaving him on the sky train to continue his journey,
I started sobbing.

Like wrinkled face, hard to catch my breath typa' tears.
As I rode down the escalator
I looked back up at the train and saw him through the window
as his train drove out of sight.

I know it sounds like a melodramatic movie scene.
To me too!
This is new to me.
We've said goodbye, or "see you soon," a thousand times.
I've prided myself in not needing to talk every day,
or being able to go weeks without seeing him
and not really missing him.
But since little bun has been in the oven,
things are so so different.

I missed him for the last two days that we were together,
knowing we would be leaving.

I want to be with him all of the time.

I don't want to miss out on this special time together;
your conversations with him,

reading to him,
checking in on him,
or just resting your hand on my belly as we drive.
Also, just how special I feel when we're all together,
the way you love me and care for me in this whole new way.

And perhaps a part of me knows that after bub comes,
things will never be the same.

Of course there will be a trillion times more love,
but it's not just us anymore.
It's not us
doing what we want
when we want
and how we want.
It's not me and you as the center of our love story.
Everything is changing,
and I want to hold on to this time forever.

In a way, it almost feels like a death.
I'm afraid I'm gonna miss it:
miss the us
that we were
before babe was here.
Miss the era,
the life that was before.

And I love you no less, little one.
You're making everything more special.

With more love there is more heartache,
because the heart opens to feel it all.
It's heartbreaking
and so beautiful
all at once.

PRENATAL TESTING

Several common prenatal tests are recommended to pregnant women as routine procedures—though many women forget they have the power to say "no" to these tests if they believe it is not best for themselves or their baby. Medical procedures have their place, and every circumstance is different. Depending on your unique pregnancy, your medical history, your family health history, and your personal preferences, you may decide that certain tests will benefit you, though you may also decide that some of them do not. Make sure you are informed and educated on the process of these tests, the possible risks and complications, the benefits, and the potential reasons for doing them.

Prenatal tests to research and make decisions about include ultrasounds, chorionic villus sampling, amniocentesis, maternal serum alpha-fetoprotein screening, screening for gestational diabetes, group B strep, and prenatal rhoGAM. It can be confusing for a pregnant mama to familiarize herself with all these medical procedures, and many mamas end up just deferring to the recommendations of their care providers. Ina May Gaskin's *Guide to Childbirth* gives a comprehensive guide to prenatal testing, summarizing the medical procedures and listing the possible benefits, risks, and complications, and I highly recommend it for women who are deciding which prenatal testing to consent to.

PREPARING YOUR ENVIRONMENT

CHOOSING WHERE TO BIRTH YOUR BABE

There are three common choices when considering your birthing location: at home, at a birth center, or at the hospital. Each of these environments has pros and cons. Envision where you will feel the most relaxed, as you will give birth with more ease wherever you feel the most comfortable.

Wherever you choose to birth your babe, the birthing space should be as soothing to vata as possible. Create an environment where you feel completely at ease, with the right people, dim lighting, soft music, and anything else that makes you feel at home. Find ways to bring in warmth, both emotionally and in temperature. Traditionally, caregivers would light a fire in the corner of a delivery room. Adding softness, heaviness, and oiliness to the birth experience will calm vata and assist the downward energy (apana vata), crucial to the delivery of your little one.

Throughout labor, your fight-or-flight response needs to be essentially turned off so that you can drop into a space of inner connection and trust. Your body has natural systems in place that will actually stop the process of labor if there are any perceived threats. *Ina May's Guide to Childbirth* explains that throughout history, only women were allowed to be present during labor and birth. When male doctors started to deliver babies, the presence of an unfamiliar man in the room would observably cause a woman's labor to slow, reverse, or stop altogether. Factors such as people in the room whom you are uncomfortable with, a space you are unfamiliar with, bright lights, loud and unsettling noises—any of this within your birthing environment can slow or stop labor if it makes you feel uneasy and your body registers it as a "threat."

A home birth is a suitable birthing option if you are healthy, low risk, and live in an area that is close enough to easily transfer to a hospital in case of an emergency. Birthing at home has many obvious benefits: the setting is intimate, familiar, and cozy; your family can be present and involved in the birth if you wish; you can be the director of your birth experience; you can feel more in your element rather than unfamiliar with your environment; and, after the birth of your babe, you can relax and rest in your own bed.

Medically speaking, home births have lower risks of medically unnecessary interventions; they have lower rates of forceps or vacuum delivery, emergency C-sections, episiotomies, and so on. It has been proven that every intervention during labor (starting with the intervention of leaving your home to go to a new space with loud noises and bright lights) begets another intervention. If you are considered to have a healthy and low-risk pregnancy and you and your baby have no underlying conditions, you and your baby may greatly benefit from giving birth at home. I would highly recommend looking into this possibility. Along with works by Ina May Gaskin, books by the board-certified family physician, midwife, and herbalist Aviva Romm are great sources for learning about statistics surrounding the safety of home births.

Birthing centers are a good option if you live too far away from a hospital to transfer easily in the case of an emergency, or if you would not be fully comfortable at home but still want to have a mostly natural birth with few interventions.

Consider a hospital birth if you have a high-risk pregnancy or if you go into labor early. Hospitals are best equipped to deal with medical emergencies and to keep mama and baby stable throughout labor and birth if there are any underlying conditions. You may also benefit from giving birth at the hospital if you tend toward having anxiety and feel safer being close to medical resources during your labor and birth. For some mamas, this safety net allows them to relax and have an easier labor.

NESTING

During the last month of pregnancy, your mind may shift into nesting mode. The old wives' tale advises that once the nesting impulse starts, labor is not too far away. Nesting is a biological response that all mammals have to prepare for the birth of their babe—it reflects an instinctual need to prepare not only your home, but also your body and mind to welcome your little one into the world.

If you wake up with an out-of-the-blue desire to scrub your floors, tidy up your baby's dresser full of onesies, and repack your "just in case" hospital bag for the—ahem—eighth time, the sweet maternal phenomenon known as "nesting" might be upon you. Regardless of your energy levels during pregnancy, there may very well come a time when you suddenly get bursts of energy and focus that seem almost superhuman. This surging vitality and sense of mission is nature's way of getting you ready to care for your little one: an increase in the amount of adrenaline coursing through your system generally around week 38 or 39 of your pregnancy. Some researchers have suggested that the nesting urge arises from a somewhat programmed adaptive human behavior stemming from our evolutionary roots to prepare for and to protect an unborn baby. At its core, nesting is about doing everything that you can to prepare your inner and outer environment to assure that you are as ready as you'll ever be.

In the weeks before my baby was born, I had the walls in my house painted, got new curtains for the bedrooms, completely redid our birthing room (we had a home birth), and got new furniture for the living room. I did laundry, deep-cleaned the refrigerator, decluttered every nook of the house, and put everything in its place. I had this feeling that I could not settle until everything was just right. I could then hunker down and really focus on the task at hand: birthing my baby and caring for him once he came.

As productive and fruitful as nesting can be, that kind of busyness may also be a way to distract yourself from any feelings that are coming up around this huge life transition and your upcoming birth experience. Nesting can be categorized as a vata activity, as there is excess energy, activity, and movement. As you now know, when vata is high, your activities can stem from an experience of feeling unsettled, anxious, fearful, and unprepared rather than from a productive, grounded, and even-minded place.

If and when you notice the nesting instincts, be mindful of the following:

Think about what you need in order to feel completely ready to birth your babe. What do you need in order to feel totally prepared to put everything else aside and just take care of them? Make a list.

Create a nesting plan. That way, you won't feel rushed to do everything all at once.

Take time to close your eyes and feel. Are there any underlying emotions that are moving you to become busy in order to distract yourself from honoring the big changes that are happening and the emotions that are coming up around them?

Do you feel nourished? Supported? Focus on what you need as well. Take time to nurture yourself as you prepare for childbirth.

Practice trust; let go of the need to control; know that your baby will come at the right time and that you will be ready. More than any external preparations, it is that inward ability to *trust* that allows for ease and connection in the process of birthing, regardless of the externals.

Nontoxic DIY House Cleaner

Essential oils are Mama Nature's gift to us. They are the aromatic compounds that serve to protect a plant from predators or other threatening influences, as well as strengthen the plant's system to assure healthy reproduction. Ayurveda teaches that by observing nature, we can utilize her gifts in a way that supports us in similar ways without any toxic side effects.

There is no need to pull out your rubber gloves and surgical masks when you clean your home. It might surprise you to know that you can concoct simple and inexpensive nontoxic cleaners from ingredients already available around your house. The oil blends listed below are naturally antiseptic, antibacterial, and antifungal. Using essential oils to create your own cleaning spray is not only uplifting for the environment, but it creates a safe, chemical-free environment for you and your little one as well. The following spray is perfect for cleaning all surfaces throughout your home.

Ingredients

¼ cup white vinegar

1¾ cups water

30 drops essential oils chosen from the following blend options: 15 drops each of lavender and lemon; 10 drops each of eucalyptus, peppermint, and wild orange; 30 drops doTERRA On Guard blend; or 15 drops each of grapefruit and doTERRA On Guard

Instructions

Combine all ingredients in a 16-ounce glass spray bottle. Shake thoroughly. Spritz on surfaces and wipe clean.

PREPARING YOUR BODY

Ancient Ayurvedic teaching suggests many ways to keep your body balanced and prepare it for labor and birth. Ayurveda offers daily routines to follow during your last weeks of pregnancy—focusing on the importance of building ojas—and emphasizes the value of preparing your vaginal tissues for birth. The teachings also provide nutritional recommendations for supporting your body in preparation for delivery.

The last month of pregnancy is all about supporting the downward flow of energy (apana vata) and preparing the passageway. The best way to do this is to really focus on a vata-pacifying diet and lifestyle in the weeks before your due date. Below are some simple yet powerful practices that will support you in preparing your mind and body to welcome your little angel into the world.

DAILY RITUALS

Eat sautéed and stewed apples in the morning to support good digestion (see page 296).

Aim to walk three to five miles per day. This gentle movement warms up the body, increases circulation, and allows for the free flow of vata.

Perform daily self-massage (see page 66).

Avoid caffeine, as caffeine constricts the channels and reverses the downward flow of vata.

Drink warm water or warm teas throughout the day to allow the channels of the body to be open and soft.

Drink a hot milk tonic in the evenings (see page 290).

Be asleep no later than 10 p.m. each night.

Connect with your baby and visualize an ease-filled labor. You and your baby are in this together! Tell your little one about the birthing experience coming up, what it might feel like for them, and that you will be right there on the other side to hold them and help them feel safe.

As a preparation for meeting your baby, consider reading Frédérick Leboyer's *Birth without Violence*—a powerful book that will help you to understand what your baby experiences during labor and how to support them throughout the process.

PERINEAL MASSAGE

One common fear pregnant women tend to have about the birth process is that the tissues of the perineal area (between the vagina, or vaginal opening, and the rectum or anus) will tear. An increasingly common recommendation is that a pregnant woman begin about a month before her estimated due date to massage or manually stretch the tissues of her perineum to reduce the likelihood of perineal lacerations and other trauma during birth. The stretching massage action will soften the muscles, connective tissue, and skin of the area, making the pliable tissue less likely to tear and reducing the likelihood of ongoing perineal pain. The perineum is also the perfect place to apply oil to ground and reduce excess vata dosha. You can use plain sesame oil or licorice-infused ghee. (See page 287 for a recipe for making ghee.)

Perineal massage is typically performed to the edge of comfort—until a slight burning or numbing sensation occurs. This may help you become more familiar with the sensation of a baby's head crowning, so that when you feel crowning in labor you are more likely to relax into it and less likely to panic and tense up, or to panic and push too hard and fast, which may cause tearing. Follow these steps to give yourself perineal massage:

Create a safe environment where you will not be interrupted.

Wash your hands thoroughly and trim your fingernails.

Use a safe lubricant (sesame oil or ghee are good choices), with a towel under your bottom to catch dripping oil.

Place one or both hands over the vulva and perineum with gratitude and honor your baby's gateway into this world.

Insert one or two fingers (or thumbs if that feels best) into your vagina up to one or two knuckles, whatever feels comfortable.

Apply downward pressure (toward your anus) for a few minutes. Slide back and forth between 9 o'clock and 3 o'clock. Note any sensation. Apply pressure to one side and then the other for several minutes.

Breathe deeply and practice fully relaxing into the sensations. The massage is not only preparing the tissues, but also training your body how to relax around intense sensation and allow the tissues to stretch. The mental aspect of allowing, without clenching or tightening, is part of the preparation too.

Stop when you feel you have had enough.

Place your hand over your vulva and perineum and send your gratitude again.

BASTI (WARM OIL ENEMA)

Mama can do one or two oil enemas per week beginning at thirty-seven weeks—this is when baby is considered full term. *Basti* in general is the therapy of choice to eliminate vitiated vata and is one of the best remedies for reducing pain during late pregnancy and labor. Basti opens mama in a beautiful way, grounds her, and oleates and nourishes the entire pelvic bowl.

Basti therapy is simple: Pour a quarter cup of warm sesame oil (about body temperature or slightly warmer) into an enema bag or bottle. (If you'd like to create an herbal oil blend for the enema, Ayurveda recommends using ashwagandha, bala, guduchi, and rose.) Lie on your left side and administer the oil into your rectum through your anus. Hold the oil inside of you until you have the urge to release.

YONI PICCHU

Another way to prepare your passageway for birth is a traditional Ayurvedic treatment called yoni picchu. This practice involves inserting a warm ghee- or sesame oil–soaked organic cotton ball into your vagina. Do this for fifteen consecutive days (six or seven hours at a time) after thirty-seven weeks. Inserting it before you go to sleep at night is a practical time. You can wrap the cotton ball in sterile gauze to assure that no shreds are left behind. This helps to lubricate and soften your tissues, allowing them to stretch more easily. It also serves as a powerful way to ground and stabilize vata dosha, drawing energy downward into the pelvic region in preparation for delivery.

SITZ BATHS

Soften the perineum by soaking weekly or twice-weekly in a sitz bath (a basin that fits perfectly into your toilet seat, so just your groin area is immersed in the bath) or a half-filled bathtub during the last six weeks of pregnancy. Prepare the bath using one of these recipes:

Recipe 1: Steep a handful of linden flowers in 32 ounces of boiled water for ten minutes. Strain and pour into a sitz bath (or half-filled bathtub) and soak for twenty to thirty minutes.

Recipe 2: Add 2 tablespoons of heavy cream along with 2 drops each of jasmine, rose, and lavender essential oils to warm water in a sitz bath or a half-filled bathtub, and soak for twenty to thirty minutes.

SUPPORTIVE FOODS, SUPPLEMENTS, AND BEVERAGES

The following are a list of supportive foods, supplements, and beverages to be consumed daily during the weeks up to your birth.

Red raspberry tea. Starting around thirty-five weeks, enjoy several cups of red raspberry tea per day. Red raspberry leaf is a mineral-rich nutritive and uterine tonic that is said to support a natural birth with minimal bleeding. Traditionally, red raspberry leaf has been used in late pregnancy to shorten the duration of labor and to reduce complications of pregnancy.

Alfalfa juice powder. Take 2 teaspoons of alfalfa juice powder daily beginning at twenty-eight weeks in pregnancy to increase blood volume and blood health, minimize anemia, and reduce blood loss (depletion) during birth and postpartum.

Dates. Ayurvedic teachings recommend eating six or seven dates per day during the last weeks of pregnancy because this palm fruit has an oxytocin-like effect on the body, leading to increased sensitivity of the uterus; dates help stimulate uterine contractions and reduce postpartum hemorrhage in the same way the hormone oxytocin does. They also support pregnancy and delivery because their natural sugars easily break down in the body and will not spike blood sugar levels, while still offering high energy; the high fiber content of dates helps you stay full, relieves constipation, and lowers your risk of gestational diabetes and preeclampsia; they are high in potassium, which helps maintain water and salt balance in the body, assisting in regulating your blood pressure; they are high in magnesium, which supports muscular health and helps alleviate muscle spasms and pain; and they are rich in vitamin K, which maintains proper blood clotting and healthy bones. You can eat dates straight or add them to smoothies and other ojas drinks to make those beverages more palatable.

Ghee. Ghee, a low-lactose oil created by clarifying butter to remove the water and milk solids, is believed to lubricate the inner walls of the uterus, thereby aiding a smooth delivery. It is a primary ojas-forming food—one of the best ways to nourish all the tissue in your body and bring about a feeling of wellness and vitality. The butyric acid in ghee is essential for maintaining good stomach health; it supports proper digestion, absorption, and assimilation of food nutrients. It also lubricates the intestines, leading to proper elimination. (See page 287 for a recipe for making ghee.)

BUILDING OJAS

During your eighth and ninth months of pregnancy, ojas becomes unstable, moving from mother to baby. Focus on building ojas in your body, guided by the list below (adapted from the *Birthing Ayurveda* blog on www.BanyanBotanicals.com; I highly recommend reading Vrinda Devani's week-by-week pregnancy and postpartum journey on the same website).

Ingest more ghee. Start putting ghee, as much as you can tolerate, on all foods. Add it to warm milk and drink it daily. No need to be stingy; it is nourishing and supports your digestive fire (agni).

Eat ojas-promoting foods. Almonds, dates, whole milk, avocados, cashews, pumpkin or sesame seeds, sweet and juicy fruits (mangos, peaches), sweet potatoes or yams, tapioca, and rice pudding are all foods that build ojas. Make sure the foods are nourishing, fresh, and wholesome.

Eat more vibrantly colored vegetables. They have more life (prana), and will thus give *you* more life!

Get good rest and avoid overexercising.

Sleep, sleep, and sleep some more! Avoid daytime sleeping, though, as this could make you feel even more heavy.

Meditate. Increasing the sense of feeling content in life is one of the most effective ways of increasing ojas.

Laugh a lot, give a lot, and love a lot. These activities fill the heart and grow ojas.

Avoid excessive sex. Ojas is released with every orgasm.

Do a daily self-massage, if possible.

Practice pranayama (breath work). Focus on slow, deep breathing such as nadi shodhana, or alternate-nostril breathing (see page 22) or abdominal breathing.

BIRTH PLAN

I suggest taking time each day in the weeks before birth to really envision the birth of your dreams. Where are you? What is your mood? What time of day (or night) is it? Who is there? Be as detailed and as vivid as possible. There is the vision that you hold, and then there are the practicalities of the process or the details that you want to assure are implemented into your birthing experience—which is where the "birth plan" comes in. The term "birth plan" can be misleading. You cannot "plan" your birth; birth is an unpredictable—and actually quite mystical—process. But you can prepare for it!

Experienced midwives and birth workers say that women who are overly attached to their birth plan, to the extent that they try to control the process of birth, are often the ones who end up having interventions that they did not anticipate or want. Understand that the ideal experience that you are putting into your birth plan is simply a guide. From there, your deeper work is to trust in the process of birthing itself and whatever arises in that space. Communicate your vision, wishes, and goals through your birth plan, and then completely let go and surrender to the process.

Birth plans are helpful to support you in finding *your* vision for your birth and are also helpful so that your support person can advocate for you if you are unable to advocate for yourself. Furthermore, a plan can also be helpful to provide to the hospital staff so that they are aware of your wishes and do not make decisions on your behalf that you would not feel comfortable with.

On the next few pages, I offer notes my partner and I made for our home birth—specifically for my husband to have on hand so he could know what was happening and how best to support me. We also gave our midwives a copy so they could understand the mood we wanted to create.

Feel free to use some or all of the following to create your own optimal birthing experience.

DURING LABOR

EARLY LABOR: 3–6 CM DILATED

Call midwives and let them know that labor has started.

Receive an abhyanga (or do it yourself) and take a warm bath to begin stabilizing vata.

Do an oil enema (basti, page 125) to bring vata downward and lubricate the tissues.

Eat a grounding and nourishing meal.

Slow down and take this time to connect with your baby, preparing yourself and your little one for the journey ahead.

Rest between contractions, even just lying down and closing your eyes for three to five minutes. Rest is vital and will support you on your journey.

ACTIVE LABOR: 6–10+ CM DILATED

Midwives arrive when contractions are one minute long with three to five minutes between them.

Walk around the house between contractions.

Have birthing partner rub warm oil on your hips and thighs in firm, downward strokes.

When a contraction comes, try various birthing positions that you have learned, or follow what feels best in your body. Consider changing positions regularly—or as needed.

TRANSITION

Contractions are one minute long with two or three minutes between each one.

If (as often happens with mamas during transition) you find yourself saying, "I can't (or don't) want to do it anymore," take a moment to notice what you are literally doing—and change it up. For example, if you are in the birthing tub and start to feel that you can't or don't want to do "it" anymore, get out of the tub and go into your backyard. This feeling often means that baby is moving down and coming soon.

Use low-pitched noises from your gut.

Trust the position that *your* body wants to birth in.

Allow natural expulsion of baby rather than effortful pushing. Your body will naturally move your baby out of you.

Breathe more rapidly through your mouth as baby begins to crown to slow down and prevent tearing.

Place a warm compress and oil on perineum.

Eat small amounts of honey off a spoon during pushing phase.

Refrain from loud or unnecessary talking during crowning and delivery.

Allow dad or mom to receive baby.

Offer mama a spoonful of panchakola ghee directly after delivery.

ROOM ENVIRONMENT FOR THE BIRTH

Aroma: pure essential oil of cardamom

Temperature: warm

Silence/soft voices in the space

Anyone in the birthing space is fully present with mama—as her witness and support

Dim lighting

Birthing tub available

Have ready: hot water bottle or heating pad, wet and warm cloths, warm oil

Music or mantra: make playlist and make sure your birth partner knows how to access it

SNACKS/MEALS

Rice gruel (see recipe on page 277)

Cut-up juicy fruits

Blended soups

Drinks: 40 ounces per hour

Electrolyte water drinks

Warm cashew milk

Warm water

Room-temperature coconut water

Raw local honey

RESPONSIBILITIES OF THE BIRTHING PARTNER

Communicating the mama's wishes to the maternity team, and relaying their advice back to her. Support her to make decisions if things don't go to plan and speak up for her if she can't do this herself.

Have a precreated text thread to let important friends and family members know that labor has started and ask for well-wishes and blessings.

Protect mama's privacy: turn phones on silent, close the door, restrict visitors. If the room seems to be getting loud, or other people are chatting about things unnecessarily—protect the space so all attention can be focused on mama.

If you determine that there are too many people and so much external stimulation that mama isn't able to relax into her primal, birthing brain, see what you can do to bring more soothing energy to the birthing environment.

Observe/anticipate mama's needs. Do not ask too many questions.

Be fully present with your partner. Be in the experience *with* her, not trying to fix, change, or necessarily "do" anything—just let her feel that you are fully there with her, witnessing her in her profound birthing process (whether you are letting her know through your words or simply in how you are showing up to support her).

During contractions, you can talk to mama slowly and softly. Affirmations are best, such as "you were born for this," "your body knows what to do," "you are doing this perfectly," or whatever affirmations you have discussed beforehand that feel empowering to mama. Rather than talking, you may also choose to hold the space of respectful silence, simply being with her as she rides the waves.

If progress seems to stop, hold gentle space for mama and baby and let the baby know that it is safe to come now; they are so loved and so wanted. Let baby know that things may feel scary right now, but not to worry—mama is right on the other side and ready to love and care for them. You can also assure mama that she is safe, that her body was made for this, and that her body is wise. This may be a good time for a bath or massage to allow mama's body to soften into a space of trusting and allowing.

You are in the mood of a warrior, not passive. If you are there when mama is in labor, it is because you are meant to be. You have something valuable to offer her. Be present and ready to serve. Deepen your breath so that you can be alert and alive.

Make sounds with her, breathe with her, move with her, walk with her.

Give her encouragement rather than direction.

Use nonverbal signals: instead of saying "relax your shoulders," gently touch her shoulders.

Give body work: hip compress, sacrum compress, pressure points.

Apply warm oil to her lower back and thighs between contractions.

Suggest ideas like taking a bath or shower, trying change in positions, or walking, and support her as needed.

Offer sips of nutritive drinks (not just water). Choose natural sports drinks, tea with honey, room-temperature juice, warm smoothies.

Listen to what she wants. She might not always want to be touched or spoken to, but being by her side is still helpful. Do not take any rejection or reaction personally.

PAIN COPING TECHNIQUES FOR MAMA

Distract from physical birthing sensations with other senses (tastes, sounds, visuals, scents, or other sensations).

Move toward sensation rather than away from it. Be curious about the pain. Rather than constrict and tighten around it, see if you can soften your jaw and your muscles—releasing resistance to your experience.

Notice what's already working and do more of that.

Become aware of your breath. Simply watch it moving slowly in and then out, in and then out.

Remember that you and your baby are in this together. Build a partnership with your little one.

Maintain mindful awareness without judging, as if you are the witness to your experience.

Find the center of sensation (much like the emptiness/stillness in the eye of the hurricane).

Find the edges of sensation. Notice how sensation is constantly changing and follow it. You are not stuck or stagnant. Sensation isn't rigid; it's fluid and always shifting.

Try bathing in warm water, whether it is a shower or a bath—or use a heating pad.

Try changing positions, really listening to your body and feeling into how your body wants to move and what position feels right, right now.

Massage with warm oil.

Make low-pitched sounds.

PLANNING FOR A HOSPITAL BIRTH OR HOSPITAL TRANSFER

Along with creating a plan for our home birth, we printed out a detailed set of notes to have ready in case a hospital transfer became necessary during the birth. A similar plan could be used when the intention from the start is to have a hospital birth. Feel free to use some or all of the instructions and reminders from the "Hospital Birth Preferences" chart below, and give a copy to your nurses and doctor upon arrival at the hospital. (Please note that none of the information in this hospital plan is medical advice; it simply reflects the conclusions and choices that we came to as a family after doing the necessary research.)

I'd like to preface this hospital plan with a few words about informed consent. In any birth environment, you are not only part of the experience, you are in charge of the experience. You have a legal human and ethical right to have the final say in anything that happens to you, your body, and your baby. Unfortunately, some medical practitioners (commonly in hospitals, but this can occur with midwives as well) either assume consent for medical procedures (this includes cervical checks) or coerce the mother into consenting to a procedure by guilting her about her ability to be a good mother—or even threatening to call social services if the mother denies their recommendations.

Ideally, every person who is present during your labor is in full alignment with the ways that you want to birth your baby, and they are there to protect and preserve that objective. Regardless of whether you are at home or in the hospital, you should not have to put up a fight with your care providers—or even feel that you *might* have to protect your ideals—during labor or birth. In the occurrence that this isn't the case, this is one of the benefits of having a support person (husband, partner, family member, or doula) who is familiar with your birth plan and your preferences and can advocate for you during your labor and birth. A simple way to establish right from the start that you are aware of informed consent and expect to be treated not only as a birthing mother but as a capable adult deserving of respect is to put a statement of informed consent right at the top of your birth plan for your care providers to read. The physician and midwife Aviva Romm suggests the following wording: *I expect to be treated like a competent adult with the legal right to be the autonomous decision maker about everything that happens to my body and my baby.*

Questions to Prepare for Birth

Whether birthing at home with a midwife or at a hospital, mama will be presented with recommended tests and procedures during pregnancy, though also during labor and post birth. It is important to understand that you do not have to consent to anything—for you or your baby—that you do not fully understand or feel comfortable with. Following are some questions that you might ask.

TESTS AND PROCEDURES

What will we find out from this test/procedure?

How accurate is it?

What are the risks? Do they outweigh the benefits?

What will you or we do differently based on the results? If nothing, is there another reason to do it?

What are all medical and non-medical alternatives?

TREATMENTS, DRUGS, AND INTERVENTIONS

How will this be helpful?

Why must this be done now?

What might happen if we wait an hour? A week? Or do nothing?

What are the advantages, disadvantages?

This may be the treatment you usually recommend, but what other approaches can you tell us about?

If several treatment choices are possible: Is there a logical sequence in which to try the different options?

HOSPITAL BIRTH PREFERENCES

Baby's estimated delivery date:
Mother:
Father or partner:
Phone number:
Midwife/Doctor:
Phone number:
Emergency numbers:

GENERAL NOTES

- Gender is a surprise! Please do not reveal it.
- We will transfer care back to our midwives directly after giving birth for all postpartum care.
- We have been preparing for a natural birth, and our hope is for a calm and joyful birthing experience. We appreciate your support in helping us create a calm and quiet environment at all times—especially during delivery and after birth. Please use soft voices, dim lights, and keep staff visits to a minimum.

LABOR

- Cordless fetal heart monitoring only if necessary
- Birthing tub
- Freedom to choose and change positions and to guide my own labor
- Freedom to eat and drink
- No induction or pain medication (if you must induce, use Pitocin and *not* Cytotec).
- No cervical checks
- No medical interventions without fully informed consent

DELIVERY

- Partner or mother will catch baby
- No episiotomy
- No forceps
- Do not reveal gender of baby

AFTER THE BIRTH

- Skin to skin immediately after delivery
- Natural delivery of placenta (+ we will take placenta home)
- Delayed cord clamping
- Do not suction my child unless it is necessary to save the baby's life
- Do not wash baby or rub vernix off; I will clean the baby sometime later

- Delay exams for bonding (two hours) and perform all checks on baby while on my chest
- Exclusively breastfeed + no pacifier
- Do not take our baby out of my room without my or my husband's knowledge and permission

NEWBORN PROCEDURES

- No circumcision (male or female)
- No vaccines
- Do *not* give RhoGAM
- Do *not* give a vitamin K shot
- Do *not* administer Synagis to our child
- Do *not* put antibiotic ointment in the baby's eyes
- Do *not* do PKU testing

IF A CESAREAN SECTION IS NECESSARY TO SAVE MY LIFE OR THE LIFE OF MY BABY

- Please use a double stitch when repairing my uterine wall and not a single stitch, to allow for VBAC [vaginal birth after cesarean] with a future pregnancy
- Do not clamp the umbilical cord until it stops pulsing.
- Please allow my husband to hold our baby until the placenta has been detached—please check our child while the baby is in his arms.
- Please let me have my baby on my chest after the placenta has been detached, and delay after-birth procedures (see above).

AYURVEDIC HOSPITAL PACKING LIST

- Insurance card and ID
- Bluetooth speaker
- Phone charger
- Essential oil diffuser
- Cardamom + rosewood essential oil
- Alternative dim lighting
- Washcloths for mama's head, body (cooling or warming)
- Abhyanga oil
- Enema bottle for basti
- Heating pad, hot water bottle
- Electric water kettle
- Thermos
- Eye mask
- Fluffy socks
- Hair ties
- Labor clothes
- Comfy clothes to nurse, sleep, and go home in
- Belly wrap
- Dad clothes, deodorant, toothbrushes

EAT | DRINK

- Honey for spoonfuls during pushing phase
- Panchakola ghee for two spoonfuls right after delivery
- Mini Instapot (Rice Gruel recipe, page 277)
- Additional Instapot for warming oil
- Rice, spices, sukanat for mama meals (see Kanji recipe on page 292)
- Fresh spring water for drinking

Last night as your daddy was rubbing my belly
he looked at me and said, "We're going to die one day."
"Yeah," I said. "What made you think of that?"
"Don't you want this to last forever?"
"Yeah . . . yeah I do."
As tears gently rolled down my face
and I soaked in the beauty of the moment a little more deeply,
hugged him a little more tightly,
stayed awake a little bit longer
because the beauty of remembering how temporary it all really is
makes me want to love a little more fully,
be a little kinder,
and not let a moment pass me by without feeling deeply
into its beauty.

So grateful I found a love like this.
A love story I wish could go on forever and ever.

Sometimes I think I shouldn't be sad
or that I should not cry,
because I know you feel everything I feel, little babe.
But then I remember:
the heartache is so beautiful actually,
because sadness
is a symptom
of a heart that has loved.
Sadness might be
just the other side.

ŚOSYANTĪ HOMA: ANCIENT RITUAL FOR A SAFE DELIVERY

In the Vedic tradition, a few days before the birth of the baby, among celebration with the blowing of conch shells, the mama is moved to her birthing room (*sutika grha*), traditionally located in the southwest part of the house, with her headboard facing east. The father then performs a ceremony called *śosyantī homa*, with the intention of bringing good health to the birthing mama and a safe delivery for their babe. Traditionally, this is a full ceremony, or *yajna*—carried out in front of a sacred fire with Vedic mantras recited by Brahmans, the local priests.

The following prayer, inspired by the translation of the traditional mantras found in Śrīla Gopāla Bhaṭṭa Gosvāmī's *Sat Kriya Sara Dipika*, has been simplified to make it accessible while maintaining the essence and bringing about the same intention. A few days before the birth of your little one, your partner might use this prayer or write their own to set the intention for a healthy delivery. This one is meant to be recited as the father (or partner) makes an offering of prasadam to the altar.

> Om Visnu
> Om Tat Sat
> On [today's date], for the safe delivery of my child I offer this nourishment.
> I offer my respects to the Earth, which supports us.
> I offer my respects to the space between heaven and Earth, which holds us.
> I offer my respects to the heavens, which give us something to reach for.
> I offer my respects to the Universe.
> O God and Goddess, please receive our offering and bring forth this child with ease and grace. May [birthing mama's name] feel the presence of the Divine Goddess supporting her as our child makes their way into the world.

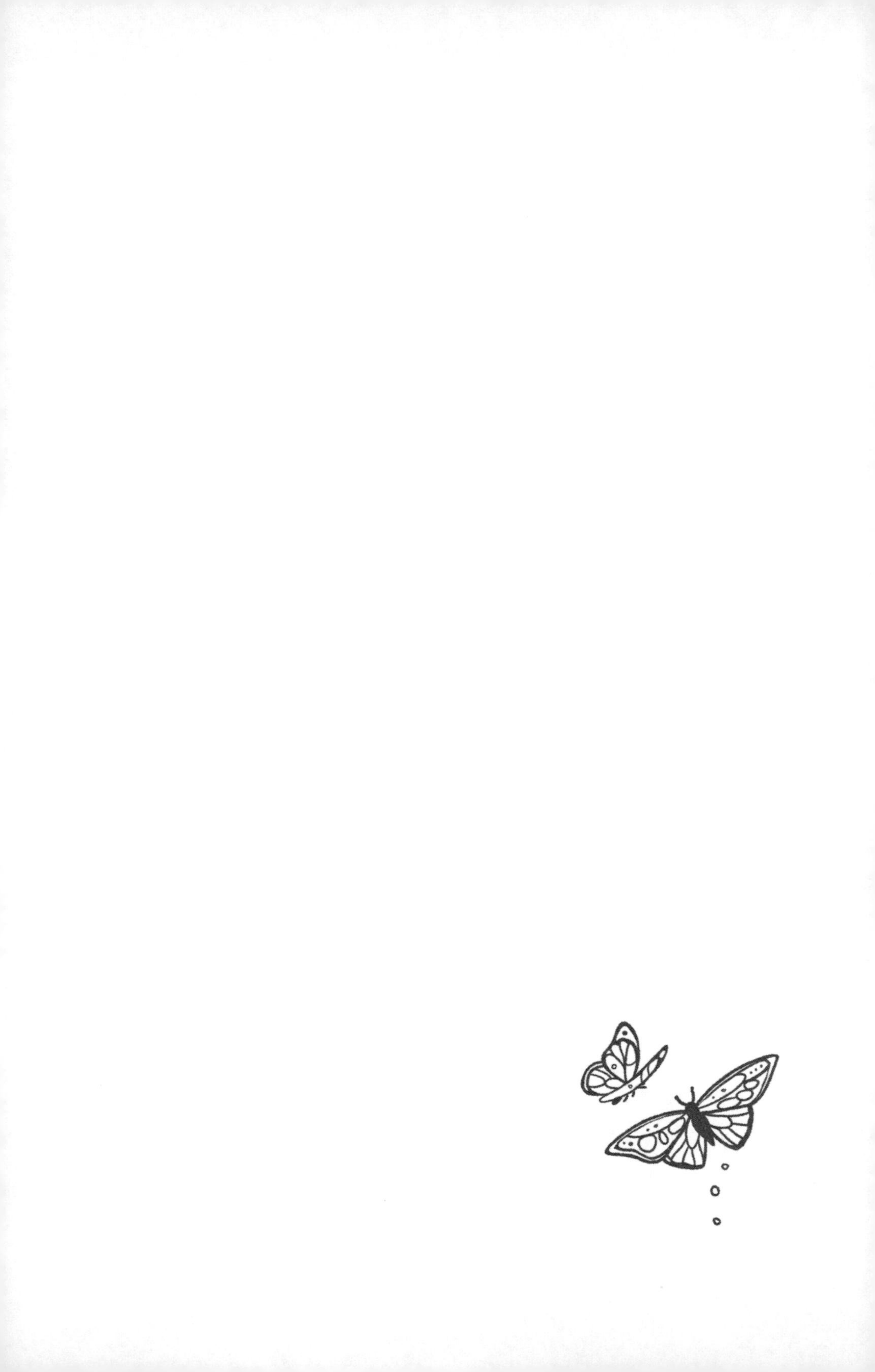

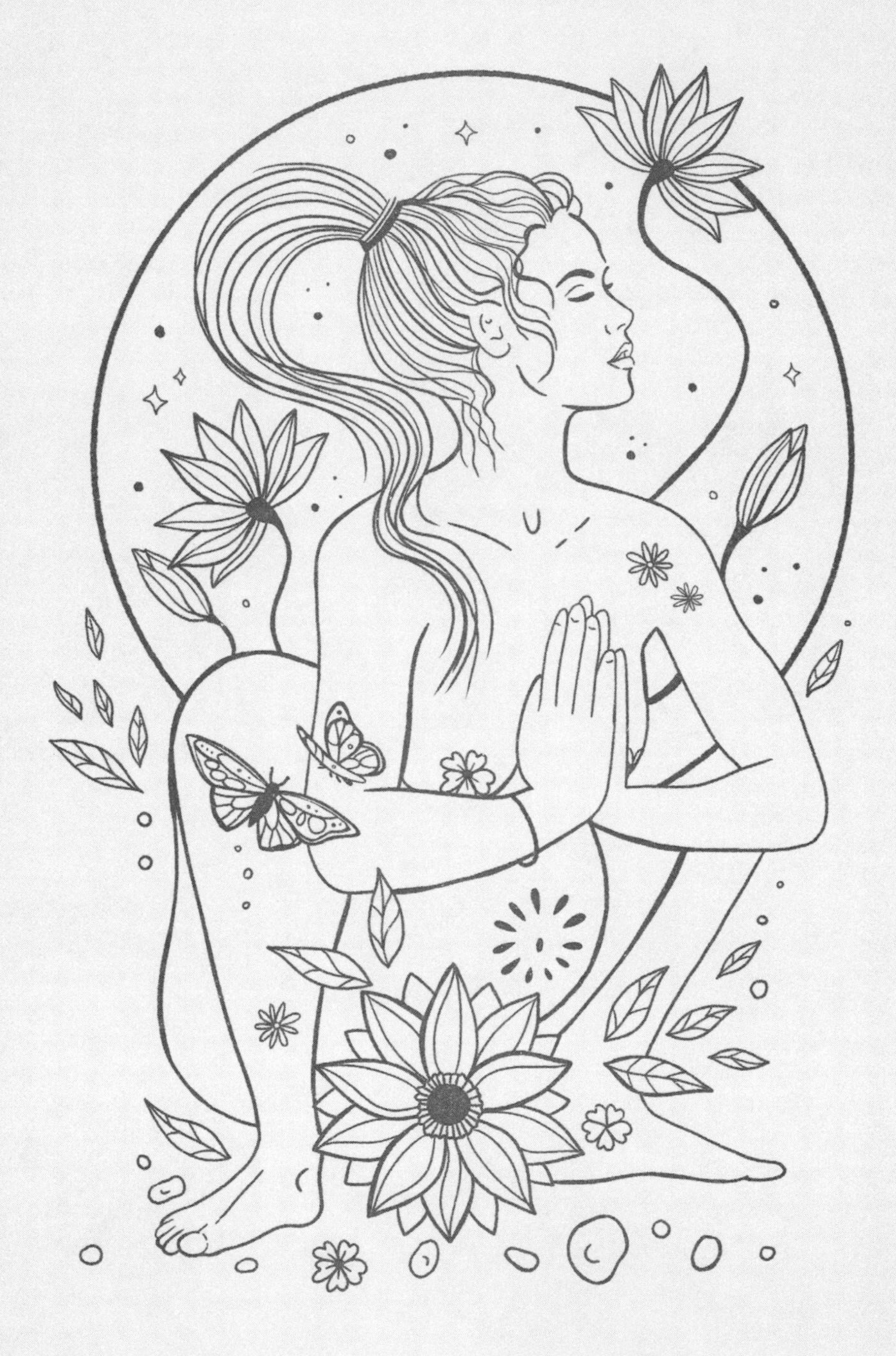

The Birth of Your Babe

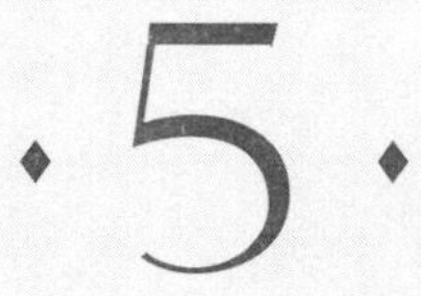

Do not let our culture take the magic and the immensity of this transition to motherhood away from you. We discuss things like work-life balance, getting your body back, having it all, bouncing back . . . but what we should really discuss is the profound portal of a woman in transition between two worlds.

—Narelle Melnick, Ayurvedic postpartum doula

No matter how much you have prepared, how many books you have read, how thoughtfully you have planned and organized and nested and gathered, there may still be a point during labor where you feel completely lost. You may forget everything you have learned and wonder if you are capable, if you are "doing" this right, if your baby will ever come out. Know that your labor is the perfect experience to prepare you, mama, for your little one. You will stretch, grow, be challenged, and transform in exactly the ways needed to mother your little angel. You will know a strength and resilience you never knew. You will give yourself completely, as you move through the profound portal that leads you toward the most selfless, unconditional love that you will ever experience.

> Your body knows what to do.
> Please trust that.
> All the ways you have prepared;
> a lifetime of experience and growth;
> everything that came before
> led you here.
> Mama,
> You were born for this.

Birth is natural. Your body was made for this. You know what to do. So much of the doing is simply getting out of the way and allowing your body to do what it does. Remember every woman that has labored and birthed before you; feel their strength and wisdom pulsating through your cells. Remember that even in the moments where you forget . . . your body remembers. Your body knows how to birth. Your baby will come out. And you? You will forever be changed.

♦

This chapter provides an overview of terms to familiarize yourself with as your due date is approaching. I also want to introduce you to the natural flow of labor and some things that you may experience, ways to know if the doshas become imbalanced and how to support them, and finally some beautiful Ayurvedic practices to support you in your birthing experience.

At the end of this chapter, I share my birth stories. I encourage you to honor your own birthing experience by writing down every detail you can remember (after the first few days of soaking up that sweet babe in your arms, of course!). This is a beautiful and meditative way to process and integrate your experience and make peace with it, especially if part of your labor or birth did not turn out the way you hoped. Every birth story is sacred, as it ends in new life—a spirit soul continuing its journey to the Divine.

I just can't believe you're a little person in there,
and I can't believe I get to see you so soon.
I wonder what you'll look like,

where your freckles will be.
I wonder what color your hair is;
if you have hair;
if it will be blond and curly like both of ours were when we were little babes.
I wonder what your temperament is;
if you're happy in there;
if you're scared at all.
I wonder if I will be able to make you feel safe;
if you'll breathe when you're out;
if you'll sleep well
and be comfortable in the world.
I wonder
if you'll remember being inside of me
and if I'll remember what it feels like.
I hope so.
Because you are truly the most magical experience of my life.

TERMS TO KNOW FOR LABOR

BRAXTON-HICKS CONTRACTIONS

Braxton-Hicks contractions are a tightening of the uterine muscles for one to two minutes and are thought to be an aid to your body in its preparation for birth. Braxton-Hicks are your body's way of preparing for true labor, toning the uterine muscles so that they will all work together, but they do not indicate that labor has begun or is going to start. Sometimes they are referred to as prodromal, or "false labor," pains, although they do not generally hurt; they are more of a feeling of tightening and then releasing of the belly muscles. They start around six weeks gestation but usually are not felt until the second or third trimester of pregnancy.

Braxton-Hicks are irregular in duration and intensity, are unpredictable and nonrhythmic, and are not usually painful. Unlike true labor contractions, Braxton-Hicks do not increase in frequency, duration, or intensity. They lessen and then disappear, only to reappear at some time in the future. Braxton-Hicks contractions tend to increase in frequency and intensity near the end of the pregnancy.

MUCUS PLUG

During pregnancy, the cervix secretes a thick, jelly-like fluid to keep the area moist and protected. This fluid eventually accumulates and seals the cervical canal, creating a thick plug of mucus. The mucus plug acts as a barrier and can keep unwanted bacteria and other sources of infection from traveling into your uterus.

As your cervix starts to soften or open (dilate) later in pregnancy (called "cervical ripening," this softening and dilation of the cervix typically begins prior to the onset of labor contractions and is necessary for the passage of the baby), the mucus is released into the vagina. You might notice an increase in vaginal discharge when this happens that can be clear, pink, brownish, or even blood-tinged. Sometimes it appears as small amounts of mucus when you wipe, or in your underwear, or it can be a bigger, thicker, jelly-like glob.

When you lose your mucus plug it does not necessarily mean that you are actually in labor; it can be anywhere between a few hours to a few weeks before labor starts. Your mucus plug may not even dislodge until you are in labor!

WATER BREAKING

In movies, a pregnant woman generally seems to experience a gush of liquid between her legs as the indicator that labor is starting. In reality, the release of amniotic fluid—"water breaking"—before labor starts only happens in about 8 to 10 percent of births. For some women, their water does not break until they are well progressed into labor, or even moments before the baby is actually delivered. On rare occasions, a baby can be born "en caul," meaning that the child is born inside of the unbroken, or partially broken, amniotic sac.

When the water breaks, it means that the amniotic sac that carries your baby has punctured, and the fluid is starting to drain. It should be clear in color and odorless. Depending on where the puncture is, the water might gush out or drip out a little at a time. If labor has not already started, after your water breaks, labor generally begins (or intensifies) soon after.

INDUCTION

Induction is the term used for artificially starting labor, either through natural methods or by using medical procedures or drugs. The reasons for induction vary: sometimes legitimate health threats to the mother or baby require labor to start immediately; other times induction is simply a scheduling convenience for the doctor or the birthing mother. Before utilizing any induction method to start your labor, familiarize yourself with the different potential benefits and risks of each method. Induction can have disadvantages to both mama and baby, and although induction may be the safest choice in some circumstances, make sure you are educated and informed of the risks.

In the medical model of care, induction methods may involve a care professional manually breaking the amniotic sac to initiate labor, or using drugs (such as Pitocin IV or prostaglandins including Cervidil, Prepidil, or Cytotec) to expedite the labor process, or both.

In the midwifery model of care, induction methods may include sexual intercourse between the pregnant woman and her partner, breast/nipple stimulation, or consuming castor oil, as well as a practice of sweeping the membranes, wherein the midwife separates the bag of waters (amniotic sac) from the inside of the cervix with two fingers.

EPISIOTOMY

An episiotomy is a medical procedure common mostly between 1940 and 1980 in the United States and, to a lesser extent, in the United Kingdom and Australia. The care provider would cut an incision into the perineal tissue of the birthing mama in order to prevent tearing and to allow for the baby's head to come out more easily during the pushing phase. This procedure is mostly outdated and should no longer be done routinely unless there is a medical reason for it, such as a risk to the safety of the baby. Care providers have learned methods of massaging the perineal tissue around the baby's head to help it come out during pushes without tearing and have found that even if the mama does tear, the perineal laceration is often smaller than it would be if an incision were made.

You are entering into the mystery.
Know that your experience will be unique,
and totally perfect
to prepare you
to care for
your little angel.

LABOR

EARLY LABOR

In early labor, you will begin to experience contractions that typically last thirty to forty-five seconds, though they might be shorter, and may be regular or irregular. They can be spaced ten or twenty minutes apart with no regular rhythm. Early labor contractions are sometimes hard to distinguish from irregular Braxton-Hicks contractions. Real labor contractions will get closer together with a more regular pattern as time goes on.

During early labor, you might experience any of the following labor signs:

- backache (constant or with each contraction)
- menstrual-like cramps
- lower abdominal pressure
- indigestion
- diarrhea
- sensation of warmth in the belly
- mucus plug discharge
- water breaking (though rupture of the amniotic sac is more likely to happen sometime during active labor)

You may feel excitement or fear, relief or anticipation. You might feel totally relaxed and ready or tense and apprehensive. All of these feelings are normal: your journey has begun! Say a prayer, create an intention, perhaps sit at your altar or in nature and connect with your Self, with your baby, and with the Divine. Sometimes early labor contractions are quite intense, but usually they will be mild enough for you to talk through them, move around the house, or stay resting in bed.

Relax as much as you can, since you may have a long day or night ahead of you. If you are tired, try to doze off between contractions, even if it is just for a few minutes at a time. If you are having a home birth with an attending doula or midwife (or both), let them know that things have started. They will likely tell you to reach out again as things progress or if anything changes.

You should contact your practitioner right away if you experience any of the following:

Your discharge becomes bright red (actual bleeding could indicate a problem with the placenta, such as placenta previa or another condition that needs to be addressed as soon as possible).

Your water breaks and the amniotic fluid is greenish.

You feel no fetal activity (though any activity may be hard to notice because you are distracted by contractions—in which case have a snack or some juice, walk a bit, even jiggle your belly, then lie down, relax, and see if the baby moves).

ACTIVE LABOR

During the phase of active labor, your cervix dilates to 7 centimeters. This is when you will head to the hospital or birthing center or call your midwife to come to your home, depending on where you are planning to give birth. Some caregivers prefer a call sooner, so clarify this ahead of time.

Your contractions will become more powerful. They become longer, typically lasting sixty seconds with a distinct peak halfway through, and more frequent, coming every three to four minutes though the pattern may not be regular.

One wave at a time;
Rest in between.
Do not waste those precious moments of ease
complaining about the past (the last contraction)
or dreading the future (the next).
Allow yourself to drop deeply
into the present moment.
Soften your jaw,
allow the weight of your body to be held by the bed,
the water, the wall, the pillows.
Relax your arms
your thighs

your belly.
Be
in your breath.
Then the next wave will begin to rise.
Prepare yourself to meet it.
Ride it.
Experience it,
and then it falls.
You have another moment to rest.

ASK FOR WHAT YOU NEED

Before labor, practice asking for what you need.

The journey is yours, and at some point you must realize that it is your work, and your surrender, that will birth your baby. Still, having the total presence and support of your birth team will allow you to feel that you are not in it alone.

Stay connected with your little one.

Breathe deeply.

Stay hydrated. This can be one of your birth partner's roles; to keep offering you drinks and light snacks without asking if you want it . . . just offer, and mama will either take it or not.

TRANSITION

During the transition from the first phase of labor (early and active labor) to the second phase (pushing), the cervix will dilate from 7 centimeters to its final 10-plus centimeters. Transition is the shortest stage, generally lasting from fifteen minutes to an hour (though it can sometimes last longer).

A person in labor may experience more space between contractions during this time and think that labor is slowing down or stalling. This is a portal where mama is between worlds. She has climbed a tall mountain and is given a moment to rest and reflect, though mostly to listen. It is said in this gap, the time right before baby comes, mama can receive messages about her little one—almost like she is downloading a manual about who they are and how to care for them. This space should be honored. Rather than having mama change positions, walk around, or start pushing, encourage her to be in the receptive space—until the urge to push comes on strong.

In the transition phase, a woman in labor is likely to be feeling intense sensations:

Strong pressure in the lower back or perineum, rectal pressure, or both, with or without an urge to push

An increase in fluid discharge

Feeling warm and sweaty or chilled and shaky

Crampy legs that may tremble uncontrollably

Nausea or vomiting (or both)

Drowsiness between contractions

Fatigue or exhaustion

Relief or anticipation

PUSHING AND THE BIRTH OF YOUR BABE

At the beginning of the second phase of labor, the pushing stage, your contractions may be a little further apart, giving you the chance for much-needed rest between them. With each contraction, the force of your uterus exerts pressure on your baby to continue to move down through the birth canal. The descent may be rapid or gradual. When a contraction is over and your uterus is relaxed, your baby's head will recede slightly in a "two steps forward, one step back" kind of progression.

With each contraction, more and more of your baby's head becomes visible. You may notice a strong burning or stinging sensation as your vaginal and perineal tissue begins to stretch. Your little one is almost here. At some point, you may have the natural urge to breathe quicker and more shallow breaths through your mouth in order to slow down the expulsion of your little one; this allows your baby's head to more gradually stretch out your vaginal opening and perineum. A slow, controlled delivery can help keep your perineum from tearing.

Your baby's head continues to advance with each wave until it "crowns"—the widest part of the head is finally visible. Generally, if the baby is in the common birth position, the head will emerge facing your tailbone. After the full head is out, the baby then turns to the side as its shoulders rotate inside your pelvis to get into position for their exit. In the same contraction, or perhaps the next, the shoulders emerge, one at a time, followed by the body.

A warm compress on your forehead or back may feel comforting.

You did it, mama.
You did it, little babe.
Welcome to the world, little angel.
You are safe.
You are so loved and so, so wanted.
Welcome, little one.
Welcome.

DELIVERY OF THE PLACENTA

The third and final phase of labor is the delivery of the placenta. Minutes after giving birth, your uterus begins to contract again. The first few contractions usually separate the placenta from your uterine wall. When your caregiver sees signs of separation, they may ask you to gently push to help expel the placenta. This is usually one short push that is not at all difficult or painful.

THE GOLDEN HOUR

The golden hour is the hour immediately following birth where mama and baby have uninterrupted skin-to-skin contact. It is a time for deep bonding and deep connection for both mama and baby and allows for a gentle welcome into the world where baby feels safe and at home—as this tiny person stays close to the only home they've ever known. There is no one poking or prodding mama or baby, and the environment stays as still and quiet as possible. If it is not possible for mama to hold baby skin to skin at this time, then the partner can take this role.

During this hour the baby's heart rate stabilizes, temperature regulates, and mother's good bacteria is passed onto baby from her skin. Signs of stress will decrease from baby as the instinctual close contact is maintained between mama and babe. Oxytocin is in plentiful supply right after birth, and this hormone—more commonly known as the "love hormone"—allows for deep bonding.

Mothers who honor this time are shown to have more successful and ease-filled breastfeeding journeys. Baby can be on mama's belly with a blanket over them to initiate the "breast crawl." All mammals (if unmedicated, meaning no drugs at all during labor), if given the chance, will slowly make their way to mama's breasts to feed. Babies are born with a "stepping reflex" that allows them to scoot up mama's chest toward the breast. Babies will try to align themselves with the nipple, and allowing them to do this on their own actually improves the chances of a successful latch. Having the baby directly on mama's belly after birth also slows down the production of the stress hormone adrenaline in the mother, so that it doesn't interfere with the production of the oxytocin and prolactin hormones that are essential for bonding and breastfeeding.

AYURVEDIC PRACTICES DURING LABOR AND BIRTH

SUPPORTING VATA AS CONTRACTIONS BEGIN

Ayurvedic tradition encourages certain practices during labor to assist in the birthing process as well as give relief and support to the birthing mama. To begin with, at the onset of contractions, someone can give the pregnant mama a full-body warm oil abhyanga—or she can do it herself—with sesame oil. Afterward mama can take a warm bath.

If desired, this bath can be infused with botanicals including herbs such as white peony root or linden; essential oils such as lavender, patchouli, cardamom, jasmine, and rose; flower essences such as Birth Formula, Peaceful Help, Rescue Remedy, and ylang ylang for surrender to a knowing that life experiences are divinely guided; or aspen and mimulus to mitigate fear.

When mama gets out of the bath, she can apply warm sesame oil around her vaginal opening and do a warm oil enema with sesame oil to nourish her whole pelvic region and help move vata downward. Use about ¼ cup of warm oil for the enema (see page 125).

MASSAGES BETWEEN CONTRACTIONS

Any support person at the birth—the partner, a friend or family member, or the doula or midwife—can offer the laboring mama relief by providing warm oil massages between contractions. Organic sesame oil is the best to use, and it can be infused with herbs such as rose and brahmi. The oil can be put into a plastic squeeze bottle and the bottle then placed in a pot of hot water to keep it warm throughout the labor. (Many mamas use some sort of slow cooker set on warm to keep the oil at the right temperature.) Warming the oil is essential, as any sort of cold applied to mama's body during labor will disturb vata, whereas warmed oil will feel nourishing and supportive. The oil can be rubbed all along mama's lower back and thighs in firm, downward strokes between contractions while she breathes and rests.

WARM NOURISHMENT DURING LABOR

In North America, hospitals routinely offer ice chips to a birthing mama and restrict all other food and beverages (an IV solution may provide hydration). In Ayurveda, this is strongly ill-advised. According to Ayurveda, if a birthing mother is given anything cold to consume, the conscious connection between her mind, body, spirit, and womb space is immediately severed.

Warm hydrating teas, soup broths, or warm nourishing smoothies are perfect to supply the mama with energy. Use the ratio of 1 teaspoon of herbs per 8 cups of water. This will keep the teas hydrating rather than drying. Hot thin soup broths make a good beverage if mama is having a difficult time eating solid foods. A little hot water can be added to any of the mama's juices or energy drinks to take out the chill, or they can be stored at room temperature (as long as they are still sealed) prior to labor. Warm blended smoothies can also be made with dates, ghee, freshly prepared nut milks, and warm digestive spices.

Consuming only hot, warm, or room-temperature food and beverages that are easier to digest is recommended during labor and following birth. One of the staple Ayurvedic recipes for a birthing and postpartum mother is a mushy, watery, sweet rice kanji (see page 292 for the recipe). This dish can be prepared by the birthing partner or doula as mama goes into early labor. She will also benefit from eating spoonfuls of kanji throughout labor. If mama is birthing in a hospital, look into their policy on eating and drinking during labor ahead of time and have a discussion with the care providers. Many other benefits of a birthing mama being allowed to eat and drink during labor can be found in *Ina May's Guide to Childbirth*.

Between pushes, while mama rests, a support person or doula can bring her a spoonful of honey. The reasoning for this is a bit mysterious but it is just one of those magical mama medicine traditions that will help her to get more effective pushes to bring her baby earthside.

According to Ayurvedic texts, mothers should have repeated inhalation of the herbs cardamom, *kustha* (costus root), *vacha* (calamus root), and *chitrak*. (Best if you can find essential oils of these herbs). Optionally have an essential oil diffuser going with cardamom and other essential oils of the mother's choice.

WHEN THE BABY IS BORN

Choosing who will catch your baby, if medically appropriate, is highly significant in Ayurvedic tradition. Some mothers choose to catch their own baby, if they are conscious and in a position to do so. Some mamas choose to invite the father or a sibling to catch the baby. Ayurveda says that the baby is highly influenced by the qualities of the person who catches them as they come out of the birth canal, as that person is their first contact with the world outside of mama's womb. The first hands that touch the baby should be the hands of a person who loves them. If you would like to catch your own baby or have a close family member or friend catch your baby, have a discussion with your doctor or midwives in advance so that they are aware of your wishes and can best support you in this. This is one benefit of a home birth, as many hospitals have policies against anyone besides a medical professional catching the baby.

Ayurveda teaches that following the delivery of the placenta, mama should consume two tablespoons of melted panchakola ghee to reignite her digestive fire (more details in the next chapter). Her abdomen can be gently rubbed with warm oil and wrapped with a belly wrapping cloth: Apply the warm oil (sesame is recommended) generously to mama's abdomen and softly rub it in with light circular motions. The cloth can then be wrapped (gently, but firmly) from her rib cage just below her breasts all the way down to her hips (see "Postpartum Belly Wrap" on page 180). This should feel supportive, as it is closing and holding the newly empty space in her womb.

The baby's head can be rubbed with warm sesame oil or ghee and then covered with a cotton or silk cap. Their feet can also be rubbed with oil and then covered with socks. This helps to stabilize vata and ground little babe into their body.

Ayurveda recommends waiting to cut the cord until it has stopped pulsing. This allows ojas to be transferred from mama to baby. All medical tests can usually wait (unless there are complications) so that mama and baby can utilize the first hour or so to simply be together. Really savor these moments, mama. Most babies will nurse within the first hour or so after birth if given the chance.

You may have the chills or feel shaky post-birth. This can be perfectly normal (as vata has been destabilized) and will not last long. Bring in warmth: warm towels, blankets, warm oil, hot porridge. If you are not chilled, you can take a shower or bath and put on fresh clothes as your partner does skin to skin with the babe. Once you are fresh and back in bed, it is a beautiful time for your birthing partner to offer you a grounding foot and leg massage as you nurse your little one.

MANAGING THE DOSHAS DURING LABOR AND BIRTH

During labor and birth, any of the doshas have the potential to become imbalanced. Below are some ways in which each dosha may display itself during labor, along with suggestions for how to pacify it.

VATA

SIGNS OF EXCESS VATA DURING LABOR

Due to the extreme work of apana vata to move your baby down and out of your womb, vata is the main dosha to be concerned with during labor. If you are birthing in a hospital, the hospital environment (cold, bright, potentially noisy) can further aggravate vata. Watch for the following signs of excess vata during labor:

Unripe cervix

Premature rupture of membranes (when water breaks before thirty-seven weeks and labor doesn't start soon after)

Irregular contractions

Malposition of baby

Start-and-stop labor

Slow or infrequent contractions

Dehydration and associated maternal fever and fast heartbeat

Fearfulness, feeling of anxiety and overwhelm

Irritable or exhausted uterus leading to lack of progress

TO PACIFY VATA DURING LABOR

Keep yourself warm with warm blankets, heating pads, or hot water bottles.

Take a hot shower.

Have a warm sitz bath or tub bath, being sure not to get chilled when finished.

Receive massages of warm sesame oil or warm castor oil.

Eat cooked, warm foods and drinks, avoid cold foods and drinks.

Keep lights turned low.

Rest frequently.

Reduce cortical stimulation (unnecessary talking, excessive vaginal exams, anything that makes you feel uncomfortable).

Minimize the number of different people coming and going from the room.

PITTA

SIGNS OF EXCESS PITTA DURING LABOR

Watch for the following signs of excess pitta during labor (and remember that sometimes vata—movement—will push pitta, so in general, pacify vata first):

Fever

Babe being born in less than three hours of regular contractions

Either a series of single contractions lasting two minutes or more *or* a contraction frequency of five or more in ten minutes

Excess bleeding; postpartum hemorrhage

Hypoglycemia (blood sugar level lower than normal)

TO PACIFY PITTA DURING LABOR . . .

Increase hydration to cleanse acidity from uterus and balance any blood loss.

Stay nourished.

Avoid overheating.

Drink coconut water for cooling hydration.

Use rosewater mist on face and belly.

KAPHA

SIGNS OF EXCESS KAPHA DURING LABOR

Watch for the following signs of excess kapha during labor:

Slow progress due to a large baby

Shoulder dystocia (one or both of the baby's shoulders gets stuck inside the mother's pelvis during labor and birth)

TO PACIFY KAPHA DURING LABOR . . .

Keep active and moving to help overcome stagnation.

Assure that partner or doula is stimulating and watchful (doing birth positions with mama, keeping her moving when she needs to)

THE BIRTH OF MY SON

It was September 23, your due date, little one. I woke up at 3:45 a.m., like I had almost every morning for the past two weeks, and got ready to head to the temple. Since your papa was going anyway, I figured there was no better way to start the day.

Hours later, we were at the DMV when I started feeling little sensations in my lower belly, like super-gentle period cramps, or maybe my belly was rumbling . . . or maybe I had to poop. They continued throughout the morning, during our business meeting, and still while having lunch.

Before heading to the springs, like we did each evening, I giddily told your papa that something was happening. A huge smile took over his face, as he announced, "We're going to have a baby!"

We drove to the springs and started timing the space between each contraction; about ten to fifteen minutes. It was around 5 p.m., and they were still gentle enough to breathe and move through with ease.

We were curious and excited. I still wasn't sure if it was real.

We swam in the cleansing turquoise waters; in through one spring, down a short river, and out the main spring. I had three gentle contractions while swimming, still unsure as to what was happening. Could he be coming?! On the way home the contractions were coming about ten minutes apart.

We were ready. All the walls had been painted, the birthing room completely redone, new furniture for the living room, kitchen cabinets thoroughly cleaned and organized, and the fridge fully stocked.

I felt like everything had to be perfect for you—as if a great soul were coming for a visit. My nesting experience was so real; like I needed to create the perfect environment and atmosphere to welcome you into—so I could focus on the task at hand: birthing and caring for you once you were here.

I went on the back porch and did some yoga. In savasana, I lay down, staring up at the sky and the leaves—and the whole atmosphere began to change.

I dropped into this realm of total presence . . . like all that existed was this eternal moment. The sun was setting, and we went on a walk to the top of the hill near our house. Everything was so vivid. The leaves in the trees—it was as though I could see each one individually moving. The blades of grass; the sounds of the birds; the colors in the sky. We laughed as I joked that it felt like we were on drugs.

As we walked back through the front door we saw that your papa's phone was flashing. It was our spiritual guide and teacher, Radhanath Swami. We could not believe it. He asked some things about the Bhakti Center, his spiritual center in Manhattan that we were directing at the time, and then he asked how I was doing.

"Well actually, Maharaj," my husband replied, "she's just starting labor."

He said that his timing is never so good, but Krishna really helped him with this one and that it must have been the reason he called. He kept repeating how auspicious it was. He asked to talk to me, as I gently bounced on the labor ball, tears rolling down my face in disbelief as he showered me with so many blessings and prayers. He said that it was going to be hard, that is why they call it labor, but it was a labor of love for a lifetime of service.

That phone call gave me strength for what was to come. He gave me strength. I felt Krishna's presence and love with me from that moment on, sent through one of His dearest devotees. Sometimes it is hard to give myself in full surrender and faith to God, so He sent His messenger, whom I have full faith in, and who has total faith in Him. I knew He was with me. It was perfect. It would all be perfect, no matter how challenging it would become.

The waves were coming about five minutes apart when we called one of our midwives and with shyness and excitement told her what was happening. She said, "This is just the beginning. Get some sleep tonight. Call if anything changes, or I'll check on you in the morning." We went to bed. I could not sleep. The excitement, but also the sensations, were keeping me up.

I went into the kitchen and started moving around the house more. I found it was much more comfortable to be leaning over when a contraction came. My breath became a lot stronger now, and my husband got up. It was around midnight.

He started preparing a feast! He knew the midwives would be coming and wanted them to have all the nourishment they needed, as well as for me to have my favorite snacks. He made a huge pot of kitchari, cut up beautiful fruits, toasted nuts, and made nourishing drinks.

I went into the bath. I remember yelling from the bath a few times, "Vira! Get some sleep!" I wanted him to be rested for when I really needed him.

The waves started coming on stronger. I sat on my knees in the bathtub with my eyes closed. Every time a wave would come I would have to get onto all fours. "Jai Gurudev, Jai Gurudev." With every wave, I called on His strength to support me. His presence was so strongly with me, and with Him, the presence of God.

A recording of Badahari's kirtan was playing on repeat. Between contractions my mind was totally, completely, 100 percent absorbed in the maha mantra like never before.

Before heading back to sleep, my husband brought me his phone and asked me to time the contractions and the space between them. As each wave approached, I would push the button. As the wave subsided, I would push it again. I did this for hours. The space between each wave felt like an eternity—an opportunity for deep, restorative rest. I could not believe the actual time was only three to five minutes.

I thought of Krishna in the Bhagavad Gita saying " . . . time I am" and saw the gift He was giving me of an extended perception of the space between.

At 4:30 a.m. I called my childhood best friend and asked her to come over. We walked beneath the moon and stars. The trees would support me through each contraction, as she listened and guided me through. I remember feeling like the baby could come at any moment.

Around 6:30 a.m. the midwife called and asked if she should come over. She arrived around 7:15 a.m. and checked my dilation. "Yup," she said, "Two or three centimeters." Only two or three centimeters?! I could not believe it. I felt so defeated. So defeated. I was up the entire night laboring, had been awake for twenty-seven hours already—the sensations were so strong, so consistent, and so close together.

"Perhaps take a walk, or maybe eat something," she said. "But most importantly, get some rest. Call me if anything changes."

My husband set up pillows on our bed, against the wall so that I could halfway sit up, leaning against them on my side. I would fall into a deep sleep for three minutes at a time, before transitioning onto all fours, which was the only position that I could move through a contraction in at this stage.

For five hours I did this: lie halfway down; fall asleep; as the wave rushed in, move onto all fours; as it subsided, lay back down. Around noon I went to the bathroom. My mucous plug came out, which marked the next stage of intensity.

Sounds started moving through me. Sounds that were moved from the deepest part of me. As my uterus would contract, my body, not me, started bearing down. It is hard to describe sensation, though easier to look at how I showed up throughout it all.

My energy, my awareness, even my eyes were totally focused inward. I knew I had to call upon a deeper strength than my own and harness all the strength that existed within me. I needed help, and also needed to know that I had everything that I needed already. I had to trust.

A wave would come. Wherever I was I would drop onto all fours, whether in the hallway, leaning against the bed, or perched near the window. My body would push as my insides were moving everything down. Down. Down. Deep within. And down. Then it would subside. Slowly. Like a wave being pulled back into the ocean.

"Rest in between," he would remind me. "One wave at time."

My body would soften, my breath deepen, as I lay back and rested into his support.

I went into the birthing tub. I asked if I was doing this right. I didn't know. Was he stuck? Why wasn't he here yet? My best friend suggested perhaps a new position—getting out of the tub so gravity could help bring baby down. We went into the bathroom, I straddled the toilet facing the wall.

Things started to slow down—perhaps nature's way of letting me rest. My midwife said that she wanted to check my cervix to see where I was at. As I walked back to the bedroom, I dropped onto all fours in the hallway. Once I made it to the bedroom, all fours again, leaning against the bed. "Why isn't he coming?" I asked. It was just after 5 p.m.

I had not slept in thirty-seven hours, had only eaten a few grapes since the night before. How much longer? The midwife asked me to get on the bed, just for a moment, so that she could check me. After a few more waves, I finally made it onto the bed.

"Oh," she said. "His head is right here!"

The relief that washed over me was like a warm blanket on a cold night. He was coming. He was going to be here. I just couldn't believe it. There was an end in sight.

The midwives took their place and got everything set up to welcome him into this world. My husband was right behind them, directly in my line of vision.

As our baby's head started pulsing out, then back in, then out, and back in, my husband was sobbing, the words "thank you, thank you, thank you" moving from his heart, and through his lips.

She told me to tuck my chin into my chest and curl myself around my baby with every contraction. My body was pushing him down and through. She suggested that my husband come sit behind me so that I could rest on him in the space between.

The ring of fire was real. I knew I had to move into a place of total surrender, complete trust, to move through it. As a wave came, my body would bear down just enough so that I wouldn't have to feel it. I told myself that the only way through, was through; and the only way he will come out is if I let go of the resistance to *feeling*—if I let go of all fear.

"When the next wave comes I will give my all," I told myself.

So I did.

"Do you want to catch your baby?" the midwives asked, as my husband took my hands and guided them down to our little babe. We pulled him to my chest, relieved to hear his sweet little cry. So attentive. His world totally changed.

His crying slowed, as he peered at us through his dark blue eyes. Just looking.

You had never seen light before and had only known warmth. You had not yet experienced the dualities of hunger and fullness, wet and dry, me and you. It would still take some time to understand that you have your own little body and are just now (at three months!) finding your own little hands.

And my whole world changed in that moment too. Rather than moving into a world of duality, like you were, I found myself moving from my world of a million priorities into a world where there was only one.

I had never known someone else's needs to be so much more important than my own. Where your happiness, your safety, your comfort, your smile, became my life's purpose. I had never known what it felt like to miss someone while they slept.

You suddenly became my everything. My dearest friend. My greatest teacher. My little angel. My heart and soul.

I showered and washed my hair. Your papa held you. The midwives cleaned up and left.

"Have you ever changed a diaper before?" I asked my husband as we drifted to sleep.

"No," he laughed.

"Neither have I."

THE BIRTH OF MY DAUGHTER

When I became pregnant with my little girl, I felt excited to start care with the same home birth midwives who supported me in birthing my son. At the same time, I felt mysteriously drawn to the idea of "free birthing" my baby—giving birth at home with only my husband present. My plan was to attend my monthly appointments with my midwives to develop a loving and trusting relationship and then see how I felt as labor neared.

As the months went on, I became internally clear that these midwives were not meant to support me in birthing my little girl. There were a lot of memories that arose around the birth of my son and a lot of healing that needed to happen around the dynamics of his birth before giving birth to my daughter. I felt anger toward my midwives around how the final stage of my labor felt suddenly medicalized. One midwife had asked me to lay on my back so she could check my dilation, as labor seemed to be slowing down. I now understand that I was in the sacred moments of transition, right before he was to come. I didn't want to lay on my back, as my body was asking to be on hands and knees for every single contraction over the last eighteen hours. I gave my power to her as the "authority" of my birth . . . because I assumed she knew better than I did, as it was only my first birth. I also now understand that there is no need to know how dilated a cervix is, as labor unfolds outside of the realm of time: mama can be 2 centimeters dilated and give birth within the hour, or she can be 10 centimeters dilated with hours still before baby comes.

Once I was on my back, she saw that baby's head was right there and suggested I stay on my back as I pushed. So I pushed—*hard* (and hurt for the next two weeks due to tearing). Everyone took their place just watching me (which feels so weird and unnatural in retrospect)—the main midwife with her sterile gloves on and all sorts of instruments laid out on a towel. She was in the place where my husband should have been as my son crowned and was birthed into the world. The midwives spoke in the sacred moments right after his birth and rubbed his body with a cotton blanket as I held him.

These things are not inherently "wrong" or "bad," though in my second pregnancy—as I began to understand the dynamics of an undisturbed birth and really dropped into the space of knowing that my body was *made* to birth—I was able to see how the midwives' presence at my first birth felt unnatural to me and got in the way of my being able to trust my body and my baby.

I truly believe that a midwife or care provider's place in birth, if present at all, should be to witness and hold the sacred space for mama to birth, interfering only if mama asks or if actually needed. They should trust mama's ability and recognize and honor mothers as the sole authority of their bodies, their babies, and their birth processes. I feel that care providers need to understand the subtleties, and thus the sacredness, of labor and the moments following birth and not interfere in those moments unless absolutely needed.

I scheduled an anatomy scan during my second pregnancy to assure that all of baby's organs were developing optimally. This is the only ultrasound I opt in for while growing my baby. At that ultrasound, the doctors diagnosed me with Marginal Cord Insertion, possibly Velamentous (VCI), which would make it "extremely dangerous" to birth at home. My heart sunk. VCI is when baby's umbilical cord inserts off of the margins of the placenta, so the exposed membranes not covered by Wharton's jelly could easily be compressed during labor contractions—causing baby to suffocate and die. The weaker bond of the umbilical cord to the placenta could also cause the cord to detach during labor, cutting baby off from their supply of blood and oxygen and causing mama to hemorrhage . . . and die. *Wow.*

In the following months I got the opinions of two other doctors and they both confirmed it was VCI. Both the doctors and my midwives affirmed that the only safe place to birth my babe would be the hospital, where they could monitor me throughout labor and assure that the umbilical cord (and thus my baby) were fine and that the placenta came out with minimal bleeding (likely with the help of pitocin).

It was two weeks before my due date. My midwives told me they would no longer attend my home birth. I was in the process of surrendering to and preparing for a hospital birth. The safest option for some mothers to birth is at a hospital; if it was truly the safest place for me to birth my baby, then it was what I was going to do. But I just couldn't see it. I couldn't imagine being in the most primal act of my life, getting into a car and driving to an unfamiliar environment and being surrounded by people I didn't know and love.

I wrote and then rewrote a hospital birth plan, and I just couldn't believe I was having to write all of these things to protect myself from other people interfering with one of the most natural processes there is. I asked and then re-asked what the consequences might be of denying procedures or leaving before being discharged, if I could be in the birthing positions I wanted to be in, if daddy was "allowed" to catch his baby.

I couldn't believe that I was going to birth in a place where the staff weren't trained in the dynamics of real, natural birth and were instead trained to interfere—where, when patients make decisions during labor and delivery that diverge from what some doctors or nurses feel is best, some hospitals threaten to report the parent to child protective services or issue court orders to coerce compliance

I couldn't believe that I wouldn't be able to go home to be with my almost three-year-old son until a minimum of twenty-four hours after the birth without signing a "Failure to Comply" agreement.

I couldn't believe I was about to birth somewhere where it was actually impossible to be the authority of my birth.

And although in some cases it may be *actually* medically necessary to birth in the hospital (and in some cases it can be an ease-filled, beautiful, and supportive experience)—I couldn't believe that *my* birth was one of them. I more and more believed that there was nothing natural about even an unmedicated hospital birth, as my body is wise and will only birth naturally—as in, how nature *intended*—in the most natural of environments. For me, that was in my home. (And, as I was to discover, it was actually outside in nature, with my body on the earth beneath an oak tree.)

I prayed. *Was a hospital birth the only safe option?* A series of profound synchronicities—coming one after the other—began giving me strength in my intuitive knowing that my baby would be birthed at home. It started with a doctor at the hospital giving me confidence that this birth would be no different than other births. Directly after, I ran into a mama whose baby's cord detached during birth and everything was totally fine. I spoke to a handful of midwives who felt fully confident in a VCI home birth. I connected with a midwife in Colorado (a woman my massage therapist suggested I speak to) who worked at a hospital and had witnessed hundreds of VCI births that were all normal births. This midwife told me, "Your body will know if and when you have to go to the hospital. As a culture, we have lost touch with our body's *knowing*. Especially as a mother—you will always *know* what is best for your baby." When I talked to one of my dearest girlfriends later that week, we couldn't believe that—out of all the midwives—that same midwife was the one who supported her during the birth of her son.

I felt that I was part of a tapestry being woven that would reveal, in time, the already destined place that my baby would be born. In my desire to do what was truly best for my little one, I was showing up and doing my part. I surrendered, open to the signs (there are *always* signs), and followed my *knowing*.

Home.

I wanted a midwife there so that if I did become nervous during labor I could lean on her wisdom and experience. I called every midwife within a three-hour radius of my home. All of them were comfortable with a VCI home birth—though with only a week before my due date, no one was available to take me on as a client.

It looked as though we were going to have the unassisted home birth that I had envisioned since the beginning of this pregnancy. I started to experience anxiety on the Tuesday before she was born. Anxiety is a rare and unfamiliar experience for me. Was a romanticized desire to have a wild and natural birth at home getting in the way of me actually understanding the severity of the situation? Would birthing at home be a decision that I would forever regret, because perhaps my child wouldn't make it . . . or I wouldn't?

"You've got me, God?!" I cried. "Let me know that *whatever* happens . . . you've got me. That it is Your divine will. *All* of it."

Three days before my due date I texted a midwife who came highly recommended by trustworthy women in my community:

I was working with midwives who are no longer willing to do a home birth because of VCI. If I go into labor tonight, our plan is free birth—though I would feel more grounded having an experienced midwife here who could monitor and hold space as needed, who knows variations of normal, and who ultimately supports me in trusting the process of birth. I've heard wonderful things regarding the space that you hold. I would love to connect about the potential of you coming to our birth.

If you go into labor tonight or overnight, call me, she responded. *I'll be there.*

I fell to my knees in gratitude. Even now, writing this, tears roll down my cheeks. I had never met or even spoken to her on the phone. She didn't ask for my insurance policy or how I would pay. She simply said, "I'll be there," in devotion to mother and the sacred process of birth.

She came over the next day—and I felt such profound shelter. A wise woman, a sister, a friend who was fully aligned with the sacred and empowering vision of birth that I held.

All was right. All was okay. I trusted that in a deep, deep way now.

I was ready to birth my baby.

♦

August 8 was my mother's birthday, and a day beyond my expected "due date." I started to feel more heavy and tired and suspected that baby was coming soon. Braxton-Hicks contractions seemed to be getting stronger, and that evening, as we were having a dinner party for my mama, they seemed to come more often.

I went to sleep that night though was awakened every ten minutes or so by stronger and stronger waves lasting for just under a minute—never too strong to get me out of bed but always strong enough to wake me up. When I got out of bed in the morning I was pretty sure I was in early labor, though I knew it could still be days before she came, as some labors come and go. I did an abhyanga and basti as my little boy and husband had breakfast. At around 8:00 a.m. I called my mom to let her know that I thought today was the day and asked her to come over to be with my son so I could be absorbed in my process. I took an outdoor herbal bath as they drew with chalk on the back porch. It was a beautiful morning.

My husband made kanji and I sat on the couch to eat. At around 10:00 a.m. the waves were getting strong enough that I had to focus on them entirely when they came. They were spaced about seven to eight minutes apart, each lasting more than a minute. I told my mom that it was time to take my little boy out and about so that I could be at home with just my husband. My husband prepared the beds and birthing tub, bathed, and did *puja* (the act of worship) in front of our altar.

By 11:30 a.m., the intensity of each wave was becoming stronger and stronger. I assumed I was still at the beginning of a long labor—considering my first experience of labor—and couldn't believe how painful these contractions were. With my son's birth, it was long and intense, but I wouldn't ever describe it as painful. With this one, I couldn't find any position that would lessen the pain. I wanted my husband's full presence now, and I wanted him to be touching me. I think I needed the warmth.

At around noon, the contractions were less than five minutes apart and lasting for over a minute—active labor.

"Help!" I cried, to my husband or to God, to whoever might hear me. "Help!" I tried hands and knees leaning against our bed; I went onto the toilet. A wave would come and bring me onto my tippy toes, holding on to the counter, and then down to all fours. I crawled into my son's playroom. *This is too intense. Something needs to change*, I thought. Between contractions, which were now just minutes apart, I walked around the house looking for somewhere or something else that might support me. I opened our back door and went outside. I dropped onto all fours beneath our kumquat tree. The earth felt like a sanctuary beneath me, the sun's warmth like a soothing balm on my back.

"I want to be near our fire pit," I told my husband as I got up between waves and walked there. I knew I wouldn't have long before the next wave came. My husband went inside to get blankets and pillows and our oil diffuser with cardamom essential oil. I told him I wanted to sleep, and I laid down beneath the oak tree and actually fell asleep—the sacred space of transition—until another wave brought me to my hands and knees. It was just after 1:00 p.m. These contractions felt different, though. They felt bearable. And suddenly my vulva was opening. It literally felt like I was blossoming, like a rose unfurling.

"Baby's coming," I said to my husband. He texted our midwife who said she would be there in ten minutes. He put the phone away and told me, "I'm fully here with you." I instinctively started breathing fast through my mouth with each wave to slow down the force of baby's head moving through me. She would pulse out, then back in after each contraction. I was in no rush. My body was opening in the most beautiful way. It was truly unbelievable.

Her head came out, facing the sky. Her eyes were closed and her face was blue. She was completely silent. We suddenly heard a voice behind my husband: "Good," was all she said. I turned around and smiled. Our birth-guardian arrived at the perfect moment—and simply watched. She knew we didn't need her, and she held the most profound and sacred space for us to feel fully confident in bringing our baby earthside. With the next contraction, baby slipped out. Daddy passed her to me between my legs. I leaned against our picnic table with her on my belly, in total awe.

"She's a little girl," daddy said.

My little girl. She's here.

My placenta plopped out effortlessly after some minutes. My midwife confirmed that it was a perfectly fine placenta (no VCI!).

We stayed outside beneath the oak tree for two or three hours. The midwife never touched my baby. My baby never left my arms. She asked if I wanted to do the standard procedures like APGAR testing, weight and length measuring, and so on. I asked, "Do I have to?" I didn't feel ready to put her down. She said, "It's your baby. You don't have to do anything." An angel. "No need, then," I said.

She left. I bathed. My husband went to pick up our little boy who was sleeping in his arms when they got home. Everything was perfect. So peaceful. Beyond what I could have envisioned for the birth of my dreams.

JATA KARMA: BIRTH CEREMONY

Jata karma is the traditional Vedic ceremony performed immediately upon the birth of your little one, before giving milk or cutting the umbilical cord. The ceremony is done right in the birthing room and is said to give intelligence to the child.

The father of the child says prayers to honor his gurus (teachers), while a young girl in the family, or another pregnant mama, grinds rice and barley into a powder with an unused stone and a washed stone slab.* The father then takes the powder between the thumb and ring finger of his right hand as he recites a prayer for God to receive and bless the grains. He mixes the powder with ghee on a golden spoon, and then places it on the tongue of his newborn baby, saying the following prayer in Sanskrit: "May the Divine God and Goddess bestow intelligence to you. Not only worldly intelligence, but also the greatest intelligence for understanding God." Once the prayers are completed, the father cuts the umbilical cord and the baby can nurse at the breast. The father bathes himself, and the ceremony is completed.

* The rice and barley are said to give sustenance, and the ghee is used to deliver beauty, memory, intellect, talent, luster, and long life.

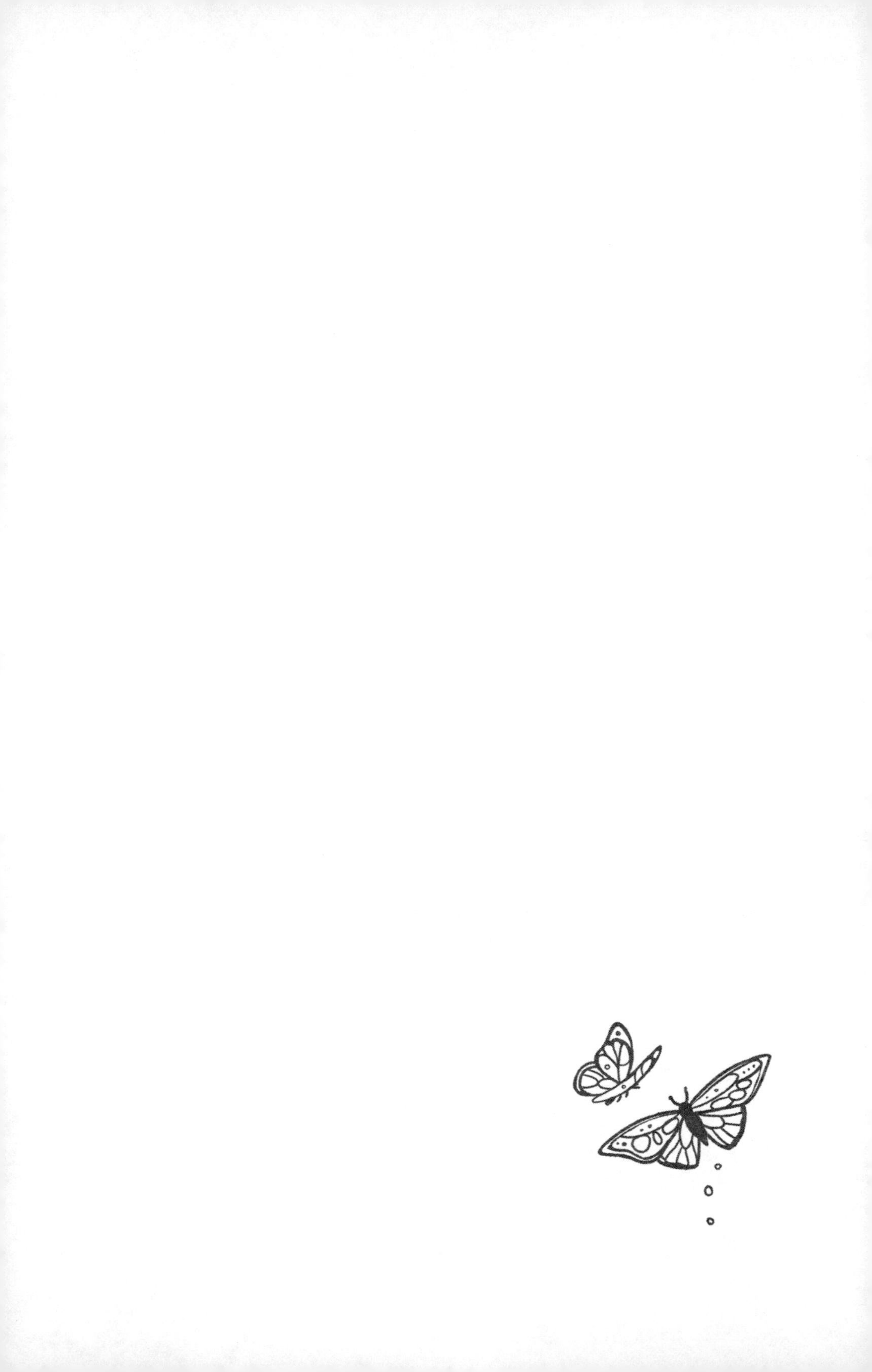

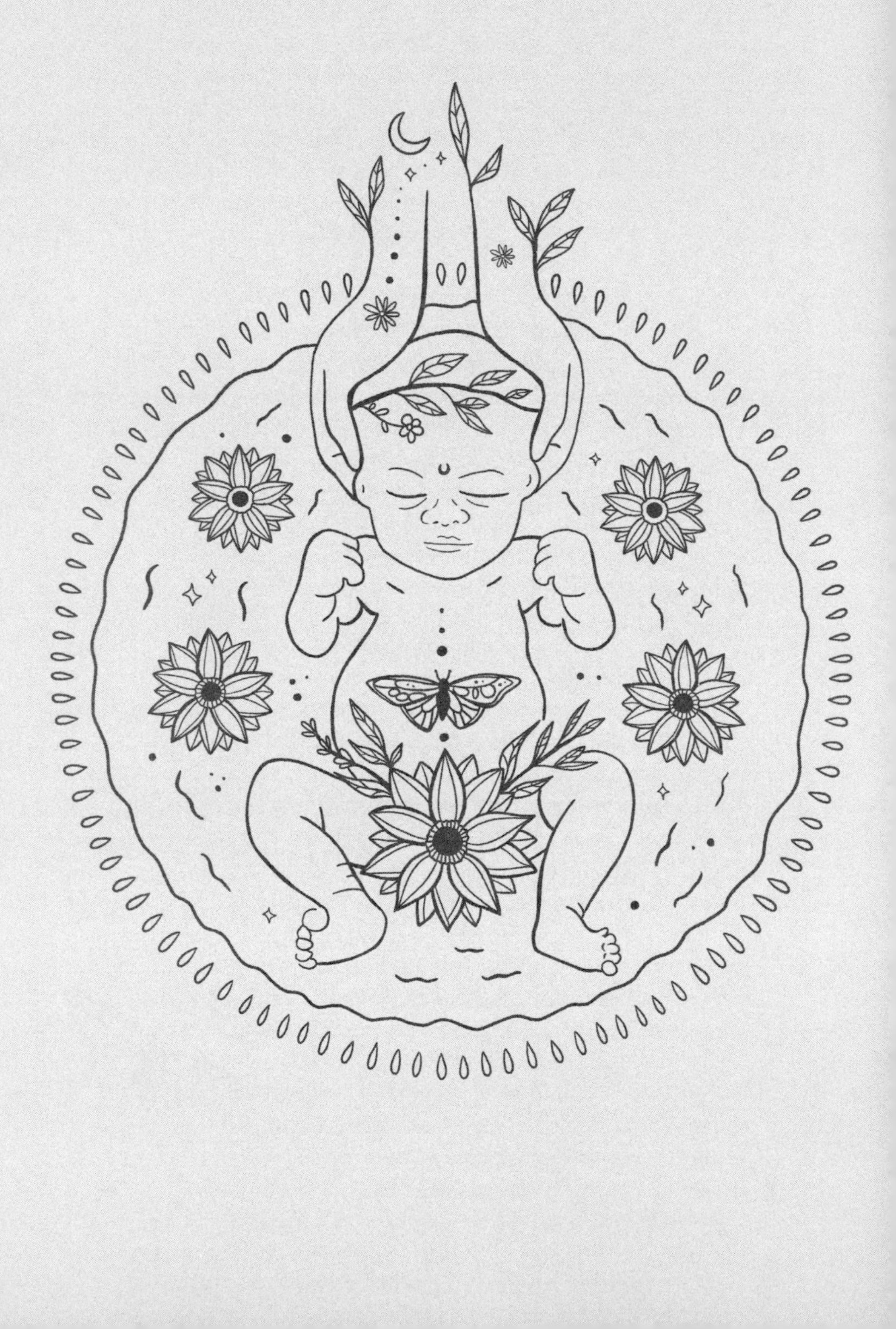

The Sacred Window

· 6 ·

After birth, there's a sacred window of time. A time for complete rejuvenation of a woman's physical, mental, and spiritual health. A time for deep, extended bonding with her newborn. The first forty-two days after birth set the stage for her next forty-two years.

—Ysha Oakes, postpartum Ayurvedic doula,
founder of the Sacred Window School

The postpartum window is a unique period of transition in a woman's life. In just a few weeks, as she recovers her strength and learns to mother her new baby, a woman's body and mind undergo changes of unparalleled intensity. She enters a rite of passage which literally changes who she is, and learns many things about life and herself in the process. She also begins a relationship with her newborn which will be a template for the baby's trusting relationships with other human beings, in a bond which will last their lifetimes.

—Jenny Allison, *Golden Month:
Caring for the World's Mothers after Childbirth*

Many cultures have traditional practices surrounding the first six weeks following birth. The traditions tend to have similarities that include a period of rest and care for the new mama; warmth; easy-to-digest, oily, and simple foods; a time away from those outside the immediate family; and the assurance of a peaceful and controlled environment. The weeks after a baby is born represent a “sacred window”—a time to rekindle the digestive fire, balance and stabilize vata, and rewire your entire system for a lifetime of love and service. Witness yourself becoming more replenished, healed, nourished, and whole than you ever were before.

For these first few weeks, babies do not yet know themselves as separate. They *feel* everything, and their sense of self is built on their surroundings. You want to create the most safe, nurturing, and predictable environment for your babe so that they know this world as safe and, although unpredictable, fundamentally good. After forty-two days, your baby will have learned what love means and will now be ready to learn about the busy, bright world outside.

Your body was the baby’s body for so long, and they still depend on it for regulating their temperature, their heart rate, their emotions, and their breath. If you are nourished, your baby’s body, heart, and mind will respond accordingly. The calmer and more relaxed you are, the calmer and more relaxed your baby will feel. Through the Ayurvedic postpartum practices described in this chapter, you can bring more ease and comfort to your little one; avoid postpartum depression, depletion, and overwhelm; avoid low milk supply; preclude the chance of your baby being gassy or suffering from colic; and more.

The sacred postpartum window is also time where you can honor your shift from maiden to mother, or mother of one to a mother of two (and so on), without distracting yourself with the busyness of everyday life. Birth changes you. In the words of Osho, “The moment a child is born, the mother is also born. She never existed before. The woman existed, but the mother, never. A mother is something absolutely new.” During the sacred window you are able to slow down enough to notice what is different and how you’ve been changed. It is a time to discover (as well as re-create) who you are, now. Big transitions in life—whether it’s your child’s birth, a big move, a loved one’s death, or something else—need time to integrate. Change can be uncomfortable, so often after a huge life shift we just want things quickly to feel “normal” again—hence the rush of many new mamas to enter back into the world. Ayurveda urges you to slow down and to allow the changes in your life to change you; it asks you to honor and acknowledge the ways you are changed and to allow yourself the space to come into this new version of yourself in a conscious and natural way.

Special things happen during this sacred window. Deep healing, deep grieving, deep connection, deep integration, and a deep inner stillness all allow for a deep rewiring of the psyche. I became a mother in that window, redefined and ready to enter into the world in my new role—like a butterfly out of her cocoon.

I was told
that as soon as little babe came out
I would feel the deepest,
most explosive love that
I'd ever experienced.
My experience was different though.
I loved this little person already,
though it was not a feeling that felt "new" or so different
than any other love I had experienced before.
And then I came back to the teaching
that love is not a feeling.
Yes,
it is something you feel.
Though the feeling is never the foundation of love.
The feeling is not where it is born
or how it grows.
Because feelings change,
and real love
is everlasting
and ever expanding,
when the foundation is established properly.
The feeling
is the fruit
of the expression of love.

What is different about this experience of love
is that I would do anything for this little boy.
I would stay up all night
and bounce him for hours
and check to make sure he is breathing
a zillion times each day.

I would go out of my way
and beyond my own needs or comfort
to make sure this little person feels safe.
Real love
is experienced,
is felt,
is grown
through service.
Through showing up
even when it is challenging,
And seeing how the heart expands.

POSTPARTUM FOCUS

Mothers who have just given birth are reborn with their babies. According to Ayurveda, mama is basically as fragile as her baby. In the traditional way, mama is meant to have her mother there, holding her and supporting her throughout this transition. She is meant to be mothered herself, and when she has that type of care, she is able to bond deeply with her baby, as well as heal and rejuvenate in a deep way. The Ayurvedic postpartum doula Sarva Blackwell says that a mama's greatest need during the sacred window is to herself "be mothered with the type of mothering that is a true expression of unconditional love, where she is completely held, completely safe at the deepest levels, and completely nourished with exactly what she needs for her deepest healing." But our society has become quite disconnected from an understanding of this need. Even if you do have your mother there to care for you, it is likely that she never received the type of care that she needed postpartum in order to pass the wisdom on to you—so she may not actually know how to show up and support you.

During pregnancy, there is a feeling of fullness. Quite literally, your body is completely filled! Then, through the process of labor, apana vata works hard to move your baby downward. Once your baby is in your arms, you are left with a lot of newly empty space inside. Wherever there is space, air will move into it, making the postpartum body the perfect home for vata dosha.

Vata is also superabundant postpartum because mama has lost a great deal of fluid during birth, and she continues to lose fluids through the discharge of lochia (the blood, mucus, and uterine tissue shed from the womb after childbirth) and through breastfeeding. She is going through many changes in all aspects of her life, including a redefinition of who she is, her relationship, her purpose, and her role in the world.

As explored in chapter 1, an increase in vata dosha comes with dryness, coldness, loneliness, anxiety, fear, restlessness, fatigue, insomnia, constipation, isolation—all the symptoms of "postpartum depression" and the most common postpartum symptoms we hear about. Nature would not have designed the life cycle in a way that would see a mother go through the deepest and most transformative experience of her life only to feel depleted, disconnected, and unwell. Though because as a culture we have become so separated from Mother Nature, this letdown is what many mothers end up experiencing.

If, however, you are nurtured in the ways that nature intended for you to be after giving birth to your little babe, you will heal and thrive in ways you never knew possible. After childbirth, your body is more open than it will ever be. Because of this, ancient traditions suggest that you can heal deep-rooted illnesses—even from childhood—through proper care. If you nourish yourself, focusing on pacifying vata for the first forty-two days after birth, the postpartum window can be the most rejuvenating time of your entire life. Your organs and tissues have to go back into position *anyway,* your relationship will continue *anyway,* your life keeps moving forward *anyway.* So rather than just leaving it all up to chance and hoping that everything works out well, Ayurveda encourages us to hold the intentional, nurturing, loving, warm, and caring space for life to come back together in the most optimal way. To balance an excess of vata, the focus of these first forty-two days will be oiliness, warmth, rest, support, and stability.

I wrote this poem after the birth of my second child, during my sacred window:

I can't tell you how many hours I've spent looking at pictures and watching videos of my older boy these last days.

Ooh my heart

The Sacred Window. Gosh, it's deep.
It's a time of becoming, a time of celebrating
. . . though I'm also realizing what a time of grieving it is.

Grieving what no longer is.
What had to die for this new life to be born.

Grieving the life that I've left behind
and what will never ever be again
. . . because such is time.
It changes everything.

Celebrating this new life.
Honoring her with every ounce of my being,
as my heart aches to be with my little boy.

Lying in bed as often as I can to allow my body its much needed rest,
as my heart yearns to play with him.

Staying home for too many days,
when all I want to do is hop in the car with my little man and head out on an adventure.
Just the two of us.

Wanting to turn back time,
or fast forward till it all feels normal,
though knowing that *this* is the sacred window.
It's a time to feel.
A time to *honor*.
A time to grieve.
A time to understand and integrate and *be in* the discomfort of change,
rather than rush through it or distract myself from it.

Because then it'll pass,
like everything does.

My heart feels totally split in two.
and of course there are magical days or magical moments where it all feels so right,
though there are also these moments where my heart really, really hurts.

Ooh, the sacred window.
A time to honor
Life,
Death,
and the space in between.

POSTPARTUM ESSENTIALS CHECKLIST

The following list collects suggestions for supportive items to have on hand during the postpartum window:

Thermoses to keep your hot tea warm at your bedside to drink throughout the day

Hot water bottles or heating pads for warming the belly, lower back, and feet

Long cotton cloth for belly wrapping

Peri bottles in each bathroom

Electric water kettle for making tea throughout the day

Pressure cooker for easy, yet nourishing home-cooked meals

Homeopathic arnica tablets for aches and pains

Your go-to, comfy, all-day, nursing pajamas

Breakfast-in-bed fold-up tray

Rescue Remedy Bach Flower Essence to take every few hours to ease stress

Herbs, ghees, and oils such as those mentioned in "Sacred Window Basics" (this page), "Postpartum Herbal Supports" (page 212), and "Beneficial Herbs and Essential Oils" (page 301)

SACRED WINDOW BASICS

Ayurveda identifies four pillars of postpartum care as essential for the healing of the mama, an ease-filled transition for the baby, and well-rounded integration of such a profound life change:

PILLAR OF REST

New mamas need forty-two days of rest after the birth of their babe to heal, integrate, and *become*.

- Stay reclined or horizontal for the majority of the day, especially for the first ten days. Then, gradually add gentle movements such as walking around the house (with socks or slippers, even in the summer months!) or a bit of light stretching. First and foremost, mama has to be able to relax. When the body is relaxed, healing happens naturally.
- Ideally, mama stays in the house (or not farther than the backyard) for the full sacred window, forty-two days postpartum—without traveling to less-predictable environments or driving in the car, which will both be overstimulating. When provided with the right environment and the proper nourishment, the body knows how to heal. After giving birth, the less activity for the first forty-two days, the better, to help bring vata back into a state of balance.
- Baby should be close to mama at all times, ideally with skin-to-skin connection.
- The environment should be warm, cozy, predictable, and low lit, with low stimulation, no drafts, and pleasing to be in. Invite as much *beauty* as possible.
- Limit guests. The people in the environment create the energy in the environment. In general, limit guests to only close friends and family members for the first forty-two days, and visits to only fifteen minutes at a time. This assures mama won't be depleted by too much interaction, and that conversational topics do not stray from the important and sacred experience that mama is currently in. Everyone who comes to visit mama should come in the mood to support her, rather than to be hosted as a guest. Rather than coming just to see the baby, they should ask mama what she actually needs. Oftentimes mama wants to be as close to her babe as possible (rather than to pass her little one around), though she might appreciate someone playing with her older child or helping with laundry, dishes, meals, and so on. Or perhaps what she needs is a shower—or to spend quality moments with her older kid(s)—and for someone to hold her little one during that time.

PILLAR OF DIET

During the process of labor and birth, a mama's digestive fire goes completely out. The postpartum diet focuses on gently rekindling this fire with nourishing yet easy-to-digest foods and eating practices.

- Eat at regular times throughout the day, assuring that you are sitting down, focused on eating, as peaceful as possible, and chewing your food thoroughly. Having someone lovingly prepare your meals and teas and bring them to your bedside at the proper times is one of the most nourishing ways of being "mothered" so that you can focus on mothering your little one.
- Have simple, easy-to-digest, warm, well-cooked, mushy foods with digestive spices (such as cumin, coriander, fennel, ginger). Gradually increase the complexity of meals throughout the six weeks to assure digestion stays balanced.
- Add a couple of tablespoons of ghee to every meal to support digestion and elimination, pacify vata, and remove ama (toxins) from the system.
- Stay hydrated! Achieve hydration during the postpartum window through mineral-rich sources such as soups, stews, broths, herbal infusions, and warming elixirs. Hydration is crucial for encouraging regular bowel movements; drinking warm prune juice as needed will also support elimination (best after lochia discharge has slowed).
- Full details for a postpartum diet are provided in chapter 8.

PILLAR OF HERBS

Among the many herbs that can be supportive to a postpartum mama, the following are some Ayurvedic staples that you will want to have on hand for daily consumption.

- Panchakola ghee. Panchakola ghee is infused with five spices (pippali, pippali root, ginger, black pepper, and chitrak) that help to increase agni (digestive fire) and decrease ama (toxins). It should be mama's first food after delivery; then use 1–2 tablespoons of this ghee on each meal for the first ten days.
- *Dashamula* tea. Dashamula is a combination of ten roots that work together synergistically to pacify vata and ground, warm, and nourish

mama during her postpartum window. It is a tonic that removes vata from the nervous system and womb, supports digestion and elimination, reduces pain, and creates a calming effect on the mind. Drink in the morning and evening (see recipe on page 287).

- Milk tonic. Milk tonic (see recipe on page 290) soothes nerves, encourages healthy digestion and elimination, and restores strength and vitality; during the weeks postpartum it also helps build a healthy milk supply. Drink each night before bed.
- Ginger tea, CCF tea (see recipe on page 288), and fenugreek tea. Drink these teas throughout the day for digestion and lactation support.

PILLAR OF BODY CARE

Postpartum body care is focused on moving excess vata from the body by deeply nourishing mama and providing her with warmth, oiliness, stability, and love. Some days it may feel overwhelming or impractical to include all this into your postpartum care. Know that it is not "all or nothing." Sometimes if we can't do it all "perfectly" we may think, "What's the use of doing any of it at all?" Of course it is best if you can do the following each day, though know that any amount is beneficial. Be as steady and consistent as possible for the full six weeks.

Postpartum belly wrap. Traditionally, a postpartum belly wrap is made with a long piece of cotton cloth, wrapped many times around your entire torso and hips. This secure container supports your organs in returning to their prepregnancy size and position, helping you to heal faster and more completely. It also brings a feeling of emotional and physical stability and support. You can make a wrap yourself with a long piece of cotton cloth or you can purchase one online. If you are making your own, choose a natural fiber such as cotton or cotton muslin. Look for the softest, thinnest natural-fiber fabric you can find. Choose fabrics that are not stretchy or only slightly stretchy, about 1 foot wide by 24 feet long.

Peri bottle after (and while!) using the bathroom. A peri bottle is a plastic squirt bottle that can be used to clean the perineal area, greatly reducing stinging during urination. You can use water or your sitz-bath tea (recipe on page 126). Dilute the tea by one-half with clean water and fill the bottle.

Daily abhyanga (warm oil massage) followed by a shower or bath. As noted in chapter 2, a basic of Ayurvedic body care is abhyanga, or warm oil massage. In the postpartum period, rather than doing the massage yourself, consider hiring an Ayurvedic massage therapist or an Ayurvedic postpartum doula, if possible, for at least the first two to six weeks. Your friends, parents, or partner can also learn how to do this, which can be a sweet bonding and nourishing time for all of you. It is quite simple, actually! For postpartum massage, use at least a cup of warm sesame oil—optionally infused with any combination of brahmi, ashwaganda, bala, and rose—and rub gently and lovingly onto your body with repetitive strokes: long strokes on the long bones, circles around the joints. Massage for thirty minutes to an hour to really absorb the oil, keeping the oil on your body for thirty minutes to an hour afterward. Abhyanga is simultaneously cleansing and nourishing; it moves stuck emotions or stagnated energy, boosts the immune system, enhances digestion, soothes the nervous system, quiets the mind, and helps the postpartum mama feel cared for, confident, and loved. Ideally, you'll take a warm shower or bath afterward.

Herbal baths at least four times per week. Many herbs can help soothe tender perineal tissue, heal tears and episiotomies (yes, you can take herbal baths if you have had stitches!), reduce inflammation, and even shrink hemorrhoids after a vaginal birth. Taking herbal baths at least four times a week can also soothe the nervous system, give space for mama to process her birth experience, lighten depression, calm anxiety, improve sleep, and bring strength. Use any combination of plantain leaf, yarrow, calendula, lavender, sage, marshmallow root, and witch hazel to create healing and rejuvenating baths (see "Guidelines for an Herbal Bath" on page 92). An herbal bath can be taken as soon as an hour after a vaginal birth as long as mama is healthy and there are no signs of infection. If you do not have a tub at home, a sitz bath can be used instead—though Ayurveda says full body immersion will give you much deeper benefits.

Hot pack. Place a hot pack on your belly and lower back for at least thirty minutes daily. The warm quality helps to pacify the coolness of vata. The hips and pelvis are also known to be the main site of vata. Applying warmth to these areas will support healing and help with lower back pain or postpartum contractions, as well as help you feel nourished, stable, and warm.

Basti. Use a warm oil enema, or basti, for seven consecutive days, starting after two weeks postpartum, to deeply nourish your pelvic region and assure that vata dosha is stable. Use ¼ cup sesame oil mixed with ¼ cup warm water.

How to Wrap the Belly the Ayurvedic Way

Sarva Blackwell of Inner Sun & Moon School of Natural and Holistic Therapeutics, which offers an Ayurvedic doula training, provides the following instructions for a postpartum belly wrap.

Start with one end of the cloth at the side of one hip and wrap diagonally up toward the opposite ribs.

Bring the cloth straight across the back to the other side of the ribcage and then cross in front, back toward the opposite hip from where you started. Continue in this crossing pattern, occasionally twisting a single twist at the sides of the body to give extra support and to help the cloth angle diagonally more easily.

Wrap from the hips up to the bra line. Experiment by wrapping until you find a way of doing it that feels most comfortable and supportive to you. The wrap should be simultaneously firm and gentle—you should feel firmly supported but be able to breathe and move around easily.

Think of it as wrapping a sprained wrist with an ace bandage.

You can wear the belly wrap as much as 24/7 during the six weeks postpartum if you like. Consider wearing it ten or twelve hours a day to start and see how it suits you. If you want to belly bind daily for six weeks, you will want to have three to five cloths on hand. You can use a belly wrap if you have had a cesarean birth so long as it is comfortable—you're the one who needs to decide when you feel ready. If you are worried or it feels uncomfortable for you, wait until the stitches are starting to dissolve.

It is especially beneficial to massage the belly with warm oil before wrapping—it's so good for the skin after going through pregnancy! Sesame oil herbalized with brahmi and rose is amazing for healing up stretch marks and helping the skin recover its elasticity.

GATHER YOUR TRIBE

Ask for help! This was one of the hardest things for me to do once my husband went back to work. I needed help with everything, but I didn't want to burden my friends or my sister, since there was nothing I could do to reciprocate. I would find time to eat, then have no time to do my dishes. I would somehow get my laundry into the washer, and then be unable to put it in the dryer or fold it. I would walk past piles of my folded clothes in the living room but not have time to put them away. I would say thank you a million times when someone would watch my baby when I showered, and later realized it was because I felt so guilty burdening someone with my responsibilities. I broke down one day in tears, feeling the huge burden I had put on myself by my inability to ask for the support that I needed. My friends and my sister were grateful, because they wanted to help, but just did not know how to.

Give yourself permission to need someone. Give yourself permission to receive. And perhaps, before baby comes, let your friends know that it might be hard for you to ask for help . . . but that you are really going to need it.

SIMPLE WAYS FOR OTHERS TO HELP

Doing laundry: washing, drying, folding, and putting away

Holding your baby while you bathe and eat

Playing with older siblings so that you can rest with baby

Holding baby so that you can give your full attention to older siblings

Grocery shopping or other miscellaneous errands

Washing dishes

Cooking

Tidying up your room

Bringing warm drinks and nourishing snacks to your bedside

The less you have to think about your own nourishment, the better. You will need someone to "mother" you as you are learning to mother your little babe. If you can hire a postpartum doula or if you have a friend or family member who is willing and able to help during this time, embrace this precious support.

It's hard to find the words.
Or perhaps
it's hard to find the time to capture them.
Redefining myself;
my offering;
who I am now and how I show up
—because it's changed.

I climbed the tallest mountain
and I made it to the other side
knowing
that things would never be the same.

I have been changed.
You have grown me.
Though it is hard to find the words—
or perhaps
hard to find the time
to capture them.

For Those Around the Mama: Bring Beauty

Whatever is done with attention and intention has an aspect of beauty infused into it. When something is made beautiful, you can actually feel the heart that was poured in. During the sacred window, mama is vastly more sensitive to the subtleties. This makes her postpartum time the perfect opportunity to invite more beauty, ritual, and ceremony into her life, really honoring this profound rite of passage that she is in, as she will be deeply, deeply moved by it.

If you are going to be cooking for her *anyway*, please know that the mood you cook in is being infused into the meals and that she will feel it. Cook with love.

If you'll be bringing a meal to her bedside *anyway*, serve it on a beautiful plate, perhaps garnished with edible flowers—and her tea in a beautiful crystal goblet or at least her favorite mug to enjoy.

If you'll be drawing a bath for her *anyway*, why not light candles, add rose petals, and turn on soothing music?

Infuse mama's space with as much beauty, and thus as much intentional loving action, as possible. It does not necessarily take more time, simply more love—and it will go a long way in nourishing mama during this sacred window of time.

GUIDANCE FOR YOUR PARTNER

The following pages are written for you to share with your husband or partner. They may be finding it difficult or confusing to understand the entirety of your experience. The process of becoming a mama is a huge internal shift! You are changing mentally, emotionally, physically, and spiritually. Sharing this letter will help your partner understand your experience, so that they can give you the support, love, and care that you need.

Dear Partner,

Wow, we did it. We made it through pregnancy and birth together, and we now have our little angel in our arms! I have gone through a lot and can still use the same (if not more!) support that you have given me during pregnancy and birth.

You may not know, but all around the world, cultures have ancient postpartum traditions that are passed down from generation to generation. Within these cultures, mamas have healthy postpartum experiences and enjoy the bliss of connecting with their new babe. In our culture, the postpartum window is often the beginning of chronic health issues for some women. It can also be the beginning of marital issues and emotional problems that can last well past the six weeks of healing.

Ayurvedic postpartum care is not in place to make me feel pampered or spoiled; these practices are essential to my healing. Otherwise, the results of my feeling unsupported or uncared for during this time can be detrimental to my health for decades to come. The six-to-eight-week window following pregnancy and birth gives an opportunity for complete rejuvenation of my body on the deepest levels; or, if not honored properly, for rapid aging, anxiety, worry, depression, digestive issues, fatigue, and pain, among other things. Every tissue and system in my body is in a state of transition for these six weeks. I must be deeply nourished in order to heal.

Birth is a tremendous, powerful act that does not go unnoticed in my body. I might be feeling open, tender, and vulnerable. Please be sensitive to this. The metabolic principle that governs all movement and change in the body (including neural, circulatory, elimination, respiration, speech, and childbirth) is heavily affected by pregnancy, labor, and delivery (vata dosha). And because vata dosha is so high in my body now, it provides a rare opportunity for change. Care for me, as I am caring for your child, and you will watch as I transition into a beautiful, nourished, and vibrant mother.

I am grateful for your support in this time, and always. Your love and care now will set me and our child up for a lifetime of good health. Your support, love, and care are an invaluable part of this experience.

Love,
This Newborn Mama

The Ayurvedic postpartum doula Ysha Oakes, founder of the Sacred Window Studies School, was fond of reminding partners that this is an important time for their relationship with the new mama: "Because her heart is so open to service, her body has the guidance and opportunity, with support, to restructure in the direction of maximum ability to love and serve." These are simple ways you can help:

- The birth of a new baby is a huge transition for your family. Be in the experience *with* your partner as you come into new rhythms together.
- Try to take at least two weeks off work if you can, not only to support your partner in all the big and small ways but also to create the space in your life to honor this new little person who has come in.
- Greet visitors and remind them of the ethics of visiting a newborn mama as well as the simple things like washing their hands before visiting mama and baby.
- Oversee visits, making sure the visitor is being helpful and respectful and doesn't stay too long (mama may feel tired even after someone visiting for 15 minutes). Be the host so that she doesn't have to be.
- Arrange for someone to keep up with household chores. If you need to and are able to, hire someone during this time to keep the house clean. It will be worth it to allow for the extra space to create the rhythm of your new life as well as time for you and mama to relax and get to know your new babe.
- Encourage mama to rest and to allow herself to be served. She may be feeling guilty about needing so much help. Now is a great time to voice your support to her, as well as to thank her for how much she is showing up to care for your newborn.
- Keep the house warm and cozy. Bring her warm fuzzy socks or blankets if she needs; fluff her pillows so she is comfy in bed; bring flowers to her bedside.

- Initiate the baby massage routine before bedtime. Use this time to bond with your baby, and allow mama to take some space to herself (or to be with your older children).
- A partner's support is said to be one of the most important factors in successful breastfeeding. Be encouraging if she is experiencing challenges. Bring her water or snacks while she is nursing your baby. Breastfeeding gives health benefits for mama and baby for years to come.
- Make sure mama always has drinks by her bedside and that she is receiving enough nourishing foods throughout the day.
- Remember that mama and baby are sensitive to their environment now. Opt for reading with a background of soft relaxing music in the evening rather than TV or news.
- Spend time with your older children while mama and baby rest.
- Spend time with baby so mama can spend time with the older one(s).

THIS ONE'S FOR MY HUSBAND

There are so many ways that partners can help during the postpartum window. I share the below note that I gave to my husband to offer a window into the more personal ways that a partner can support.

I have a million reasons to be grateful for you, though here I'll name just a few.

Thank you for . . .

making sure my peri bottle was always filled with nourishing herbs to help me heal

doing a gazillion loads of laundry during our postpartum weeks

cleaning and tidying the house every single day

making my herbal teas each morning before I wake up

cooking me Ayurvedic postpartum breakfasts and lunches for twenty-eight days straight and for providing superfood baked goods each evening

keeping me hydrated with water, electrolytes, and teas constantly by our bedside

giving me an oil massage four days a week, and hiring my dear friend to give massages the other three days cleaning and drawing my bath every eve and lighting the candle every time (love is in the details!)

stocking the house with groceries and getting roses each time you go out

. . . not to mention all the ways you show up for this little chub.

Sometimes in relationships
we only love someone
when they are acting the way we want them to act.
Or we only care for them
when they're giving us what we need to feel cared for.

Often, our love is built on conditions,
that unless met,
constrict our heart's ability to deeply care
and to really love unconditionally.

I am learning what it means to love,
because you are the easiest person to care for.
Not that it is always easy
—but that there is never any hesitation
to show up and serve you.

It is easy
to put your needs in front of mine
and to remember how to let myself be cared for
so that I can keep showing up for you.

It's easy
to give myself completely
without needing anything in return;
To love you when you are fussy
or tired
or in pain.
It's easy to love you all of the time,
and to show up and care for you no matter what.

It's easy,
because it feels so natural.
Because it *is* natural,

for our heart to love like that.
#motherhood #aspiritualpath

It is so important for you and your partner to feel connected with each other: to know that you are never in it alone, to feel supported, appreciated, valued, and seen. But nurturing that deep connection in your "new" life is not always so easy! Three things have been game changers for my partner and I:

1. Being affectionate with each other. At least one long, long hug or some eveningtime cuddles with just the two of us is so sweet and important.
2. Appreciating each other. We are a team! See what your partner is doing—see the little things—and let them know how much you appreciate them. Say "thank you" often. It keeps the love flowing . . . it really, really does.
3. Checking in with each other daily. After babe sleeps, we have a cookie and milk date on the couch. We check in about how the day went: where we can use more support, what can be done differently, what was really hard, and what went really well.

That is what it is, having a little babe:
we are serving together.
We are no longer the center of our relationship.
There is a higher principle
that we both agree upon
that we are showing up for
fully.

Thirty-nine days with you,
and we're slowly expanding our bubble just shy of our forty-two-day sacred window.
Papa goes back to New York City this Friday,
so we're testing the waters to see how you do out and about
—in a car seat, with more noise and more people, in a less predictable environment.
And I get to see how I mother out and about
—in a less predictable environment.
Where it all seems so new and so different
and I forget what I know
and suddenly feel like it's day one again.

This window has been so special.
Developing your nervous system with a stable and steady foundation.
A nervous system that knows that the world is fundamentally safe
and a little hunny that knows that he is fundamentally okay.
Loved.
Cared for.
For a mama to build her confidence in this new role.
To know that she is capable.
And to heal her own stories,
her own nervous system,
so that she knows that she is fundamentally okay.
Loved.
Cared for.

A window that has taught me how to turn inward
in search of my strength,
my healing,
my ability,
my resilience
—when my habitual instinct would rather distract.

The forty-two days reminds mamas to go within
—and we need that reminder.
Especially now.

LIGHT ON THE SACRED WINDOW*

At the time of conception, a woman offers her body as a vessel to bring a soul into this world. In complete surrender, she allows her body to be the vehicle in which a new soul grows and flourishes. It is as if she gives up all rights of ownership to her own body and fully offers it up in service. Her body may take on many challenges; even in the healthiest of pregnancies, the body undergoes dramatic change. At the time of labor and delivery the mother must surrender all control and allow herself, as the vessel for bringing new life into the world, to open. In those moments, she becomes a gateway between the heavens and the earth. As this process unfolds, whether it is her first or ninth child, she changes—and will be forever changed.

This transition is *sacred.*

And to be sacred means it is to be honored.

Healing is not something that has to be earned. Nurturing and nourishment through childbearing is not a luxury, or to be seen as pampering; it is an essential birthright of every woman. In our modern world we have forgotten the art of sacred rituals. We have all but lost the wisdom of our ancestors. We have adopted the habit of moving too quickly past these moments of deep transformation in our lives, allowing them to pass us by without so much as bowing our heads in reverence.

Every culture around the world has specific traditions, rituals, and recipes that are in place to honor the postpartum window. Many cultures around the world mark this time as sacred. It is up to you to reclaim the ancient traditions of your heritage and deeply honor the process of conception, pregnancy, birth, and the weeks postpartum.

Ayurveda is the science of life. It is not specific to one race, one culture, or one country; it is ancient knowledge that applies to all beings on earth. In addition to the Ayurvedic practices you have read in this book, I encourage you to inquire within your own family and your own heritage, to learn the traditional postpartum practices of your culture. So many cultures are rich in wisdom surrounding the sacred window if you dig deep enough.

---

* **This section is contributed by Krsna Jivani, a botanical Ayurdoula, herbalist, and mama.**

If you are not called to find ancient traditions to honor your sacred window, I encourage you to create your own rituals and infuse them with deep intention. In any form, choose your way to honor this time for your healing and transition into motherhood.

The Ayurvedic concept of postpartum practices may seem drastically different from what is common in Western society. In North America specifically, it is recognized even among medical professionals that there is a lack of awareness surrounding postpartum care. Women are pressured to return quickly to their pre-baby lifestyles and "get back on their feet," literally. When a woman is not properly supported and cared for postpartum, it shows up as "postpartum blues," depression, anxiety, overwhelm, fatigue, issues bonding with her baby, and other chronic health issues. Naturally, when the mother suffers, her baby also suffers.

Ayurveda refers to certain times of a woman's life as a *kayakalpa* or "body time." These are special windows of time that offer the opportunity for complete restructuring of a woman's physiology. These times offer renewed energy, youthfulness, growth, and expansion, as if the aging process has been reversed. The kayakalpas that occur in a woman's lifetime are her first menstruation, commitment in marriage or to a lifetime partner, menopause, and of course, the sacred postpartum window.

The sacred postpartum window is a kayakalpa of deep cleansing and nourishing that heals mama on all levels. It is a time best spent surrounding yourself in a sattvic environment and consuming sattvic sounds, tastes, sights, textures, and smells—just as is recommended during pregnancy. This is important not only for your healing but also for the nervous system of your newborn baby.

According to Ayurveda, it is ideal that your baby stays within your auric field—that is, the field of energy emanating from and surrounding mama's body—for several weeks, never going too far from you. During this time you can continue to act as the filter you've been for your baby for the past forty weeks, nourishing them with an environment that teaches them the qualities of goodness so that they can feel safe, supported, and peaceful in the world.

It's not in an instant that you become a mother.
It does not happen the moment you become pregnant, or the moment you give birth.

It happens over a collection of moments.

It happens when you're sitting in your bath after finding out you are pregnant, and grieving over the loss of your youthful body that is about to change in many (and some unspeakable) ways.

It happens as your consciousness shifts from "me" focused to "we" focused.

It happens in the bittersweet times of pregnancy when you want to savor the moment but simultaneously want it to end.

It happens as your baby grows and one day you realize you've gotten to know their likes and dislikes, their temperament and their sleep patterns, before you have even seen their face.

It happens during labor, when it's the hardest thing you have ever done, but you find the strength to do it in the best way you can manage, for the health of your baby.

It happens the first time you see their face and their little fingers and toes and you stare at each other with complete wonder and curiosity.

It happens in those first few days postpartum when you can barely walk and your body is sore and exhausted but you don't even realize because your only concern is that your baby is comfortable sleeping on your chest.

It happens when they start to recognize your voice and stop crying when they hear you close by.

It happens over millions of tiny decisions that you make during your day, knowing that every small decision impacts their experience of life.

It happens the moment you realize that this tiny little being loves you more than anything in the whole world, because you are their whole world and all that they know.

It is still happening, every day, as my heart grows to love her more and more with every noise she makes, every smile that appears on her face, even every time she cries out.

When a baby is born, a mother is born with them. And together they grow in their new bodies, their new experiences, their new world.

So no,

You don't just wake up one day as a mother.

The seed of mothering is planted deep in your being. And it sprouts,

And grows,

And blossoms,

And changes with the seasons.

THE UNIVERSAL MOTHER PRINCIPLES

When receiving care throughout your postpartum window, remembering these principles and applying them to every aspect of your day will help bring awareness and a deeply nourishing mood to support your healing. Some things to aim for:

Simplicity: Simple things will feel nourishing. Place a fresh rose by your bedside each day, drink warm water, change into clean pajamas or even a comfy dress. Notice how these simple actions nourish you deeply.

Listening: Listen to your body. Listen to your baby. Do you feel overwhelmed and overstimulated? Take a step back. Rest. And listen to what your body and your baby are telling you.

Grounding: Literally, stay grounded. Meaning, stay at home as much as possible. Make your home as cozy as ever and nest, nest, nest.

Intuition: It is easy to get overwhelmed with what you "should" do or how others perceive you as a mama. Tune that out. Mama knows best.

Nonjudgment: Avoid judging yourself at this time. You are learning and growing so much.

Flexibility: Be flexible with yourself and your baby. This is your permission to throw "timed feedings" and "timed naps" out the window. The postpartum window is a time of adapting to frequent change and getting to know your little one. What works for you and your baby may look different from what works for someone else.

Compassion: Be compassionate with yourself. You are doing your best. You are an amazing, competent, caring mother, and most importantly, you are the perfect mama for your babe. It's true.

As a new mother, you will spend every ounce of your energy and every minute of your day caring for your newborn baby. This little soul is depending on you for full support to maintain her life. She breathes because she hears you breathe, her heart beats rhythmically because she feels your heart beating. In order for you to be the best mother you can be, you must allow yourself to receive mothering care from loved ones around you. If you do not allow yourself to receive nurturing during this time, you may feel that you have no nurturing to give. Therefore, it is essential for the health of your baby that you fill your cup first by allowing others to support and care for you.

PREPARING FOR THE POSTPARTUM WINDOW

"Preparing for postpartum" is not a phrase we commonly hear in our society. We hear "preparing for labor," "preparing for birth," and "preparing for the baby"—but when, if ever, do we hear a pregnant woman say she is preparing for postpartum?

Most women in North America associate the word "postpartum" with things like postpartum depression, postpartum anxiety, or sleep deprivation. Many women have no concept of what to expect during the postpartum window due to the lack of education and conversation around it in our culture—if that's you, it's okay! You're not alone. We are here to help.

Considering that the postpartum window is such a significant time in a woman's life that it can have effects on her mental and physical health for decades to come, it is an absolute necessity to properly prepare for it. There are common postpartum experiences that you may encounter in the days or weeks following the birth of your babe. Many women are shocked at these unexpected occurrences and think, "How come no one told me about this!?" A wide range of feelings and physical experiences are completely normal. Don't be surprised if you experience any of the following:

You may be bleeding for several days up to several weeks; if you overexert your body, your bleeding can increase or come back.

You may have cramping pains during breastfeeding as your uterus shrinks back to its normal size.

You may need help getting out of bed to go to the bathroom or shower. Try not to get out of bed for any reason other than these for at least the first five days.

You may feel weak. Very weak. Perhaps weaker than you have ever felt before.

You may feel more vibrant and powerful than you have ever felt in your life.

You may not have an appetite, or you may forget to eat.

You may feel hungry and have a huge appetite!

You may feel guilty for needing so much help. ("Can you bring me some water?" "Can you help me into the shower?" "Can you plug my phone in?" "Can you help me sit up and fluff my pillow so I can breastfeed?" "Can you bring me some lunch?") *Allow* yourself to ask for help.

You may have pain or a feeling of heaviness in your pelvic floor if you are standing for too long, especially if you have stitches.

You may feel out of breath, even after going for short walks around the house.

You may feel strange in your body, as it has adapted to pregnancy and is now suddenly not pregnant anymore. Your bones may have shifted; your weight may be carried differently; your posture may feel different; your breathing may feel different.

You may feel restless, like you want to get out and do things or get up and clean the house (. . . don't).

It might hurt to pee or poop.

It might not hurt to pee or poop, but just the idea of it can feel scary!

You might be overwhelmed with feelings of love toward your baby right away! Or it may take time for the love to grow. It will.

You might grieve the life you've left behind.

During the postpartum window, all kinds of feelings, emotions, thoughts, experiences, pains, joys, and realizations may arise. You may not have thought that your body would need *time* after birth to heal. Do not hesitate to reach out to your care providers, friends, or family members if you are not sure if what you are experiencing is normal. Hearing reassurance from others who have been there before can be a huge relief!

When preparing for your postpartum window, educate yourself on what to expect and how to navigate it. This can turn a potentially challenging time into one of the most blissful times of your life.

My sacred window was the best few weeks of my life: it was a time of resting in bed with my sweet, soft, cuddly baby and spending every moment soaking in everything about her; having a support person who was prepared and ready to serve my needs and be at my side for help, cooking all my Ayurvedic meals, teas, and snacks; resting mostly at home for six weeks alone with my family in order to adjust to our new baby; receiving abhyanga massages from an Ayurvedic massage therapist and dear friend; having a meal train set up so that friends and local wise women could deliver daily meals for my family and me; and generally honoring the sacred window by simply giving myself the time and space that I needed to heal. This type of experience takes preparation and planning, gathering of resources, patience, and dedication to achieve.

Before the baby is born, your natural nesting instincts will have you planning and preparing, organizing and gathering. Use this energy to plan your postpartum window. Clear your schedule for six weeks after the birth as much as you can. Make arrangements for work leave, older children's schedules, pets, house cleaning, meal preparation, and any other responsibilities you may have. The more you think of now, the less you will have to worry about when all you want to do is stare at that sweet baby in your arms!

Gather some recipes you will want cooked during your postpartum window (see chapter 8 for some staples) and buy the dry groceries in advance. Make a grocery list for anything you cannot buy in advance and leave it accessible for your support person so that they can go to the store for you when needed. If your support person is unavailable, look into ordering from online grocery delivery services. Print out the recipes so someone can cook them for you. Deep-clean your house just before your due date (including doing *all* the laundry) so that you can enjoy a clean, peaceful, sattvic environment with your newborn baby. Consult an Ayurvedic postpartum doula—someone who is educated and trained to help you prepare and navigate your postpartum window following Ayurvedic guidelines. You will already have a lot on your plate with preparing for birth and your baby. Adding the element of Ayurveda to your planning may seem overwhelming, especially if it is unfamiliar. Talk with an Ayurvedic postpartum doula to explore what your personal needs are for your postpartum window and how they can best support you.

Ayurvedic postpartum care is needed for every mother, though it can sometimes be quite costly. A traditionally inspired blessing way or a baby shower—or maybe both!—can be a great way for your tribe to support your postpartum healing. A blessing way is a celebration of the journey into motherhood, but instead of showering the baby with gifts, friends and family shower the mother with love, support, and blessings in her transition into becoming a mama. A baby shower or a blessing way can include opportunities to prepare for the postpartum window:

- Start a "postpartum care" fund where friends and family can make a donation for your postpartum care instead of buying a gift. This can help pay for doula care, massages, or hiring extra help like cleaners and childcare for your older children.
- Start a meal train so friends and family can sign up to bring a postpartum meal.
- Put postpartum care items on your baby registry, such as a pressure cooker; a thermos; hot water bottles; a postpartum belly wrap; organic sesame oil; herbs like dashamula, fenugreek, and fennel; organic dates; basmati rice; and ghee.

- Create a sign-up sheet for friends and family to take on different support tasks postpartum, such as grocery shopping, giving older children rides to and from school, catching up with dishes, doing laundry, or tidying the house.

Postpartum-Prep Activity for Your Blessing Way

1. Gather various organic dried herbs and oils from the directions below and have them arranged in separate jars on a table. Provide your guests with string, scissors, labels, markers, empty paper tea bags, and jars.
2. Explain to your guests that the herbs have healing benefits for a postpartum mother, and that you will use what they make during your postpartum window to support you in your healing.
3. Allow each guest to make as many items as they wish (or as you have supplies for).

Infused Oils

Your guests can choose any of the dried herbs listed below, place them in a jar, and pour sesame or sunflower oil over them. Ask them to label the jar, and then you can save it for when you need it! You can place the filled jars on a windowsill where warmth from the sun will pull the medicinal qualities of the herbs into the oil. After six or eight weeks, strain out the herbs and keep the infused oil to use as needed for support postpartum.

Three potential combinations:

- hemorrhoid relief oil: sesame oil with St. John's wort, yarrow, rose
- nipple soothing oil: sesame oil or ghee with comfrey, calendula, plantain, chamomile
- abhyanga oil: sesame oil, rose, jasmine, lavender, calendula, chamomile

Herbal Tea Blends

Provide empty paper tea bags for your guests. They can choose any combination of the following herbs and place them in a bag. Label these along with what they are used for and save them for when you need them most!

Herbs for nervous system support:

- chamomile
- lavender
- licorice

Herbs for digestive support:

- coriander seeds
- cumin seeds
- dried ginger
- fennel seeds

Herbs for lactation support:

- chamomile
- fennel seeds
- fenugreek
- licorice
- red raspberry leaf

Epsom Salt Soaks

Guests can mix Epsom salts and herbs in a jar and add a couple drops of essential oils for added benefits and scent. Label the jars, and when you are ready to use them, pour them into the bath (or place them into a large tea bag or sock to keep the herbs from getting stuck in the drain). Epsom salt soaks can be made with any of the following herbs:

- calendula
- chamomile
- comfrey
- lavender
- rose
- rosemary
- sage
- yarrow

Herbal Baths

Guests can choose a combination of herbs and place them in a jar for you to use in making herbal baths. Share the following benefits of each herb with your guests so they can craft a bath for you with deep intention and healing energy. They can write a little note on the jar sharing the benefits of the herbs or expressing their blessings and wishes for your postpartum healing. Following "Guidelines for an Herbal Bath" on page 92, a lovely bath can be created from any combination of the following herbs:

- ashoka: Ashoka is perhaps Ayurveda's most supportive herb for the female reproductive system. It is also said to remove sorrow and grief that is hidden in the womb.
- calendula: Calendula is a powerful healer of scars and wounds, making it very supportive for mamas who experience perineal tears during birth, have had stitches, or underwent a C-section. It also can help prevent infections.
- chamomile: Chamomile is gentle and calming. It relaxes the entire nervous system and can reduce muscle tension and cramping. It is gentle enough for newborns as well, making it a great option for mama to bathe with her babe.

- dashamula (cut): Many of the herbs in this list can be too cooling or drying when used on their own, or in excess, during the postpartum window. Dashamula is deeply grounding and warming, making it an important addition to any postpartum herbal bath formula.
- hibiscus: Hibiscus is a sacred flower often used in devotional ceremonies. It also helps to balance the first and second chakras (root and sacral chakras).
- lavender: Lavender is deeply restorative to both the mind and body. It can ease anxiety and depression and be a wonderful sleep aid. It is also gentle enough to bathe with baby.
- linden: While linden is also soothing to the nervous system, it holds a particularly divine feminine energy, bringing calm and beauty into the heart. It is said that linden removes obstacles in the heart that get in the way of unconditional love.
- oatstraw: Oatstraw rejuvenates the nervous system and rebuilds and restores reservoirs of energy within the body. It is the perfect herbal ally for when exhaustion sets in. It can also restore peace of mind after a traumatic or shocking event, and therefore it is beneficial for mamas who experience birth trauma.
- rose petals: Rose is the queen of all flowers and a deep ally for feminine healing. Rose soothes the emotional heart by comforting and then releasing grief and sorrow.
- witch hazel bark: Witch hazel bark is soothing and healing for inflamed, damaged tissues. It can also be supportive in slowing down lochia (postpartum bleeding) and soothing hemorrhoids.

THE DOSHAS DURING THE POSTPARTUM WINDOW

POSTPARTUM AGNI AND AMA: According to Ayurveda, the strength of an individual's agni—the digestive fire—will determine not only their ability to digest food but also their ability to digest and process life experiences. When rapid transformation happens (as during the birthing process), the fire of digestion is completely put out. It is absolutely essential that this fire is rekindled, tended to, and nurtured in order for you as a postpartum mama to assimilate into your new experience of motherhood. Otherwise you risk becoming overwhelmed, withdrawn, depressed, distant, or anxious, and you may experience many of the other common feelings women have when they cannot process the experience of birth and early motherhood. During the early days postpartum, your body will be healing and your baby's body will be constantly growing and changing. Every day feels different and adjustments need to be made. With strong agni, you will be able to adapt to your new role as a mama and tend to your growing baby with ease, confidence, and grace. You will also be able to digest your food properly so that babe is able to easily digest your breast milk. Chapter 8 offers a list of specific ways to assess the strength of agni, starting at page 270.

Ama is what is left in your body or mind when agni cannot properly digest the food or experience. The material gets stuck in your body, where it can clog channels and create imbalances. During pregnancy, your body builds many tissues. After the delivery of your baby, your body still holds on to much of what it has built up. Tending to balance involves releasing what has built up while simultaneously restoring the depleted tissues.

The only way for ama to be released from the body is for it to be digested by agni. The postpartum weeks are a time of rekindling and tending to the fire of digestion in order to release what is built up from pregnancy while also nourishing and restoring the body. This process is easily supported by following the Ayurvedic dietary and lifestyle recommendations mentioned earlier in this chapter (see "Four Pillars of Postpartum Care" on page 177).

POSTPARTUM VATA: Vata dosha is the combination of air and space elements within the body. The moment your baby is born, your previously full womb quickly becomes empty. That large empty space in the center of your body fills with the air element. Vata qualities of dry, light, cold, rough, subtle, mobile/quick, and clear are balanced by their opposites of oily, heavy/solid, hot/warm, smooth, gross (as in solid material), stable, slow, and cloudy/viscous. Every postpartum mother will have excess vata. Because of this, the entire Ayurvedic postpartum regimen is intended to reduce vata and bring these elements back into balance by bringing stability, nourishment, hydration, warmth, and oiliness to the body of the mother. Vata appears in a newly postpartum mother in the following ways:

feeling cold, especially right after birth

shaking after birth

feeling depleted

having a limited milk supply

experiencing indecisiveness
having the urge to do a lot of activity
feeling anxious or unsure
having a sense of fragility, being easily upset
suffering from constipation, gas, or difficulty digesting
worrying or experiencing disturbing thoughts
experiencing insomnia and sleep disturbances
retaining lochia
being dehydrated
lacking appetite
having afterpains/cramping

To reduce excess vata, follow the vata-balancing guidelines of oiliness, warmth, rest, and quiet found on page 21, and in particular focus on these vata-balancing approaches:

Rekindle the digestive fire with ginger, lime, and salt before meals.
Drink cumin, coriander, and fennel tea.
Drink fenugreek tea for lactation support.
Hydrate with warm, mineral-rich teas and broths.
Follow guidelines for an Ayurvedic postpartum diet.
Eat regularly.
Use oil basti (oil enema) to balance the pelvic area (the seat of vata).
Receive daily abhyanga massages.
Use a heating pad or hot water bottle on your belly and lower back.
Use a belly wrap.
Drink dashamula tea daily for four to six weeks (see the recipe on page 287). It calms the pelvic area and rejuvenates vata's downward energies.

POSTPARTUM PITTA AND KAPHA: Excess pitta during the postpartum window can display itself as excessive blood loss, hot flashes, skin rashes, diarrhea in mother or baby, irritability, or anger. To soothe pitta, avoid too much spice or excess heat. Use pitta-soothing guidelines from page 25 while also respecting the vata-balancing regimen, remembering that sometimes vata pushes pitta, causing it to flare up. You can also use pitta-soothing teas.

Excess kapha postpartum is evident when baby has mucus symptoms or there is a lack of uterine involution (called "boggy uterus"). Mama may also be experiencing heaviness in her mind, emotions, and body. To reduce kapha, reduce dairy and heavy foods while respecting the vata-soothing regimen, stimulate uterine contractions with uterine massage, and drink kapha-soothing teas.

With any postpartum imbalance, consider consulting an Ayurvedic postpartum doula to support your unique experience.

COMMON POSTPARTUM IMBALANCES

Various imbalances can arise during a newborn mama's sacred window. If you experience any of the symptoms or imbalances described below, always come back to the sacred window essentials: Are you resting every day? Is your environment peaceful? Are you following Ayurvedic diet guidelines? Have you been receiving (or doing) your abhyanga massages? Have you been taking your herbal teas and panchakola ghee? Do you feel supported? Oftentimes, the imbalances can be solved by tending to those simple aspects. After coming back and checking in with the main pillars of postpartum care, then you can look for further remedies for the following imbalances if you still need them.

CONSTIPATION: Constipation can be intimidating for new mamas. After everything you just went through, you may experience some PTSD the first time you sit back down on the toilet—I know I did! Eliminating body waste can also be painful due to the vulnerability of the tissues in their current state—especially if you had stitches!

Prepare for TMI here—the first time I sat on the toilet after giving birth and having a third-degree perineal tear with stitches, I could not have been more grateful that my poop came out soft, supple, and pain free! I knew that this was thanks to the watery, soupy, oily rice pudding I ate as my first postpartum meal and for the following three days. Diet is crucial here. If you follow the Ayurvedic postpartum diet from immediately after giving birth, you're not likely to become constipated. If you do have trouble, however, follow these tips:

On an empty stomach, eat stewed fruits with a big spoonful of ghee on top (see page 287).

Add a couple teaspoons of ghee to everything you eat.

Drink warm, hydrating drinks throughout the day to get bowels moving.

Completely avoid iced or cold drinks and food, as well as raw food.

Drink hot milk tonic (page 290) with a tablespoon of ghee before bed.

Give yourself a warm abhyanga massage, focusing on clockwise abdominal movements, followed by soaking in a warm bath.

HAIR LOSS: Postpartum hair loss soon after the birth is a sign of vata going out of balance, but it can occur even several months after giving birth. If you are noticing hair loss, go back to the sacred window basics on page 177 and continue to nourish yourself with a vata-pacifying regimen. Extreme hair loss beyond four months postpartum may be a sign of a thyroid imbalance (see "Postpartum Thyroid Issues" at page 208). To maintain healthy hair postpartum, consider the following Ayurvedic treatments:

Do a daily warm oil scalp massage with a 3:1 mix of brahmi oil to castor oil; leave it on overnight.

Make teas out of herbs that naturally boost collagen such as *he shou wu*, calendula, nettle, mangosteen fruit, and gynostemma.

Eat fruits that are naturally collagen boosting, such as berries rich in vitamin C.

Include more ghee in your diet to help balance your hormones.

Practice a vata-pacifying diet and daily routine.

HEMORRHOIDS: Hemorrhoids commonly result from the pushing phase of labor. They may also appear after having mild constipation—if this is the case, follow the tips to alleviate constipation. To treat the hemorrhoids topically, apply a small amount of neem ghee externally on the affected area three to five times a day.

POSTPARTUM ANXIETY AND DEPRESSION: According to Aviva Romm, one in four women in the United States are diagnosed with depression or anxiety, and postpartum anxiety and depression are especially common in North America. Many factors can lead a new mother to experience mood disorders during her sacred window, including lack of support from her family, lack of emotional and psychological support, being looked down upon for parenting choices, having a history of eating disorders or anxiety and depression, hormonal imbalances, financial stress, past experience or hearing stories of pregnancy loss or sudden infant death syndrome, or history of family trauma.

All too often, mothers are told that it is "normal" to suffer during their sacred window. This mentality needs to be changed. *New mothers do not have to suffer.* Postpartum mood disorders can be managed or even prevented with the proper rest, nutrition, herbs, and most importantly, a good support system. Assure you know the following signs and symptoms of postpartum anxiety and depression so you can seek help and support from professionals if necessary:

extreme and persistent ups and downs

no happy or joyful moments

not sleeping because of too much worry

extreme worry of hurting the baby by accident or on purpose

constant anxiety or worry in general

refusal to eat

remaining in bed full-time because of lack of motivation (rather than intentional rest)

persistent need to sleep around the clock

If you do not feel right, if you are struggling, or if you feel that you are not enjoying being a new mama at all, please reach out for help and support. *Just because postpartum anxiety and depression are common does not mean that it is normal, and it does not mean you have to suffer through it.* You can get support, and you can thrive as a new mother.

Evidence shows that mothers who follow the Ayurvedic postpartum practices are less likely to suffer with severe mood disorders. Along with following the sacred window basics beginning at page 177 and the Ayurvedic postpartum diet guidelines in chapter 8, you can try these other Ayurvedic approaches to nourishing yourself to prevent or remedy mild postpartum anxiety:

Drink dashamula tea first thing in the morning and right before bed (see page 287).

Receive daily massages using sesame oil infused with rose, ashwagandha, bala, or brahmi; oil can be left on all day or overnight.

Apply 3–10 drops of warm plain sesame oil in each ear.

Take warm baths and showers.

Avoid cold air drafts or exposure to cold.

Avoid exposure to unpleasant people or violent movies.

Avoid traveling, driving, or running errands.

Use several bastis (oil enemas) as needed.

Drink a cup of room temperature orange juice mixed with 1 teaspoon honey and a pinch of nutmeg.

For postpartum depression, try these methods for support:

Have lots of skin-to-skin contact with baby.

Enjoy quality time with loved ones.

Boost serotonin and dopamine naturally with herbal allies like blue lotus and mucuna (see page 305).

Make sure to follow a well-balanced diet of whole foods that are freshly prepared and nourishing, and be sure that you are eating enough!

Either continue to take prenatal vitamins or take postnatal vitamins, as nutrient deficiencies can result in depression. I recommend (pre- and) postnatal vitamins that are made from whole foods and herbs rather than those containing vitamins and minerals from synthetic sources. Additionally, there are postnatal vitamins that are fermented with probiotics that make them gentler on your digestion and less likely to cause nausea.

Have a daily warm oil massage with herbal oils.

Try seven days in a row of warm herbal oil bastis.

If you are following all the Ayurvedic postpartum recommendations and still experiencing depression or anxiety, you may have a complicated situation where all three doshas are out of balance. Deep depression can be serious; please find a skilled Ayurvedic practitioner, Ayurvedic postpartum doula, or other skilled professional who can guide you through your healing process.

MOOD SWINGS AND IRRITABILITY: Distinct from anxiety and depression, you may experience temporary mood swings or moments of feeling extra sensitive and irritable. A new mama's heart is so tender. In these moments, check in with yourself. You may be pushing yourself too hard, or you (or baby) may be overstimulated. You may have needs that are not being met; perhaps you feel you need more support. Ask for what you need. Rest. Eat nourishing foods. Do abhyanga massage. Take a warm herbal bath.

If you're noticing that these remedies seem to be recommended for every postpartum issue, you're right—they are the pillars of postpartum care that keep you in balance. If you need additional support, here are some specifics from the Ayurvedic toolbox:

Add shatavari-infused ghee (or simply shatavari powder) to your hot milk to stabilize hormones and mood.

Wear your belly wrap.

More rose everything! Rose petal tea, rose mist spray, ayurvedic rose jam (see page 217).

Use herbal allies such as rose, jasmine, hibiscus, mucuna, vanilla, maca, shatavari, and damiana. You can make teas out of these herbs either in combination with each other or individually. You can also use them in powder form and add them to foods, warm smoothies, or hot milk. (See page 306 for a recipe for mama's mood tea.)

SLEEP ISSUES: As with many of the other common postpartum imbalances, sleep issues are a vata imbalance. Pacifying vata by returning to the sacred window basics will address the root cause of the sleep issues. Anxiety may also be causing lack of sleep—if it seems that is the case, see the tips for postpartum anxiety and depression on pages 204–206. If you need additional support with sleep, the following tips will be useful:

Apply warm sesame oil to the bottom of your feet and the top of your head before bed, cover with socks and a hat.

Use a hot water bottle or heating pad on your belly at night while falling asleep.

Drink warm liquids instead of cold throughout the night.

Wake and go to sleep at the same time every day.

Go to sleep before 10 p.m.

Use ashwagandha-, bala-, or brahmi-infused oil during your abhyanga massages followed by a warm bath daily.

Use transdermal magnesium.

Eliminate stimulants like caffeine.

Drink a hot spiced milk tonic before bed (see page 290).

Add saffron, nutmeg, or poppy seed into your diet.

Nap while baby naps to help deal with sleepless nights.

Practice yoga nidra (yogic sleep meditation) and *ujjai pranayama*, which is a breath technique used for gently warming the body, calming the mind, and soothing the nervous system. In this breathing technique, you constrict the back of the throat to support lengthening each breath cycle. Each inhalation and exhalation is long, full, deep, and controlled.

Drink dashamula tea first thing in the morning and before going to bed (see page 287).

Make a tea with ½ teaspoon of ashwagandha and a pinch of cardamom and brahmi.

Drink brahmi tea, chamomile tea, or lavender tea before bed.

Make a tea or milk tonic (see pages 306–307) with ashwagandha, ginger, rose, passionflower, blue lotus, and valerian. These are easiest to use in powder form; mix ½ teaspoon of the powdered blend into your milk or tea. (See page 306 for moon milk tea recipe.)

Use valerian or lemon balm tea or tincture.

POSTPARTUM THYROID ISSUES: Feminine problems including infertility, miscarriage, fibrocystic breast disease, ovarian fibroids, cystic ovaries, endometriosis, PMS, and menopausal symptoms are usually caused or aggravated by hypothyroidism. The thyroid is a gland that regulates metabolism, heart rate, cognitive function, moods, hormones, breast milk production, digestion, immune system function, and healing. Postpartum thyroid issues are common but often overlooked by health professionals because they are mistaken for other common postpartum challenges.

You may have increased risk of thyroid imbalances postpartum if you have elevated thyroid antibodies or if thyroid problems occurred during pregnancy. Thyroid issues can also show up postpartum due to hormone and immune changes. There are two types of thyroid imbalances: hypothyroidism (underactive thyroid) and hyperthyroidism (overactive thyroid). Symptoms of under- or overactive thyroid, or a combination of both, can show up anywhere from the first few weeks to eighteen months postpartum or even beyond.

SYMPTOMS OF POSTPARTUM HYPOTHYROIDISM

Slow cognitive function, severe brain fog, extreme “new mama mind” or “milk mind,” forgetful and unfocused thinking

Constipation

Depression

Weight gain or no weight loss after giving birth

Muscle loss

Fatigue

Severe hair loss past four months postpartum

Difficulty with breast milk production (even after using herbs, lactation aids, and troubleshooting)

Skin problems (redness, acne, dryness, etc.)

Hypothyroidism comes with symptoms that may make you feel slow and lethargic, so to treat it with stimulating herbs could help temporarily to get you out of your "funk" and get through the day (such as by drinking coffee, chai, matcha, or green tea). But in the long run, caffeine will burn out your adrenal glands, and if the underlying issue is hypothyroidism, stimulants won't solve that problem. Hypothyroidism is better treated with a proper diet, and the condition can be supported with vitamins and herbs such as transdermal magnesium, transdermal vitamin D, and transdermal ashwagandha. Be sure to get thyroid levels checked before using stimulating herbs.

SYMPTOMS OF POSTPARTUM HYPERTHYROIDISM

Metabolism and energy on overdrive

Wired feeling/inability to sleep

Weight loss and then some, within weeks

High elevated moods/extreme feeling of "doing great" to the point of burnout

Frequent or extreme postpartum anxiety

Constant need for the bathroom, to poop a lot

Depression (Although it seems counterintuitive, depression can arise in combination with any of the above symptoms. This type of depression may display itself as feeling unsatisfied, no longer being motivated to do things you love, not enjoying motherhood, and so on.)

Herbal remedies for hyperthyroidism, to support the nervous system and help to calm your body and mind, include the following:

ashwagandha	lavender	transdermal magnesium
chamomile	lemon balm	vitamin B complex

If you suspect you have a thyroid imbalance, visit your ob-gyn, midwife, or family doctor and ask to get your thyroid levels tested. Ideally you'll test once, wait two weeks, and then test again. The levels can fluctuate, and you want to be sure there is an imbalance before treating it.

If you are suffering with any of these symptoms and they are getting in the way of quality of life, caring for your baby, or feeding your baby, do not accept the response "It's because you're a new mom—it's normal." If that is a reply that you get from a medical professional and your intuition tells you otherwise, I would recommend getting a second opinion.

For more information on naturally treating postpartum thyroid issues, read *Natural Health after Birth* by Aviva Romm and *Healing the Thyroid with Ayurveda: Natural Treatments for Hashimoto's, Hypothyroidism, and Hyperthyroidism* by Marianne Teitelbaum. I also highly recommend Dr. Teitelbaum as a practitioner who can guide you on healing your thyroid using natural remedies. See "References and Suggested Reading" at the end of this book.

BALANCING PRACTICES POSTPARTUM

The following are practices that will support your postpartum healing.

POSTPARTUM PRANAYAMA: One of the most simple and effective methods of generating sattva during the postpartum window is by practicing pranayama, or conscious breathing techniques. At any time throughout the day, sit quietly and notice the flow of your breath going in and out of your body. Simply by bringing awareness to the breath, peace and calm is brought to the mind, body, and emotions. For a more formal practice of pranayama, practice either nadi shodhana or ujjayi breath any time you feel the need for calm, balanced, clear energy. It is not necessary to sit up straight on a meditation pillow to practice these techniques. They can be done while lying horizontal, or even while nursing, snuggling, or walking your baby. Pranayama is effective not only throughout the sacred window but through a mother's entire life.

Nadi shodhana, or alternate-nostril breathing (described in detail at page 22), is a stabilizing breathing technique that can be practiced as often as needed, with as many repetitions as desired. After a few days of practicing using your hand to close the nostrils, you can continue this practice without the hands, using your consciousness to direct the prana alternately in and out of the nostrils in the same pattern. Prana (life force) flows where consciousness directs it. This pranayama is the ultimate balancer, balancing all the hormones in your body.

Ujjayi breath—the "ocean-sounding breath" practiced during many yoga asana classes—is a calming breathing practice that enhances prana in the body. This pranayama technique simply involves taking a deep inhale through the nose then exhaling out the nose with a slight constriction at the back of your throat. Your inhales and exhales will sound like soft ocean waves.

MAMA MARMA THERAPY: *Marma* therapy (*marma chikitsa*) is Ayurveda's pressure-point healing system, an ancient bodywork technique that accesses marma points—the anatomical locations where muscles, joints, ligaments, bones, nerves, and veins meet—through touch. Marma points are also the intersecting points of the more subtle channels in the body that carry mental and emotional impressions. They are access points into the flow of consciousness, where mind-body connections take place. These points, which are located on the skin, are used for communicating with deep tissues and organs. The thumb (relating to the element of ether and thus limitless consciousness) is used to apply pressure to specific points to treat different diseases ("dis-eases") or imbalances in the body.

Marma is especially useful postpartum when abhyanga massage is contraindicated. Special circumstances where you would receive marma instead of abhyanga would be strong emotional shifts, respiratory congestive issues, and cesarean sections. In these cases, marma would be more rejuvenating, restoring, and healing for mama than abhyanga oil massages.

You may have heard postpartum women talk about frequent crying. Crying a lot (from emotions such as grief, frustration, or anger) is an indication of excess vata or pitta carrying the emotions to the surface. If this is the case, marma therapy will encourage deep rest and restoration.

Marma can be given by an Ayurvedic practitioner or an Ayurvedic postpartum doula, or it can be self-administered.

POSTPARTUM HERBAL SUPPORTS

The following is a deeper look at some of your postpartum herbal supports, as well as a few important additions to your list.

PANCHAKOLA GHEE: *Panchakola*, meaning "five spiced," is a traditional herbal formula made by infusing ghee with black pepper, ginger, pippali, pippali root, and chitrak. A heaping spoonful of this medicated ghee should be taken immediately after giving birth as the first food that you eat. The combination of the spices stokes your digestive fire, and the ghee allows the medicine to penetrate into the deep tissues of your body.

This ghee should be served on top of every meal for at least the first ten days of your sacred window, starting with 2–3 tablespoons per meal and slowly reducing the amount over time as your digestion increases. Panchakola ghee can be prepared by your Ayurvedic postpartum doula; otherwise, check the resources list in the back of the book for places to order online.

DASHAMULA TEA: Dashamula, a tea made of ten roots, is used in Ayurvedic postpartum care to alleviate vata dosha in the nervous system. During your sacred window, dashamula helps your body to digest ama, increase strength, relieve pain, reduce tension and anxiety, promote calm, and generally restore health and well-being. Dashamula also aids in strengthening the uterus after childbirth. Take it as a strong tea, twice a day, every day for forty-two days. You can find the recipe on page 287 and information on where to order dashamula in the resources list at the end of the book.

SWEET WATER LACTATION TEA: Sweet water lactation tea is a staple beverage used in traditional Ayurvedic postpartum care practices. This simple formula can be started immediately after birth and drunk every day for the entire sacred window. It can also be supportive beyond the sacred window in times you may feel your milk supply dropping. The tea is simply ⅔ teaspoon fennel seeds and ⅓ teaspoon fenugreek seeds in 8 cups of water—according to Ayurveda, fennel and fenugreek are some of the best herbs for supporting lactation. Bring the water to a boil and let the seeds simmer for five or ten minutes. The seeds can then be strained out and the tea can be poured into a couple of thermoses. Keep these thermoses near your bedside table and nursing station, and drink them throughout the day.

HERBAL CHEWING MIX: Many digestive spices are likely to already be in your kitchen cabinet: chapter 8 gives directions for an herbal chewing mix created from fennel seeds, sesame seeds, unsweetened coconut flakes, turmeric, cardamom, clove, ginger, and mineral or black salt (see page 289). These are all known to support good digestion, and thus overall well-being for mama and babe. Beginning two or three days after the birth and continuing for forty-two days (or as desired), take a teaspoon of this mix after savory meals twice daily.

GARLIC: Garlic, well roasted in ghee, supports agni, and thus appetite, digestion, lactation, grounding, and immunity. It also greatly minimizes the risk of infection and generally speeds up the post-birth recovery process. See the "Garlic Chutney" recipe on page 289.

SHATAVARI: The herb shatavari (described more in chapter 9) is a beautiful post-birth breast milk enhancer that also rejuvenates the body in a deep way, strengthens and nourishes the tissues, and balances the hormones and moods/emotions. Shatavari is traditionally used to maintain the healthy production of female hormones. It supports a healthy immune system and assists in both physical and mental digestion. It is sattvic (pure, harmonious) in nature, calms the mind, and promotes love and devotion.

You can add shatavari to milk tonics (see page 290), warm smoothies, or any cookie or *laddu* recipe—half a teaspoon is a sufficient serving. Begin using shatavari eight or nine days after the birth, when digestion is stronger, and enjoy for the rest of the postpartum time or longer.

SPECIAL CIRCUMSTANCES

CESAREAN BIRTH: Everyone and every body is different, so the time frame for a mama's sacred window is simply a recommended amount of time. But as a general rule, in the case of a cesarean birth the mother will need extra care and longer time to heal than with a vaginal birth—after a C-section, the postpartum window traditionally extends to eight weeks.

Ayurvedically speaking, when thinking about the healing needed for the mother, we look at the qualities of the birth. A cesarean birth has increased exposure to an environment that aggravates vata. The operating room is cold and bright; the surgical instruments are cold, sharp, and penetrating;

air can become trapped in the abdomen; and the hospital setting can be unfamiliar, and therefore unsettling.

Being mindful of the fragile state you may be in after this type of birth, the following are considerations about "extras" to keep in mind for your care:

Extra fragility. After undergoing a major abdominal surgery, you will be in an especially vulnerable state. Following a cesarean birth, you can receive marma therapy for the first two weeks, and then abhyanga massages can begin, avoiding the incision site until it is fully healed.

Extra mobility support. Especially within the first few days, you may need support walking, sitting up, holding your baby, getting out of bed, sitting on the toilet, getting into and out of the shower, and any other necessary movement.

Extra nutritional considerations. Rebuilding agni is essential after a cesarean, as it is for all postpartum mothers, but following a C-section, the amount of fat and oil (ghee) in agni-building recipes should be reduced. Excessive oleation can inhibit the reconnection of the tissues at the incision sites.

Extra care for mentally digesting the experience. Come to peaceful terms with your birth story. This is especially necessary for mothers who have undergone an emergency C-section rather than a planned one, but it is relevant for all postpartum mothers. Share your thoughts and feelings with your support person.

Extra attention to swelling. IV fluids can sometimes cause extra swelling in the body, and this is especially common for mothers after a C-section. Gentle massage of the lower legs and feet can help relieve swelling. Drinking coriander tea will also aid in eliminating excess fluid. Adding ¼– ½ teaspoon *gokshura* herb to your milk, dashamula tea, or soups can reduce fluid retention.

Extra attention to warmth on the abdomen. As the abdomen specifically was exposed to the vata-aggravating qualities mentioned before, it will need extra attention. Applying warmth through the medium of warm water bottles or bags on the abdomen will bring vata into balance. After a couple of weeks, a cloth soaked in castor oil placed on the skin will reduce discomfort and heal the tissues.

Ayurvedic recommendations for enhancing mama's physical well-being after a cesarean birth include these other tips:

Use a warm water bottle over your incision site.

Put 1–3 drops of lavender and helichrysum essential oils on the bandage or incision site (after removing the bandage) one or two times daily to prevent infections and speed healing.

Use a hot water bottle to relieve the shoulder and mid-back pain that may occur five to ten days after delivery.

Wait ten to fourteen days before starting abhyanga massage.

Receive marma therapy treatments until massages begin.

Use less oil, fat, or ghee in all your recipes until the incision site has knitted back together.

Use a belly wrap.

Use silicone strips for scar healing.

Watch for candida/thrush—reduce sugar to prevent this.

Take a probiotic (mama and baby).

Take homeopathic arnica tablets to help with soreness and pains.

Avoid full baths for six weeks; shower instead.

Use the herbal bath recipe on page 92 to wash over your incision and pat dry after showers.

Eat stewed prunes, with a pinch of cinnamon and cardamom, to support elimination.

Eat almond-date laddus for connective tissue rebuilding (see recipe below).

Almond-Date Laddus

This recipe for nourishing fruit and nut balls (*laddus*) comes from Ysha Oakes and appears in her postpartum cookbook *Touching Heaven.* These almond-date laddus build ojas and support the regeneration and strengthening of connective tissue. Once agni is strong—usually after about eight days postpartum—eat one of these laddus in the morning and one in the afternoon.

Ingredients

1½ cups blanched almonds

1½ cups unsweetened fine shredded coconut flakes

⅓ cup gum acacia resin (not powdered)

3 tablespoons ghee

2 tablespoons succanat or rapadura sugar

⅛ cup milk or almond milk

1 teaspoon saffron threads

½ cup Medjool dates

1 tablespoon ginger powder

1 tablespoon shatavari powder

1 tablespoon cardamom powder

1 tablespoon cinnamon powder

Instructions

1. Blanch the almonds by soaking them overnight, then pour boiling hot water over them and let them sit for a few minutes. Strain the water out, and peel the skins off. They should slide right out of the skins. Discard the skins, then place the almonds in a food processor and grind into a coarse almond meal.
2. Roast the shredded coconut in a heavy-bottomed large pan until slightly golden. Set aside in a large mixing bowl. In the same pan, gently roast almonds until lightly golden. Stir frequently.
3. In the same heavy-bottomed pan on low heat, gently roast the gum acacia in 1 teaspoon ghee until the gum acacia uniformly puffs up. Set aside and let cool. Once the gum acacia is cool, grind it in a food processor with the sugar until the mixture is a fine powder. Sift the powder through a mesh sieve to separate any remaining hard pieces, or use your fingers to feel and separate the hard pieces. Combine gum acacia powder with almond meal and coconut flakes. Mix until uniform.
4. Bring milk or almond milk to a simmer, turn off heat and add saffron threads to steep, then add pitted dates to soften in the warm liquid.
5. Warm the remaining ghee in pan, then ginger and shatavari. Stir and cook until you can smell the essential oil of the ginger releasing, then add the remaining spices—cardamom burns easily, so watch closely! Once the cardamom and cinnamon begin to release their aromatics, add the milk, saffron, and date mixture, warming the dates until soft.
6. Transfer the paste to the food processor and blend until smooth.
7. In a mixing bowl, combine the date paste into the dry mixture; blend with your hands until the mixture is well combined. Form into one-inch balls and store in the fridge. Eat two laddus per day at room temperature.

MISCARRIAGE, STILLBIRTH, ADOPTION, OR SURROGACY: By definition, "postpartum" means the time following birth. Many doulas and practitioners also believe that the time following pregnancy should be honored *especially* when a child has been lost in the pregnancy (because of miscarriage or stillbirth, for example) or placed in a different family after the birth because of adoption or surrogacy arrangements. The woman's body during pregnancy begins undergoing changes immediately upon conception, and she will need physical and emotional healing and restoring after loss no matter the circumstance.

Looking at it through an Ayurvedic lens, vata will be increased due to the empty feeling that comes with the loss or absence of a baby you were carrying. Some believe that these circumstances are even more reason to honor the postpartum window, as there is an emotional heaviness that comes with any experience of loss. You will need time to grieve your child, even if it was your choice to give up the child for adoption or abort the fetus for any reason.

If you are grieving the loss or absence of a child, you need time to process your deep sadness, and you may need ways to cope with any accompanying insomnia, anxiety, anger, apathy, disassociation, or depression. Agni and appetite may be very low. Incorporate as many of the postpartum basics from this chapter as possible, as well as the remedies listed throughout. Some additional, grief-specific Ayurvedic remedies include these:

Take ashoka baths to remove sorrow and strengthen the uterus (see page 199).

Have a ceremony to honor the life of the soul you carried.

Take Ayurvedic rose petal jam (see recipe below) to support the heart.

Honoring the time following the end of your pregnancy will bring you closure, give you the space to restore your health, and provide the opportunity to nourish your body, mind, and heart.

Sun-Cooked Ayurvedic Rose Petal Jam

According to Ayurveda, rose rules *sadhaka* pitta, the aspect of pitta that governs the emotions. Rose is uplifting and healing to the emotional heart. Rose petal jam is an ancient Ayurvedic healing recipe good for any time your heart is in need of extra love. This recipe from Sarva Blackwell of Inner Sun & Moon can be used in the fourth month of pregnancy, when the heart is developing in the fetus; during early postpartum, when mama's emotions are vulnerable; or after a loss.

Ingredients

organic dried rose petals

organic turbinado sugar

Instructions

Sterilize a glass jar by heating it in the oven at 300 degrees Fahrenheit for fifteen minutes. Sterilize its lid by boiling it in water for twenty minutes and then allowing it to air dry completely. Once your jar and its lid are sterile and dry, you are ready to begin!

In the morning collect enough fresh organic roses to fill the jar (ideally collect them before sunrise, as the sun will evaporate some of the precious oil and aroma). Gently wash the roses with water and shake off any excess water. Remove the petals and pat them dry. (Optionally, spread them out on a towel for an hour or two to let a little more water evaporate.) Weigh the petals. Then, based on the weight of the rose petals, weigh out twice as much sugar by weight.

If the sun is not intense where you are, use a clean coffee grinder or food processor to grind the sugar into a powder. If the sun is intense where you are, you can leave the sugar as granules. Fill the clean dry jar with the rose petals and sugar. Stir well with lots of love, prayer, and intention. Put the lid on the jar and set the jar in a sunny windowsill for the rest of the day.

The next day, the rose petals will have wilted and will no longer be filling the jar to the top. Repeat the same process as the day before, collecting enough new fresh roses to fill the jar the rest of the way up again. Wash them as before, shake out the excess water, remove the petals, pat them dry, and weigh them. Fill the jar to the top with the new rose petals and twice the amount of sugar by weight as the weight of the petals. Stir well with love, prayer, and intention, put the lid on the jar, and set it in a sunny windowsill for the rest of the day. Continue this every day until the jar is still completely filled to the top when you check on it the next day. Then, continue to leave it in the sunny windowsill for three or four more weeks. Every day, open it up, stir it well with love, prayer, and intention, then close it back up again.

After three or four weeks you will have a beautiful rose petal compote with a jam-like consistency. Store the jam in the refrigerator and use it as a spread the way you would use any jam or eat spoonfuls of it on its own.

Notice the effect it has on your emotions, mood, and heart.

Mothers often call their children "my heart outside my body."
I thought I knew what that meant;
I thought it was just a way to express
how much they love their children.
Ayurveda says that from the fourth month of pregnancy, the mother has two hearts:
her own and her baby's.
I thought I knew what that meant;
I thought it meant the heart is formed in the fetus, so the mother has two physical hearts in her body.

So simple. So obvious. I thought.
But now I know what it truly means.
From the very beginning of motherhood I felt the *duality* of reality become intensified.
And I realized
I am feeling what it is like to have two hearts.
One heart is excited to experience the world and grow and learn together,
while the other laments the passing of time and sweet, sweet moments that are just too short.
One heart loves connecting with others, and forming bonds and relationships,
while the other heart feels the separation from the times when it was just you and me.
One heart feels proud of developing independence and new skills,
while the other heart simultaneously wishes you
would only need me, forever.
At first I was confused
constantly feeling my heart completely torn apart by the duality of every experience.
But now I understand.
It's not my heart, it's you.
I feel not only what I am feeling,
but also what you are feeling.
From the fourth month of pregnancy,
your heart was formed.
And so, all the duality I felt,
it was you.
Your desires, your wishes, your emotions
Your experiences.
As you grow I feel what you feel
and I also feel what I feel.
So now I know,
a mother has two hearts.
One lives in her,
and the other,
Is you.

Niskaraman Samskara: Welcoming Baby to the Larger World

After the sacred window, the first place mama and baby visit leaves a strong impression in the mind. The Niskaraman Samskara is the intentional first outing beyond the family home. Rather than your first trip out of your house being to the grocery store or to run errands, let it be to a thoughtfully chosen place that feels sacred to you.

In the Vedic tradition, the mama and babe remain in the birthing room (*sutika grha*) for ten to thirty days. After that time period, she and the newborn child can leave the birthing room, though they continue to remain indoors until the third lunar day of the third waxing moon after the birth.

On this day, the baby is bathed in the morning. Then, at sundown, the parents take the baby to the temple of the Lord. Standing in front of the deities with mama on the father's left side, holding the baby in a clean cloth, mama hands the baby to the father. She then walks behind the father to stand on his right side, still facing the Deity. The father then recites the following prayer:

> I pay respects to the all-pervading Lord who existed before the material creation, from whom emerged the protector of the worlds, and into whom the worlds merge at the time of destruction. O all-pervading Lord, may misfortune not come to my child.
>
> The Lord, who is the giver of consciousness, giver of strength, whose order all beings in the universe obey, whose very shadow is immortality, who is death to death personified, whom we should worship with fine offerings. Therefore O Lord, death of death personified, may misfortune not come to my child.
>
> May Nara Narayana, the Lords of protection, bestow to the child, and to me, the good fortune that mother and child not be destroyed.

After this, the father shows the child to the deities, while chanting a Vedic mantra. He continues singing as he hands the baby back to the mother, and they all return home together.

After three more waxing moons, on the third lunar day, the father returns to the temple. He goes to the deities and offer flowers three times, saying this prayer:

> The Lord, to whom no living being is superior, who has entered the worlds as the living entities, is the Lord of the living entities, but is intimately united with them. All-knowing Visnu, pervading all, may harm not come to our child.

After he returns home, singing Vedic prayers, the ceremony is considered complete. Now baby and mama have ceremoniously honored their sacred window and are ready to gradually rejoin the world.

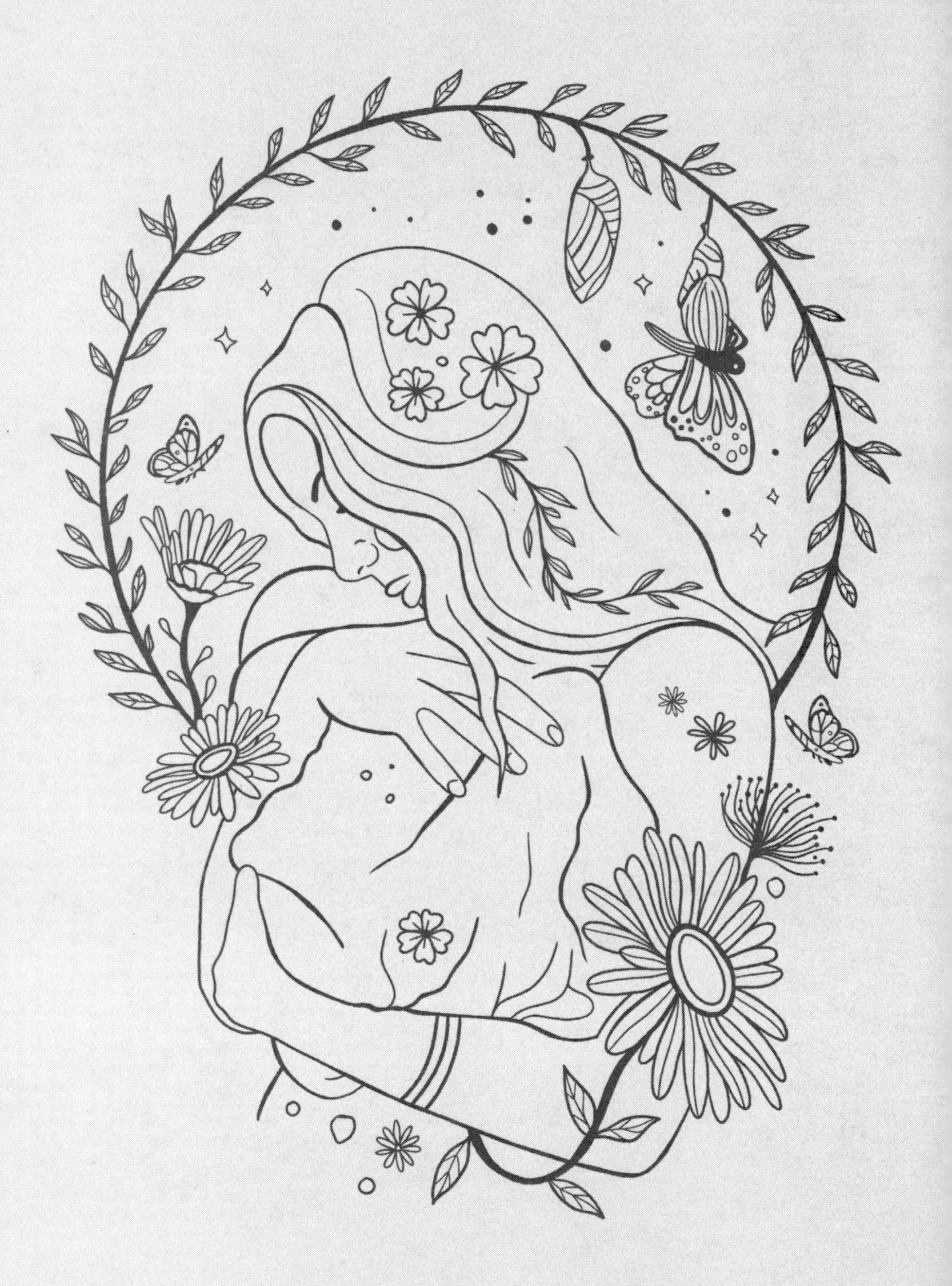

Newborn Mama

· 7 ·

No parent is ALWAYS conscious, gentle, positive, peaceful, and authentic. We have to choose to be and practice moment by moment, day after day. The more we practice, the stronger we grow.

Lelia Schott, certified parent and family wellness coach

You have tilled the field, planted the seed, nourished your little one with all the love, care, and attention you could offer. You have been mothering your little angel since the moment they arrived in your womb, and now you have birthed them into the world and are mothering in a whole new way. You are learning how to be a mama to your little one.

With all the attention on your newborn baby, let us not forget . . . you are a newborn mother! Even if you have had children before, every child brings new experiences, new challenges, and new parts of yourself to discover.

In this chapter you will find insights into how to mother with self-awareness, gain understanding of (or refresh your memory of) newborns and newborn essentials, learn about common newborn challenges and natural solutions for them, and discover Ayurvedic approaches to common issues with breastfeeding.

I was such a newborn mama when I had my first little babe; I literally knew nothing. I felt like any other mama with a little more experience than me could be a better mother to him than I was. I felt that other mamas would know how to rock him, when to feed him, how to help him stop crying, or even know why he might be crying . . . when I was just figuring things out as we went along. *What are his needs? Why might he cry? What do I do with him when he's awake? What if he is in pain? How do I know? What do I do?!*

Then I realized that he and I were figuring it all out together—it was his first time too. I was figuring out how to put him to sleep, as he was figuring out how to fall asleep in my arms. I was learning how to feed him, as he was learning how to eat. I was discovering who I had become, as he was discovering who he was. We were both in a brand-new world, both newly born, and discovering everything . . . together.

The main realization I had in my newborn mama days was that as long as I was showing up with presence, attention, and love, I was offering what was most valuable to my little one. Mother Teresa taught that the greatest suffering in this world is the experience of feeling alone. When my little one had nights of tummy pain, I was with him, holding him, so that he knew that he was safe and so loved. When he would cry, I would never abandon him; I would hold him and love him so that he deeply knew, from his earliest experiences, that he is never, ever alone.

This chapter is one that I wish I could have read before giving birth to my first baby. It would have helped me to feel a little more prepared for what might come up and equipped me with natural solutions to have on hand to deal with the things that did. I didn't know how much I didn't know, and many of you may be way more experienced than I was, but for those of you who are in the same shoes, I hope this chapter will be an amazing support for you, if and when you need it.

Our first weeks together . . .
I remember it being hard, but I don't remember why.
I think the main thing was the transition into a whole new world,
from literally one moment to the next.
Where suddenly I wasn't the center of my life,
and my desires weren't first,
in a way that is so real.

It's hard to even understand what that meant before him.
Suddenly this little being was the center of my life,
my constant meditation
and my sole responsibility.
Though I read many (many!) books,
they must have left out the chapters called *Vira Chandra*—
how to take care of *him*.
Because it all felt so new
and I felt I didn't know anything
and we were figuring it all out as it came.
And that's what felt hard.
Or different
than usual.
Because nothing was predictable,
and I had no idea what was to come.
And then it passes.
Time moves.
Suddenly it's all just a memory.
forgotten . . .
unless remembered.

MOTHERING WITH SELF-AWARENESS

Being a mama is full on. Having your heart beating outside of your body, as your precious little babe, is no small feat. Motherhood is a spiritual practice. Entering into it with awareness and the readiness to be transformed will help you to heal past patterns and revise conditioned beliefs, allowing you to expand in ways that you never knew possible.

The practice is to be steady internally; to notice your mind and emotions, but to not let your actions stem from them. Your mind may say, "I don't have time for this," or "Why isn't he listening?" and your automated emotional response may be to become impatient and frustrated. Then you act from that place: you yell, close down, or unconsciously move toward whatever learned behavior you have habituated. These are conditioned responses: responding to the current situation based on your past experiences in life. Although it may not seem like it at the moment, how you respond when you are impatient or frustrated is a choice.

As a mama, you have to notice when you become triggered: when you are frustrated that he won't sleep, angry that she won't stop crying, pulled out of your center by the myriad of ways that he may or may not be acting. Believe it or not, your baby is not conniving. He is not trying to disrupt your harmony. She does not know that what she is doing or not doing is causing you distress.

We have all developed programmed reactions (or coping strategies) that come along with uncomfortable emotions that we'd prefer not to feel. When we have an automated response to an internal experience, it keeps us from actually feeling what is happening inside and thus responding in a present and conscious way. What we do not allow ourselves to feel lodges itself in our body and begins to contort and control the way we *are* in the world. What we do not allow ourselves to feel creates a lens through which we experience life.

Because we have all been hurt in the past, we do everything that we can to not have to feel similar, uncomfortable feelings. We protect our emotional triggers by turning on autopilot: reacting to the present experience based on learned responses from the past, rather than feeling into what is arising in the present and choosing how to respond with more awareness. Because it is so easy to go on autopilot, we end up missing out on the very opportunities that could help us heal and help us grow.

Rather than using anger to express condescending words, you can *choose* to use that same energy to bring clarity and direction in a respectful way. When you feel disrespected, rather than withdrawing your love, you might use the feeling as an opportunity to connect more deeply with your child. Rather than hurting them if they hurt you, you might tap into how you can show up for your little one and lead by example. Rather than instilling within your little one your unconscious, learned reactions that do not ultimately serve to uplift your relationship, you can impart within them the greater vision of how to be a loving, respectful, kind, and conscious human being.

It's not my child. *What is this bringing up in me?* As mamas, we have to take responsibility for our inner experience. If I feel undernourished and overwhelmed, I am much more likely to get annoyed with my child for acting in a certain way. If in the same circumstance I felt nourished and connected, I would be able to be present and even enjoy the experience. As you become present to what is arising within you, notice your impulsive desire to act in a certain way. Instead, pause. Take a deep breath. Become present to the part of you that is steady beyond the emotion. *How do you want to show up for your little one?*

As much as possible, let your actions come from this steady place within you, where you can choose how you want to respond, rather than projecting your unhappiness, frustration, or dissatisfaction onto your babe. From that steady place, show up with the love and attention that instills healthy beliefs and progressive opportunities for your baby to thrive. As you respond to your little one with more consciousness and love, you heal your own past as well; you rewrite your own stories and beliefs around discipline, teaching, and the role of a caregiver.

When my little guy is melting down, every part of me may want to let him know that it's not okay to scream like that—though that goes against what I actually want him to know: I want him to feel safe expressing his feelings to me. I want him to know that none of his emotions are too big for me to handle. I want him to know that it is okay to *feel*. My ability to stay centered and hold loving space for my little one's big emotions helps him to regulate. Often, our children are frightened by what they feel, not having the ability to understand the big energies moving through them. You are your little one's safe place, mama. You are their anchor. Though if you show them that you are unable to stay calm in the midst of their storm, they'll feel that they have nowhere to land, which produces even more fear, overwhelm, and anxiety for them—and likely more impatience and frustration for you.

If you are unable to hold calm, loving space for your child, likely at some point in your own upbringing you learned that it wasn't safe to feel. Some emotions, yes. The pretty, happy, lovely emotions were all welcomed—though you learned that it is best to tuck away the other more "ugly," needy, big ones. So you end up rejecting parts of yourself, parts of your own experience, and therefore reject that same part of your child. If you are unable to hold that calm, loving space for your child, it is because their innocent actions touched a part of *you* that needs to heal. And until that part of yourself is given the attention and acceptance that is needed, you will be unable to feel calm in the midst of their chaos. To see your little one as a *whole human* in a tiny body—fully deserving of respect—and to respond based on your *values* rather than from the emotions that arise from your *conditioned worldview* is what it means to mother consciously.

You can improve your ability to pause in the moment, take a deep breath, and practice acting from a nontriggered place by better understanding your own triggers. Reflect on the following:

How did your parents discipline you? What were their patterns?

Did they react to you based on their emotional experience rather than respond from a centered and loving place?

What beliefs and patterns of reaction have you taken on because of your parents' behavior?

How is the energy *behind* your words and your actions shaping your child's views of themselves?

Does the way that you show up for your child teach them that they are welcome to communicate with you?

What beliefs are you imprinting upon them that were imprinted upon you from your parents? Do these beliefs serve?

♦

The real work of a mama is the inner work.

Especially in the moments that you feel depleted, undernourished, or disconnected from yourself, it will be easy to get triggered by the monotony (or unpredictability!) of your days. As with all close and conscious relationships, the relationship between you and your little one refines you. It will stretch you to become patient by giving you opportunities to practice patience; to become more loving not because you want to be, but because any other response will leave you more frustrated; to see all the patterns of reaction that you have learned throughout your life and to exercise your ability to respond with more kindness, more awareness, and more love.

It is important to mother purposefully, with intention and love, rather than acting and reacting from an unconscious place. Your actions in the first years are being soaked up by your little one's psyche and forming their views of themselves and the world around them. They are learning in every interaction: Am I worthy of love? Can I give love freely? Is it okay to ask for what I need? Will my needs be met? Am I safe? Is the world safe?

According to Ayurveda, the element of ether is heightened in a baby. They are connected, tuned in; they feel everything. They can feel subtle energy, and if you pay close attention, you will notice that they behave and act differently based on the subtleties of their environment. They feel if there is hostility. They feel when your actions are coming from a place of love or when they are coming from a place of anger, resentment, or frustration. The underlying energy of all your actions instills foundational beliefs within your little one, and therefore how they learn to interact with the world.

I remember when my little guy kept biting me when he first got his two bottom teeth. Every few minutes while nursing he would chomp down on my nipple. I started to feel frustrated, feeling like he was doing it on purpose. From this frustrated place, I put him down on the bed, moved to the other side of the bed, and turned my back to him.

Suddenly, I realized what I was doing.

Oh my God.

I turned and looked at his little face and he looked stunned, studying my own face to know how he should feel. My pattern throughout my life was to close down and withdraw my love when I was hurt so that the other person would know that they did something wrong. I probably did this with my dad when I was young; I have done it with my husband; and now, there I was, doing it to my little son. I learned it from my own mama, who I am sure learned it from hers.

I thought I had healed that pattern years ago through the work I had done in my relationship with my husband. But here I was, being refined by my little one, seeing the parts of me that still had not healed; the parts of me that were still unable to love; the parts of me that were still triggered, and thus attached to a story from my past; the part of me that needed to prove something in order to love or be loved. And now I was unconsciously acting out the same drama that would instill the same beliefs, and thus the same patterns, into my little one. Wow.

I noticed.

I became aware.

And that is the first step of all healing and transformation.

♦

First, check your energy.

If I am frustrated with my baby when he is biting me and I put him down to "teach him a lesson," then tell him (from that frustrated place) that what he did was not okay, he feels the frustration and also the guilt of doing something "wrong." An infant not only feels guilt, but they connect all their experiences to their value and worthiness as a person.

Next, take a deep breath.

I dropped into the boundless reservoir of love and compassion that God has gifted mamas with. I looked at my little angel in that mood, and immediately he softened and smiled. From a loving place, I let him know that biting hurts mama, that it does not feel good.

As I'm sure you have heard, it's not necessarily *what* you do or *what* you say, but more the energy that you do or say it with, that has the most effect. It is not about *not* expressing what you need, or *not* putting him down, but more importantly, *how* did you express your needs? *How* did you put him down? What was the energy *behind* your actions? As that is what is felt the most. Responding from a place of love and care creates a completely different experience for your babe.

Beneath every behavior is a feeling, and beneath every feeling is a need. Rather than responding to a baby's behavior, respond to their needs. What needs are they expressing *through* their actions? Do they need more attention? More presence? Do they need to feel more comfortable? When you meet their needs, you are addressing the cause of their behavior, rather than temporarily pacifying the symptoms.

♦

What are other, more effective ways to communicate with your little one without making them feel ashamed about who they are, or guilty for what they did? Again, your little one does not know that what they are doing is causing harm. They do not know "right" from "wrong," "good" from "bad." They are simply experiencing the world from a deep state of *being*. Our task at this time is to respond in such a way that allows them to feel safe and to let them know, through our energy and actions, that they are fundamentally cared for, valued, and worthy of love, no matter what.

How then, do you create clear boundaries without limiting their self-expression? What can you do instead of responding to your teething baby's pain with more pain? Speaking practically, you can recognize their need to bite on something and offer your finger or a teething toy instead of nursing, and then you can return to the nursing session later when they are not hurting as much. Perhaps you can voice to them with a loving yet firm and serious tone that "that hurts" and that you will not let them bite, and that you will not give them milk when they bite.

Your boundaries are important, and by no means do you have to suffer the pain of a biting baby while nursing. But instead of using punishment as a form of teaching, there are constructive ways to create the boundaries that *you* need while simultaneously letting the baby know that they can express *their* needs without being punished. The definition of discipline that Magda Gerber, a renowned early childhood educator, shares in *Dear Parent: Caring for Infants with Respect* is "training that develops self-control, character." This is in line with the actual source of the word, the Latin root *disciplina*, which means "instruction" or "knowledge." So, discipline is *educating* our children so that they understand appropriate behavior, values, and how to control their impulses—rather than punishment that makes the child feel ashamed or "bad." By cultivating the perspective that your little one is never trying to cause you stress, pain, or suffering, you can respond to them in a way that is respectful and clear, and in a way that models the behavior you want them to learn. By expressing to them that it hurts when they bite, they may learn how to express themselves when they are hurt in a respectful way; when you provide them with an alternative relief for teething, they may learn that they can count on you for support when they need you. By being clear in your energy and intentional with your responses—rather than becoming triggered and then responding unconsciously—you support them in learning how to regulate their own emotions and create the boundaries necessary for them (and you!) to feel safe.

You will feel much, much better as a mama when your actions come from a place of responsiveness, compassion, presence, and care. You will also notice that it is a much more effective way to teach your little one.

You have to be so mindful as a mama, and simultaneously so gentle, patient, and forgiving toward yourself. Mamas tend to put so much pressure on themselves to be "perfect"; but you deserve just as much grace and forgiveness as you are giving your child. You are learning. You will become triggered at some point. It is an opportunity for your growth. And like any spiritual endeavor, conscious motherhood is a *practice*.

We are all conditioned by our past experiences—by the ways that our parents dealt with us and the ways we have seen others being treated. We are affected by our friends, by the media, and by society. When you are a new mother, many new things arise that you have never experienced before and therefore may not know how to respond to in ways that are actually supportive.

Guilt is a common emotion among mamas, though rather than getting stuck in it, know that it is there to show you what you value. The experience of guilt makes it crystal clear when you have acted out of alignment with what you care about, and thus it helps you self-correct the next time around. The important part is to be able to notice the way you reacted, to become aware of the way in which you wish you showed up, and to keep refining. Children do not need a perfect mama. They need a mama who is genuine and who is committed to the work of becoming better. Apologize to your little one when you step out of line. Let them know that it wasn't okay how you spoke to them, ignored them, or touched their body. Let them know that it wasn't their fault and that there is nothing they could do to make you not love them. Take responsibility for your actions so that they eventually learn how to take responsibility for theirs. This repairing also supports your little one, from the youngest of ages, to rewrite—or reintegrate—what happened in a way that is supportive for their development.

♦

You are a newborn mama. You are learning how to love in the deepest and most profound way possible.

Swami Prabhupada would often say that the closest thing to God's love that we can experience in this world is the love that a mother has for her child. Experiencing this love from the inside out, from the heart of a mama, has revealed much to me about the way God loves us all. Wow, God loves me without reason. There is nothing I could do to make Him not love me. There is no way that I could act that would make the Divine turn away from me. I am not "good" or "bad" in His eyes. I am simply *me*, and that is perfect. How can I become an instrument of that boundless, shoreless ocean of love in my little one's life?

In the Puranas, the Ultimate Mother is known as Sri Radha. Both the Padma Purana and the Brahma Vaivarta Purana elaborate on her pastimes of love with Lord Krishna and reveal how the divine couple is the Source of all that is. Sri Radha is the embodiment of love and compassion. You can pray to her to become an instrument of divine, motherly grace: to know how to love your little one without conditions. Mother Yasoda is Lord Krishna's mother. You can pray to her for the wisdom of how to raise your little one with devotional love. Goddess Bhumi is Mother Earth: the epitome of generosity, care, nourishment, and reciprocation. You can honor Mother Earth for being the perfect example of how to love no matter what.

The ancient Vedic scriptures guide us toward living a life where we intentionally support each other, respect the world, and honor God as the source of all that is. When we show up in our relationships, offering our gifts without selfish motives, without the need for validation or recognition, we will feel a deep satisfaction and fulfillment that might otherwise feel elusive. While this may be hard to conceptualize, the living example of millions of mothers gives us an insight into what selflessness really is. Devotional service is love expressed.

I remember when I was learning to love my little one: the kind of love that is beyond what I could feel, but rather a love that stemmed from learning what he needed and how I could serve him. I remember the depth of experience I began to move into as I took full responsibility of caring for him, and the realization that the experience of love is deeply enhanced through service. When you really love someone, you will naturally go out of your way to make them feel happy, content, and at peace. It will give you the greatest joy to see them joyful, and the greatest satisfaction to know they are satisfied.

My first experience of loving him was a knowing that there was nothing I would *not* do to protect him. There is nothing I would not give up or give away if it meant that he would be safe. Through serving him, I began to know a love that I had only heard about from others. My own needs effortlessly became secondary, as the well-being of my little one moved to become my top priority—a constant meditation and full absorption. The way a mama serves her little one is unmotivated and uninterrupted, which births a love consisting of those same qualities.

un·mo·ti·vat·ed: without a reason or motive.
un·in·ter·rupt·ed: without a break in continuity.

You are here to love, and thus serve, your little one—to let them feel the way that God loves them through the way that you care. When you can remember who they really are, beyond the limited scope of "your" child, you can see the pure spirit soul within their tiny little body; this eternal spirit who has been traveling from one body into the next since time immemorial searching for the lasting happiness that can only be found in connection to their true Self and in relation with God. You can understand that the greatest service, while caring for their basic needs and loving them with attention and intention, is to raise them to know who they really are, beyond their body, mind, and emotions. Instill within them, through your own example, the real value of living a deeper life and the importance of spiritual connection.

Nama Karana Samskara: Name-Giving Ceremony

In Vedic tradition, it is auspicious for the parents to have the name-giving ceremony—*nama karana*—on the 10th day, 12th day, 101st day, or first year after the birth of their baby. After the father spends the morning bathing and worshipping the Lord with certain offerings and mantras, the Vedic name-giving ceremony is done with the father offering ghee-soaked wood into a fire while saying specific prayers.

If you will be doing a baby-naming ceremony, you can bring your own sacred intention into naming your baby. Start the morning by cleaning your house and then taking a shower. Make a small fire or light some candles, and arrange some flowers, leaves, or fruits in a mandala shape around the fire with the intention of creating a sacred space.

Say the following prayer, or a prayer that you write yourself with similar intention.

> I offer my respects to the earth.
> I offer my respects to the space between the heavens and the earth.
> I offer my respects to the heavens.
> I offer my respects to the universe.

With your family sitting around the fire, you can hold your baby in a clean cloth and sit on the father's right side. Handing the baby to their father, mama walks behind papa and comes to his left side. At this point you should be facing east. The father touches the mouth, nostrils, eyes, and ears of the baby with his right hand and says:

> Your essence is spiritual, immortal like the Lord, O [baby's name] enter in this solar month. May the Lord consign you to the day. May the day consign you to the night. May the night consign you to the day and night. May day and night consign you to half-months. May the half-month consign you to the full months. May the months consign you to the seasons. May the seasons consign you to the year. May the years consign you to long life, O [baby's name].

The father then whispers the name of the baby into the left ear of the mother, saying, "[baby's name] is your son/daughter."

The father then gives the baby back to the mother and places more ghee-soaked wood into the fire. He can end the ceremony by saying the same offering of respects as in the beginning.

He cried a lot this week.
And I bounced on the ball as I put him down for a nap
and cried too.
I begged him, or God, to just tell me what he needed.
I felt frustrated when he seemed to cry for no reason
and sometimes annoyed
by how much he needed me.
I felt like I needed a moment.
One breath.
Two seconds
for me.
The ability to shower without saying,
"I'm just showering, little angel! I'll be right there!"
To eat a whole meal in peace,
or at least sitting in one place.

And then he smiles
and my whole world melts.
My whole world
melts.

I am yours, little one.
Completely taken.

I feel like God must have given mamas super powers.
Truly.
To love like this is unreal.
And the ability to serve like this . . .
what an opportunity.

I need you too, little one.
I'm learning what it means
to love.

L. R. Knost, the author of *Two Thousand Kisses a Day* and *The Gentle Parent*, writes,

> I discovered early in my parenting journey that raising my voice might scare my children into compliance, but it taught them nothing other than to be afraid of me, to hide their mistakes and problems from me, and to raise their own voice when they were frustrated or upset themselves. Speaking quietly, though, drew them in close, quieted them down, built trust, and opened their little ears and minds and hearts to my words and my thoughts and the life lessons I wanted them to learn. Teaching and guiding and modeling positive communication skills naturally took center stage once I'd made that first discovery. Learning to control myself rather than try to control my children, to show respect instead of demanding respect, to listen instead of lecture, to communicate instead of command, to parent instead of punish, to problem-solve instead of becoming part of the problem myself, has been the journey of a lifetime. What a lifetime it's been.

As mamas,
our job is to instill within them the knowing
that there is nothing they could do
that would make them undeserving of our love.
That there is no emotional state
that we cannot hold space for with patience and attention.
There is no need
that is too big of a burden.

It's a practice,
as there are moments when I'm tested.
And I know that when I'm tested to step into something,
there lie my greatest opportunities for healing and growth.

There are moments when I feel things or want to do things
that I would never do.
There are moments when I want to shake you.
There are moments when I want to leave you crying on the bed.
There are moments when I want to avoid you or ignore you.
There are moments when it takes everything in me

to take a deep breath.
To pause.
To ask myself,
"How can I love you more, little one?"
And I feel guilty even admitting these things,
because I feel that maybe I'm the only mama in the world that ever feels like this.
Though I know that I'm not,
because this is the work of a mama.

There are moments
when I want to project onto you
what's happening inside of me
instead of taking responsibility.

These are the moments
where healing can happen.

When I don't react out of frustration or anger;
When I don't act based on how my parents may have acted;
When I choose not to act based on my patterns and conditioned beliefs;
When I instead exercise my ability to
respond
with more awareness, more love, and more kindness.

The real work of a mama is the inner work.

Where are your actions coming from?
A place of love?
A place of frustration or anger?
Because that's what they feel
and that's how they then learn
to respond to the world.

Deep breath, mamas.
It's a huge responsibility.
It's the most important work.
And I'm right here with you.

Understanding Newborns

Your newborn babe has left the warm, watery, dark, quiet, and comforting home of your womb and entered into a world that is cold, dry, bright, loud, and startling in contrast. You will notice them adapting to these changes in different ways. Their skin may become dry; their arms will reach out looking for the distinct boundary of the surrounding womb, though now they feel only space.

In order to support them in developing a nervous system that is well adjusted to their environment, it is essential to help ease their transition into the world. This is why Ayurveda places a strong emphasis on the postpartum window as a time where mama and babe stay at home. The home environment can be kept quiet, peaceful, predictable, warm, and comfortable, so that your baby can adjust well and develop a stable nervous system.

Newborn babies do not need much else besides your love and care. Generally speaking, a healthy newborn that does not have any medical conditions or temporary imbalances will cry for only a handful of reasons. If your baby seems unhappy or uncomfortable, check their basic needs first. Is their diaper dirty? Are they hungry? Are they tired? Are they too hot or too cold? Do they want to be held? Are they gassy or in an uncomfortable position?

If their basic needs are all met, check to see if it is their primary need: mama's love. Hold them close, sing to them, rock them, let them nurse just for comfort, even if they may not be hungry.

According to Ayurveda, it is best for a newborn baby to be in the auric field—the energetic field exuding from the body—of their mother for the first several weeks, no more than a couple feet away. You are their entire world—their comfort and their home. Your voice is soothing, your smell is inviting. They do not know a world without your heartbeat close by. It soothes their nervous system and quite literally stabilizes their breath to feel your warmth. Use this time to be with your little one. Do not be rigid about eating and sleeping schedules or other "shoulds." Simply get to know your little angel, and allow your rhythms to ebb and flow as you discover yourselves, together.

BASIC NEEDS

When tending to your little one's basic needs, be as present with them as possible. When you are caring for them in these necessary ways, whether it be changing their diaper, bathing, or feeding them, offer them your full attention so that they know that they are worthy of deep love and care.

Here are some details pertaining to caring for your baby's basic needs:

Diaper changes. A baby will be uncomfortable sitting in a poopy diaper, and a dirty diaper may cause a diaper rash, so change your little one's diaper right after they are finished pooping. If you are using a disposable diaper, most of them have an absorbent quality that pulls the wetness away from their skin, so it will not feel uncomfortable if the baby is in the diaper for a while after peeing; generally they can pee two to four times in a disposable diaper before they need a change. If you are using cloth diapers, the baby will likely be uncomfortable after peeing just once because they will feel the wetness. I suggest using cloth diapers as often as possible, especially as your little one gets older, to reduce waste and expense. We used mostly disposable in the early days, as it invited more ease to our early postpartum rhythm, but then we switched to using one cloth diaper per day, then two, before switching over completely.

Temperature regulation. The traditional advice used to be that parents should check the baby's hands and feet to see if they are cold. The recommendation now, however, is to feel the temperature of their chest—if the skin there is cold, they are too chilly and need some warmth. If their chest is hot, they need to cool down. A rule of thumb is for your baby to be wearing one more layer than you are, as they are likely to feel cold in the first few weeks of life (since they are used to the warmth of your womb). An infant cannot regulate their own body temperature until they are several months old, so it is dangerous for them to overheat. If they are sweating, they are too hot and probably uncomfortable. Skin-to-skin contact is a great way to regulate your baby's body temperature if they are hot, cold, or have a fever. Let them rest on your bare chest and their temperature will quickly regulate to match yours.

Nourishment. Better than creating feeding schedules and tracking your newborn's eating times is to learn your baby's cues for when they are hungry, and feed them when they cue you. If your newborn is crying and upset, hunger is one of the first things to check. Among the many hunger cues that the baby may give (moving around, looking around, opening their mouth and moving their head around, licking their lips, reaching for you, and so on), crying is the last one.

Ayurveda recommends at least two hours between feedings so that the milk has time to fully digest in your babe's stomach. However, in the newborn stage, please do not worry too much about timing, as every child's needs are different—you can feed them more often if they are hungrier or less often if they are sleeping (you do not have to wake them up to eat). During growth spurts—which happen roughly at three days, five days, ten days, three weeks, five weeks—your baby may "cluster feed," meaning that they continuously nurse on and off for what could be hours at a time. As they are constantly growing (and quickly), their schedule yesterday may be completely different from what they need today.

Sleep. Newborns sleep a lot. They need sleep to support the rapid growth that is happening in the first few months of life. Especially during growth spurts, they may need to sleep more, or their sleep schedules may change completely. Every time I thought I had figured out my baby's schedule in the first few months, it would change a few days later. Try not to get attached to a nap schedule or sleep schedule. Let them sleep when they are tired and wake up when they feel rested. You can help them to fall asleep by nursing them to sleep, walking them around, holding them to your chest while bouncing on a birthing ball, rocking in a rocking chair, walking around with them in a baby carrier, or swaddling them. Swaddling helps your little one to feel contained, similar to when they were in the womb. It brings in the warm and stable elements, helping to pacify vata dosha. Making the *shhhhhh* sound over and over again is also soothing to them, as the sound reminds them of being in the womb.

DUNSTAN BABY LANGUAGE

In June 1998, an Australian opera singer named Priscilla Dunstan gave birth to her first child and her keen ear quickly noticed five distinct sounds to her baby's cries. Pursuing Dunstan's resulting theory, that infants use these five vocal sounds to communicate before learning how to speak, researchers eventually observed over four hundred babies of varied ethnicities and backgrounds to verify her claim that these sounds are vocal reflexes used to communicate different needs. Listen carefully to a baby's cries and you will be able to distinguish what it is they are asking for. My husband and I found this especially useful, so I share it here with you:

Neh (I am hungry). Babies make the sound reflex *neh* to communicate hunger. The sound is produced when the sucking reflex is triggered, and the tongue is pushed up on the roof of the mouth.

Owh (I'm sleepy). An infant uses the sound reflex *owh* to communicate that they are tired. The sound is produced much like an audible yawn.

Heh (I'm experiencing discomfort). A baby uses the sound reflex *heh* to communicate stress or discomfort—perhaps that it needs a fresh diaper or a change of position. The sound is produced by a response to a skin reflex, such as feeling sweat or itchiness in the bum.

Eairh (I have lower gas). An infant uses the sound reflex *eairh* to communicate they have flatulence or an upset stomach. The sound is produced when trapped air from a belch travels to the stomach, where the muscles of the intestines tighten to force the air bubble out. Often, this sound will indicate that a bowel movement is in progress, and the infant will bend its knees, bringing the legs toward the torso. This leg movement assists in the elimination process.

Eh (I need to be burped). An infant uses the sound reflex *eh* to communicate that a large bubble of air is trapped in the chest, and the reflex is trying to help release the air bubble out of the mouth.

NEWBORN ESSENTIALS

The following list of baby essentials (which doesn't include the obvious diapers and wipes) are things I got the most use out of when my baby was a newborn (that is, in the first three months or more) and would highly recommend for any new mama.

Disposable and washable organic bamboo breast pads. Reusable breast pads are great for the first couple of weeks postpartum. Wear disposable pads at night, as the reusable ones may soak through after a couple of hours and waking up in the middle of the night with a milk-soaked bed is no fun! For the reusable ones, I found bamboo to be the softest and they did not make my nipples itch like some of the cotton ones with seams down the middle.

Haakaa breast pump. This pump attaches to your breasts easily and lets you express milk naturally through suction. You can put it on the breast that babe is not feeding from to catch the extra milk that comes out.

Muslin cotton swaddle blankets. Even if you do not swaddle your babe, these light cotton blankets are cozy and are the perfect small blanket for use in the house or while traveling (even if just in the stroller or car seat!).

Burp cloths. Keep these by your bed, near your nursing station, in the diaper bag, and in any common area around your house. Burp cloths are great not only for catching spit-up but also to catch any leaking breast milk while nursing!

Soft, light, bamboo pajamas for baby. Organic cotton is lovely, but there is something even lovelier about a newborn in buttery soft bamboo footie pajamas! The light fabric feels nice on their skin and can end up being what little babe wears for the first six to eight weeks of their life, if they wear anything at all!

Boppy nursing pillow. This will save your back while nursing! Even when not nursing, I would use this for my baby to sleep on me without having to use my arms to hold him. It can also be used to prop your newborn up after nursing if they are spitting up quite a bit. And finally, these pillows are useful when baby starts to sit up on their own but needs a little assistance not to fall over. *Tip:* Get an extra cover for laundry day.

Baby carriers and wraps. You will get great use out of hands-free carriers once you start moving around the house more. Baby will benefit from being close to mama's heartbeat for as long as possible and as often as possible. Again, Ayurveda says a baby should not leave the mother's auric field for at least the first six weeks, so this is a great way to keep them close.

Diaper changing pads. You will likely want some portable diaper changing pads, a plastic foldable one, and some cloth washable ones (three or four). Changing pads are great to keep next to your bed or your baby's sleeping space during the first few weeks for midnight diaper changes. And remember to store one in your diaper bag for on-the-go changes for months to come!

Baby lounger. Baby will feel so cozy napping in this little pillow anywhere around the house in the first several months. It can also be used as a cosleeper in your bed.

Baby bathtub. This can be placed right in your bathtub or sink and can be used from the first bath to the hundredth!

Washable incontinence pads. Get two to four of these and put them on your mattress under your sheets where you sleep. From postpartum bleeding, baby poop explosions, leaky pee diapers, and puddles of breast milk, these will save your mattress.

Bedside basket. Get a nice basket and place it next to your bed so that is easy to access without you having to get up when the baby is with you. In the basket put everything you might need for you and your little one—diapers, wipes, diaper rash cream, waterproof changing pads, a few onesies, and anything else that you will be using frequently.

IS THAT NORMAL?

During the early days of motherhood, you will likely find yourself repeating the phrase "Is that normal?" for just about everything.

Of course, always go with your intuition, and when in doubt, ask for guidance. Call your midwives, your doctors, your pediatrician, your doula, your lactation consultant, your mom, your mom friends, or anyone you can get advice from. It is always better to be safe than sorry and it eases worry to hear "Yes, that is normal" when you are feeling nervous.

Here is a list of questions that may come up, and I can assure you: "Yes, that is normal."

"Why is her heart beating so fast? Is that normal?" Babies' tiny hearts beat faster than ours. They commonly beat around 120 beats per minute, which will sound and feel very fast to you. It is normal.

"He keeps forgetting to take a breath! Is that normal?" After being accustomed to life in the womb, babies need time to learn how to breathe. They can sometimes forget to take a breath, for up to ten seconds. If you are noticing this frequently, keep them close to you or even on you, so that hearing your breathing reminds them to take a breath. If the suspension of breath is longer than ten seconds at a time, call your pediatrician. Otherwise, it is likely to be normal.

"Sometimes she snores in her sleep. Is that normal?" Babies have tiny noses. Sometimes they snore until they grow out of it a month or so after birth. If the snoring seems concerning to you, contact your pediatrician. If it is just due to their tiny nose, they will grow out of it—it is normal.

"My newborn's poop was black and sticky for several days and now it's watery and yellow! It looks like diarrhea!" The first few poops after birth will be a black, sticky, tar-like substance called meconium. This can pass within a few hours, days, or within the first week or so. After that, the poop will gradually become a yellowish waterier substance that may be a little mucousy. A breastfed baby may have poop that looks like it could be diarrhea, but it is just the normal consistency of baby poop. In fact, for a breastfed baby, yellow liquidy poop is healthy!

"She keeps throwing up all the time! Is that normal?" Spitting up and throwing up are two different things for babies. If your baby is regurgitating milk or even what looks like curdled milk after eating, this is spitting up and is likely to be normal. If they are projectile vomiting (the milk comes out forcefully in a straight line out of their mouth), call the pediatrician. See page 252 on "Spitting up (in Breastfed Babies)" for more info on this.

"He is constantly drinking milk! I feel like I am nursing all day long! Is that normal?" Newborn breastfed babies will drink milk every two or three hours—sometimes more, sometimes less. During the typical growth spurts—at three days, five days, seven days, three weeks, and five weeks of age—which can last anywhere from one day to several days, they may do what is called cluster feeding. Cluster feeding means they nurse constantly on and off for hours at a time. This is normal and natural, and if your baby wants to cluster feed, cozy up with a good book to pass the time. They will benefit from the nourishment of the extra milk, so best to allow them to eat when they are hungry and stop when they are full.

"His skin is peeling. Is that normal?" Newborn babies' skin goes through a lot in the first few weeks. Peeling is a normal occurrence, as their skin is used to the watery womb, and our world in comparison is dry and cold. Starting with baby abhyangas after the umbilical cord falls off may help with peeling skin. However, it is nothing to be concerned about and is totally normal.

"Her poop is green!" Yes, green poop is normal for babies! Their digestion may simply be adjusting to changes in your diet or they may be teething. In fact, almost all colors of poop can be normal for newborns. In general, the only color to call your doctor about would be white poop.

"She has blood in her diaper! Is she okay?!" Sometimes female infants will get what looks like a mini period in their diaper. It will probably only show up once or twice. This is normal spotting of blood due to the hormones in mama's milk and not a cause for concern. If it lasts more than a few days, call your doctor to be sure.

BABY BATH TIME

When your baby is first born, you may notice a whitish, waxy coating on their skin—a protective layer called *vernix*. In a hospital setting, the standard practice is to wash this coating off. Ayurveda advises to leave the vernix rather than washing it, and instead to massage it gently into the baby's skin until it is absorbed. This natural external barrier has many benefits including protecting the baby from pathogens, regulating their body temperature, keeping their skin moisturized, and balancing their pH.

According to Ayurveda, a newborn baby can have an herbal bath any time after birth. The herbs can be the same ones that mama uses for her herbal baths. Fill the bath with lukewarm water, or water just warmer than body temperature. When you add the boiling water from the herbal infusion, wait for the bath to cool before putting your baby in. Remember that their skin is very sensitive and if it feels hot at all to you, it will feel extra hot to them.

The bath given immediately after birth is considered more of a ritual than a wash to clean them off. A bath can be calming for your baby and allow them a smooth transition out of the watery womb and into the world. Once the bath is prepared with the herbal infusion and cooled to the right temperature, you can slowly lower your baby into the water feet first. You can hold your baby face up with one hand under their head and neck and the other hand under their bottom and allow them to float on their back in the water. Your baby should appear warm and relaxed; they may uncurl their arms and legs and reach out into the water. Assure that their feet are always contacting a boundary, whether it is your body or the edge of the bathtub. They are used to the boundary of being in your womb, so too much space or vastness can feel overwhelming—and even scary—to them.

The best practice for a newborn bath is to keep the baby's umbilical cord out of the water, and just allow your newborn to float on their back on top of the water—the usual Ayurvedic recommendation is to wait until the umbilical cord falls off to give baby a full bath. However, a floaty herbal bath can be a sweet, relaxing welcome into the world for your baby. The herbs have the added benefit of being antibacterial and soothing to the skin. If the cord does get wet, simply dry it after the bath and apply powdered goldenseal to the umbilical area to dry and help it heal.

After a baby's welcome bath, it is not necessary or recommended to bathe them again until the umbilical cord falls off naturally. Optimally, the umbilical cord will simply dry up and fall off on its own without any intervention. Make sure to use diapers small enough that they do not cover the umbilical cord. Powdered goldenseal applied gently around the belly button with a Q-tip once a day will aid drying and healing and help prevent infection. Until the cord falls off, you can wash the baby with a warm, clean, damp washcloth or sponge if needed, but often a baby does not need to be washed at all. After the umbilical cord is gone, you can begin to bathe the baby once every day or every couple of days in lukewarm water after a massage (see the next section).

BABY MASSAGE

A baby massage is a traditional practice that supports the health of a baby and allows for deep bonding with the parents. The Ayurvedic recommendation is to start baby massage after the umbilical cord falls off and to continue daily for at least the first year of the baby's life.

BENEFITS OF BABY MASSAGE

Activates important bonding hormones between parent and baby

Promotes healthy and nourished skin

Boosts baby's weight gain

Prevents bacterial infections

Increases circulation of the blood and the lymphatic system

Drains toxins from the body

Strengthens the immune system

Supports digestion and bowel movements

Helps with sound sleep

Strengthens limbs and joints

Soothes the nervous system

Pacifies excess vata dosha

TIPS FOR AN AYURVEDIC BABY ABHYANGA

Use organic oils only (conventional oils have many pesticides).

Use sesame oil in general. Use sunflower or coconut oil if your baby is prone to overheating or rashes.

Use the palms of your hands and closed fingers instead of finger tips in order to calm your baby, rather than stimulate them.

Take cues from your babe. If they are not enjoying the massage, you can stop or change your methods. They should appear calm or happy and not be upset with abhyanga.

On that same note, always ask permission to give the massage. You can ask by showing them your hands with the oil on it so they know the massage is coming, and wait for their positive response before moving forward. This is important even from birth—it teaches them respect for their bodies and expectations for safe touch.

Be sure that the pressure of the massage is moderate: not so light that it tickles or so deep that it hurts.

Only massage after basic needs (feeding and diapering) have been met, and wait thirty minutes after a feeding.

Massage from the heart outward down the limbs.

Do not massage if the umbilical cord has not fallen off yet, if the baby is sleeping, if it's very soon after feeding, if baby is giving negative cues (for example, crying or fussing), or if the baby is ill, congested, or has a fever.

Choose a song to sing during the massage. As soon as you start to sing, your little hunny may light up, as they begin to understand that this certain song means massage time.

One of the most important parts of baby massage is transmitting love through your hands, which means being totally and completely present with your baby during this time.

1. Warm the oil first in your hands or place the oil bottle in hot water for a few moments.
2. Place little babe somewhere cozy and make sure the room is warm. Be sure to place a sheet or towel underneath, as things are about to get oily!
3. Gently begin by applying oil to the baby's scalp, rubbing their head in circular motions with your palms.
4. Massage from the baby's heart down the arms and then the legs. Use long strokes down the limbs, and circles around the joints—making sure to really rub the oil into baby's tissues.
5. Massage baby's abdomen in a large clockwise motion, using a gentle touch with little to no pressure.
6. Turn your baby onto their belly or side, and massage their back and bum.
7. Let baby soak in the oily goodness for ten or twenty minutes. Make sure your little one stays warm!
8. Bath time!

Ayurvedic Baby Soap

Ayurveda recommends using a soap made from the following recipe for the first year of your baby's life. (You can also use this soap yourself after abhyanga massages!) This homemade liquid cleanser is gentle on the skin and removes excess oil without being drying. No other commercial soap is necessary for your little one.

Ingredients

1 tablespoon chickpea flour

½ teaspoon sandalwood powder

½ teaspoon rose water

⅓ cup milk (can substitute milk with coconut milk or water in vegan households)

Instructions

In a small saucepan, mix the chickpea flour and sandalwood with enough milk to form a paste. Mix well and then add the rest of the milk. Cook on medium heat, stirring constantly with a wooden spoon. When the mixture begins to bubble and thicken, it is ready. Make sure the soap has cooled before applying it to your babe's skin. Since it is made with milk, this soap should be made fresh before each bath.

COMMON NEWBORN CHALLENGES

If your babe is experiencing an imbalance in the newborn phase, it may be a result of mama having an imbalance. Mothers and babies are so intrinsically connected in those early days that the health of the mother directly affects the health of the baby. Not only your diet but also your mind and emotions affect your little one. As Ayurveda emphasizes, most imbalances and disease in the body and mind can be treated with diet and lifestyle alone—so Ayurveda recommends evaluating mama's diet and lifestyle, as well as the energy in the environment that is surrounding mama and little babe, before treating baby.

Please be assured, however, that sometimes babies have minor imbalances that are *not* due to mama's diet and mood. My little one got a heat rash a few days after his birth. At the same time, he had really wet, yellow poop. These are usually obvious signs that there is too much heat in the body, so my husband and I both felt an urgency to lower the baby's pitta. I felt added pressure to make sure I was not eating too many heating spices, along with guilt that something I was doing (or not doing) could be harming my babe. Every time I ate, I would be worried that it would affect him negatively. Feeling like I could be the cause of his suffering due to my diet or emotions did not feel good! Then our midwife came for a home visit, looked at his poop, and laughed: "That is what normal baby poop looks like!" She also told us our house felt way too warm and to open the windows to allow some cooler air in—oh, okay, so simple!

The following is a list of what might arise in your newborn days, and Ayurveda's approach to what to do if they do.

COLIC

Colic is not a diagnosis but rather a description of symptoms. When a baby is "colicky" they usually exhibit a combination of fussing, crying (for hours at a time), and gassiness. If little babe curls their legs into their chest, turns bright red with tense limbs, and cries inconsolably, your baby may be experiencing the abdominal pain associated with colic.

According to Western medical science, colic is something that just happens sometimes with no apparent cause. According to Ayurveda, the cause of colic in a breastfed newborn is the diet of the nursing mama. Colic takes three weeks or more to manifest with symptoms, after poor eating habits have accumulated. Before colic manifests, you will see symptoms of gassiness in your little one; if mama's diet is not altered, after several weeks, you may have a colicky baby. Often when certain foods are removed from the nursing mama's diet, the baby's symptoms improve. Common foods that cause colic include wheat, dairy, soy, and peanuts—but really any food that mama is unable to digest properly will affect the quality of her breast milk and thus disrupt her little one's tummy (hence the importance of slowly rekindling mama's digestive fire with proper foods after giving birth, as taught in the next chapter). Caffeine, chocolate, cruciferous vegetables, onions, and raw garlic are among the other foods Ayurveda recommends removing from mama's diet. In general, make sure mama's digestion is balanced and that she is able to digest her food efficiently without feeling gassy or bloated. (See the food guidelines in chapter 8 for supporting mama and babe.) Once you put these changes in place, your babe may take a few days to a week to show significant progress, but it will come.

Most of the time, colic will disappear on its own as the baby's digestive system matures (around four months old), though watching your little one in extreme discomfort or pain can be heartbreaking, and trying to care for a colicky newborn can be exhausting. Below are some other remedies that may help. If symptoms persist, consult a lactation specialist or pediatrician.

REMEDIES FOR COLIC

Empty one breast at a time when breastfeeding. Your baby may be getting too much lactose in the foremilk and not enough fatty hindmilk. Make sure the baby is nursing on one side until the breast is fully empty before switching to the other side.

Herbal teas for mama. Make a tea with any combination of caraway, cumin seeds, chamomile, catnip, fennel, dill, or anise to sip on while the baby is nursing. The herbal remedy will transfer to your breast milk and ease your baby's digestive system.

Herbal tea for babe. Fennel seed or dill seed tea is helpful for relieving gas and intestinal cramping. This can be given directly to the baby. Bring 1 teaspoon of seeds to boil in 1 cup of water; steep and strain. A few drops may be all that is needed, but a small bottle is fine if your baby wants more.

The colic hold. Lay your baby with their belly across your forearm and your hand supporting their head and chest. Keep the baby's head slightly higher than their feet. This may relieve some of their discomfort.

Burping. Burp the baby with gentle pats on the back after every feeding to reduce gas buildup in your little one's stomach.

Take a warm herbal bath together. Make an infusion with chamomile and lavender and add it to your bath water. Hold your baby to your chest for skin-to-skin contact while relaxing in the warm water.

Baby abhyanga. When your newborn is relaxed and calm but not asleep, gently massage the baby and rub sesame oil in clockwise circular motions around their belly using your first two fingers with gentle pressure.

Eliminate stimulating substances. When mamas smoke or consume caffeine, the stimulant can pass through breast milk and lead to colic.

Add probiotics to your diet. Add yogurt, kefir, or lactobacillus capsules to your diet.

Essential oils. Put a few drops of chamomile, fennel, or lavender essential oils in warm water, soak a washcloth in the water, squeeze it out, and then wrap it gently around your baby's abdomen.

Homeopathic treatment. Colic Calm is a homeopathic remedy found in most pharmacies. I highly recommend having a bottle of this at home just in case it is ever needed. It eases babies' discomfort almost immediately.

CONSTIPATION

A breastfed newborn will generally poop daily, if not several times a day. According to Western medicine, it is normal for your baby to start going several days without any bowel movements after six weeks of age, and as long as there is no pain or cramping associated with the constipation, baby will eventually have a soft bowel movement and all will be fine. However, according to Ayurveda, everyone—including infants!—should have bowel movements at least once per day and anything less than that is considered constipation.

Again, as long as your baby is not uncomfortable or in pain, mild constipation is common and nothing to be concerned about, but if you want to help get your baby's bowels moving, Ayurveda recommends changing your diet to include more warm, oily, watery foods—specifically focusing on stewed fruits (recipe on page 296) for breakfast each morning until baby starts pooping daily. You can also drink warmed prune juice so that baby receives those benefits while nursing or put a little bit of ghee on your nipple for your baby to ingest while nursing. Another Ayurvedic folk remedy is soaking a Q-tip in olive oil or ghee and gently inserting it a quarter-inch into your baby's anus. They should have a bowel movement shortly after! If you are concerned that your baby is in any discomfort or pain from constipation, always consult with your pediatrician or midwives.

SLEEP "SCHEDULES"

A newborn baby's sleep pattern does not seem to have much rhyme or reason. Keep in mind that just about any schedule your baby has for sleeping is probably normal: They can sleep all night and all day. They can sleep all day and be awake all night. They can sleep all night and be awake all day. They are adjusting to the rhythmic patterns of day and night, and that takes time. Furthermore, they need a lot of sleep to continue growing. Remember that newborns will go through growth spurts every several days for several weeks and then every several weeks for several months. All the growing that their brains and bodies are doing is exhausting!

As a general rule of thumb, a baby's "wake window" (the time that they can tolerate being awake between naps or before bed) will start small and gradually increase over time. After the first few months, you will likely start to see a rhythm regarding what time baby wakes up for the day, when their first nap is, how much time they can be awake before the next nap, and what time they generally fall asleep for the night. As their wake windows naturally increase, the number of naps they take each day will decrease.

Rest when the baby sleeps so that you can care for them when they are awake. If they are tired, let them sleep. If they are awake all night, try not to get overwhelmed; their schedules are changing from day to day and it is only temporary. If you are exhausted and need to rest, ask for help! You can only care for your baby if you are in good health. If you are confused about their sleep schedules and nap times, talk to other moms in your community; they will all have advice for you. As you will learn, every baby is different, and you will get to learn your own baby's patterns and schedules over time.

That being said, if you are struggling with sleep deprivation, you do not have to suffer through it silently. In the early days, there is not much you can do about adjusting a baby's schedule, but you can ask other adults for support. Take turns with your support people, whether that would be your partner, family members, friends, or doula, and ask them to care for your baby while you rest. After your baby is a few months old, you can adjust their sleep and feeding schedules to become more regular so that you (and they!) can sleep for longer stretches of time. And of course, if you feel that something is wrong, always follow your intuition and consult your care providers.

THINGS THAT SUPPORT RESTFUL SLEEP

Drink your hot milk tonic each night!

Diffuse lavender or roman chamomile essential oil.

Use a sound machine in baby's room.

Use a weighted blanket or weighted onesie that is appropriate to your baby's weight.

Swaddle your baby to help calm their dispersed energy if you notice their hands are flailing and their breath is fast. Swaddling will also keep them from waking themselves up.

Give baby a massage and bath before bedtime.

Make the baby's sleeping area as dark as possible, and during their waking time, let it be light. This helps them to adjust to the time of day.

SPITTING UP (IN BREASTFED BABIES)

Spitting up—several times a day—is a common occurrence for a newborn in the early days. Projectile vomiting, however, can be a cause for concern and is a reason to call your pediatrician. One common reason for spitting up is reflux—when the baby's stomach acid flows back up into the esophagus. Reflux is something that should be diagnosed by your pediatrician. Supplementing breast milk with formula or feeding your baby cereal mixed with breast milk is often recommended by Western medical practitioners, though studies have shown that neither of these treatments improve reflux;

in fact, they may even worsen it. In some cases, making changes to your diet may help the baby's symptoms. Reducing dairy and following the other Ayurvedic postpartum diet recommendations in chapter 8 is a good place to start.

Another common reason for spitting up is an oversupply of milk or a fast letdown (when your milk is released forcefully). When your baby is still only a few days or weeks old, they may not be able to handle the amount of milk that is coming down if you have an abundant supply. Too much milk volume can lead to your baby nursing less or for shorter periods of time, turning away from the breast as a source of comfort, or refusing to nurse at all, so try to resolve an oversupply issue early. As with all breastfeeding concerns, it is best to consult a lactation specialist who can determine your personal situation and provide the best and easiest solutions. If your newborn is spitting up due to oversupply, you may see some corresponding signs from them:

- struggling at the breast
- choking with milk letdown
- spitting up a lot of milk
- having green, frothy stools
- nursing for short periods of time
- pulling off the breast soon after letdown
- having bouts of unexplained crying
- not settling into a feed

For solutions, pay attention to the following details:

Baby's latch. A good latch will help your baby control the flow of milk. (Support from a lactation consultant can help you learn how to improve your child's latch.)

Baby's position. Try having your baby's head higher than your breast.

Patterns of nursing. Switching breasts too quickly can lead to baby getting too much foremilk and not enough hindmilk. Try allowing a longer time for feeding on each breast before switching, or offer the same breast for a few feedings in a row.

Burping. For some moms, the solution is as simple as remembering to burp the baby after every single feed and between switching breasts.

Frequency of feedings. If your baby is going too long between feedings, they may be overly hungry and try to drink quickly. Watch for and learn your baby's early signs of hunger, such as eye movements, small sounds, and body movements.

Draining the breasts. Empty one breast at a time at each feeding. This will regulate the supply of milk. Do not pump extra milk, because it will cause your breasts to fill quickly again.

Herbal supplements. If you are taking herbs to increase milk supply, stop—and that may help solve the issue. Some herbs—including peppermint, sage, and parsley—are considered antigalactogogues (they decrease milk supply). Making these herbs into a tea may help in reducing milk supply.

Oversupply can cause a mama to have sore nipples, plugged ducts, mastitis, thrush, or breast pain. If you have tried all the above solutions and nothing seems to be working, I recommend consulting a specialist. Your baby's symptoms of oversupply can also be signs of low supply, but you can usually tell the difference by whether the baby is gaining appropriate weight or not. Breastfeeding issues can sometimes be solved by simple changes that you may not be aware of, so experts can be a tremendous help.

NEWBORN SKIN: CRADLE CAP, DIAPER RASH, AND HEAT RASH

Within the first couple of weeks after birth, your newborn's skin may go through several different changes as they adjust to life outside of the watery womb. Some skin rashes and conditions are normal, and some may be uncomfortable or irritating for your baby.

You may see "stork bites" (red dots on the back of the baby's neck or between their eyebrows), dry or peeling skin, baby acne, milia (little white bumps on the cheeks), or swelling in the baby's face (from the birth experience) that will go down within a couple of days. All this is normal.

Other common occurrences that may arise are cradle cap, diaper rash, and heat rash. Although these are mostly harmless, they can be irritating or uncomfortable for your babe, and of course, as a mama, you will want to help your baby be as comfortable as possible. Neem-infused ghee is a great Ayurvedic remedy for baby rashes, baby acne, and peeling skin. The resources section at the back of this book has suggestions on where to order some.

Cradle cap is a yellowish crust that can sometimes appear on a baby's scalp, forehead, or eyebrows. It does not need treatment and will go away on its own eventually, but if you want to remove it you can gently massage the area with ghee or coconut oil and allow it to soak into the skin overnight. Optionally, you can add essential oils of lavender, frankincense, or tea tree (or a combination). In the morning, the skin with cradle cap will be soft, and you can gently pick off the crust and comb or brush it out of the baby's hair with a baby brush. Be gentle when picking the crust off, as baby's heads are delicate. The cradle cap should come off almost effortlessly and not break the skin or disturb your babe at all.

A red, sore rash on a baby's bottom, known as diaper rash, occurs for several reasons. Sometimes baby has a skin sensitivity to chemicals in wipes or disposable diapers. Or they could be having a reaction to the detergent used to wash their cloth diapers. Often, rashes are caused by sitting in a dirty or wet diaper for too long (even a short time if their skin is sensitive). Other causes are yeast infection, reaction to antibiotics, or a reaction to the nursing mama's diet. To prevent diaper rash, or to help remedy it if necessary, the following approaches can help:

Elimination communication. Watch your baby's cues for when they have to pee or poop, and take them to use the toilet (from birth!) instead of using diapers. Eliminating diapers would, of course, eliminate diaper rash.

Daily abhyanga massage. Nightly baby massages with sesame oil, followed by using coconut oil where the rash is, will often soothe and heal diaper rash quickly. A combination of lavender and tea tree essential oil mixed into the coconut oil is also soothing and healing for your baby's skin.

Soaking up sunlight. Lay your naked baby in some indirect sunlight daily.

Hygiene awareness. Use the cleanest diapers, wipes, soaps, and detergents: unfortunately, commercial baby products can sometimes have highly harmful chemicals in them. Do your research to choose high-quality body products or laundry soaps for your baby. Avoid Vaseline as well as fragranced soaps, detergents, shampoos, diaper creams, and talc powders.

Change soiled diapers immediately. If you spend a lot of time with your baby, you will always notice when they poop. Change their diaper right after they are finished. You may want to wait about ten minutes from when you first notice them pooping to make sure they are fully finished, then put the baby in a fresh diaper right away. If your baby has sensitive skin, you may also want to use a dry cloth and pat the bum dry after a cleanup, to make sure baby is completely dry before putting on a new diaper.

Change your diet. Think about whether the diaper rash might have appeared when you introduced a specific food into your diet, and try eliminating it to see if the rash goes away. Diaper rashes resulting from diet will be accompanied by a red or irritated anus on your baby.

If diaper rash persists, you might be dealing with a yeast infection. Susun Weed's *Wise Woman Herbal for the Childbearing Year* discusses yeast infection diaper rashes and how to treat them with home remedies.

Another type of rash that is not uncommon in newborns is a heat rash. A heat rash can be identified when you see tiny pink bumps, mainly on the neck, chest, and upper back. Babies can experience heat rash anytime they are overheating, whether from the temperature in the house, from the temperature outdoors, or simply from being overdressed. Ayurveda adds the perspective of heat rashes being a sign of excess pitta (fire) in the body, which could not only be an effect of the temperature but also an effect of the nursing mama's diet and emotions. Eating spicy foods or foods that contain too many warming spices could cause excess heat, as well as a mama's emotions "heating up" through anger, frustration, irritability, or resentment.

Heat rashes, as in all pitta imbalances, simply need to be cooled. Sometimes all it takes is applying a cool washcloth to the skin or turning on the air conditioning in the house. If heat rash is more serious, mama may need to change her diet—especially avoiding spicy foods or foods that have too many warming spices—in order to see improvement. Some other Ayurvedic solutions you can try to remedy heat rash include these:

Give baby a lukewarm bath using the Ayurvedic baby soap recipe on page 247. Chickpea flour, sandalwood, rose, and milk are all cooling to the skin.

Use the essential oil solutions described in chapter 9.

Drink cooling teas or infused waters made with things like cucumber, watermelon, fennel, hibiscus, or rose.

Drink fresh coconut water.

Gosh . . . the ways I love you.
It actually, literally hurts my heart.
And sometimes it's scary to love this much.

You were in bed crying the other afternoon.
I was exhausted, dizzy, and lying next to you.
"Please just close your eyes."
"Go to sleep, you can do it on your own"
. . . even though you've only ever done that once since you were a newborn,
and you've only ever known to fall asleep in our arms.

I felt frustrated with you, for the very first time.
I got up, bounced you on the ball, and you fell asleep almost immediately.
And then the first wave of guilt I've felt as a mama.
"He needed me, and I let him cry."
Tears rolled down my face as I looked at my little man.
"I love him too much," I thought,
and it didn't feel safe.
The same feeling that has come up for me in all my relationships.
Because to love too much means that
eventually
I'll get hurt.
Though with this wave
it was the acute awareness of time
and how time washes away everything that we love in this material world.

That one day I won't be here,
I'll have to leave him.
I won't be able to take care of him
or to love him.
Or worse,
the f*ed-up reality that sometimes our children leave us too early.
I feel so sad about that
and so angry about the way this world is set up
and so frustrated that we learn how to love here,
but then are forced to let go.
And hopefully
rather than protecting my heart and limiting my experience of love,
that realization can urge me to love much more deeply,
in every moment
that we're here.
Because time passes
and nothing here
lasts.
You're a little heart doctor, my angel.
And you're teaching me how to love.
Because with you,
the walls that I've built to protect my own heart
become so clear.

I might blame you
or get frustrated with you for a moment,
before realizing
you just *need* me . . .
and *my* inability to show up for you
makes me frustrated.
***My* idea of what you *should* be doing (but aren't)**
makes me frustrated.

What do you need, my angel?
How can I show up for you?

Just one tiny lesson in love
out of the billions you've already given me.
Thank you, my little love.
These months with you have been profound.

BREASTFEEDING: MOTHER NATURE'S PERFECT DESIGN

Ayurveda teaches mamas to be totally and completely present while feeding their little ones. Nursing at the breast is potent medicine and, simultaneously, a powerful medium of communication between mama and babe. It is how your bodies communicate.

We know that a baby receives antibodies from their mama's milk, strengthening the baby's immunity to any germs or viruses mama has been exposed to. Also, baby's saliva tells mama's body what antibodies to create and then deliver through her milk, based on anything that they have been exposed to!

But deeper levels of communication are also happening: not only physiologically but also emotionally, psychologically, and spiritually. This profound exchange of energy will leave both mama and baby feeling deeply nourished (more than just a full tummy for babe!) if feeding your little one is approached with deep love, care, and presence—and is really respected as sacred, quality time.

BALANCING VATA DOSHA AND NOURISHING RASA DHATU

According to Ayurveda, breast milk is the by-product of healthy rasa dhatu, or plasma. Rasa dhatu is the first tissue to be nourished after the successful digestion of whatever you eat, mama. Remember, there are seven tissues that make up your physiology—and to the extent the first is nourished, the second will be, and so on. Breast milk being a by-product of the first tissue (rasa) means that nature designed for baby to receive the initial nourishment from whatever it is that you eat! With the surplus of nutrients left over, the rest of the tissues in mama's body are fed. If mama isn't nourishing herself properly with the right quality and quantity of food, she will quickly become depleted—there will not be enough nourishment to fuel her own body as well as her baby's. Mama needs to conscientiously feed herself with easy-to-digest yet deeply nourishing foods so that whatever is not transferred to baby through her breast milk can continue to nourish her.

Because the postpartum window is already a time when vata dosha is high, and dryness is a quality that is exacerbated with high vata, mama needs to be nourished in all the ways that pacify vata: warm oil massages; warm, cooked, oily meals; lots of love and affection. When mama is nourished, her love overflows from her breasts in the form of milk, and baby will be nourished as well.

Breastfeeding mamas require more calories than the average woman and should take care to consume plenty of warming, nourishing foods to satiate her body and buffer the stress of breastfeeding. Ayurveda is concerned with assuring not only that the quantity of mama's milk is sufficient, but also the quality. When you eat foods that are similar to the qualities already inherent in rasa, the quality and quantity of your breast milk will increase. Rasa dhatu is liquid, and thus nourished by foods and drinks that invite more liquidity and nourishment. (Rasa is also nourished by seeing beauty and by feelings of gratitude and joy.) Foods valued for enhancing lactation and nourishing rasa dhatu include:

- Oats
- Soaked and husked almonds
- Raw dairy, especially cow's milk and raw butter
- Ghee
- Roasted garlic
- Fennel seeds
- Fenugreek seeds
- Shatavari
- Sesame seeds
- Saffron
- Juicy fruits and sweet, fresh fruit juices
- Dates
- Well-cooked leafy greens

FROM BREAST MILK TO SOLID FOODS

Ayurveda recommends that babies exclusively breastfeed for the first five or six months of their lives and be breastfed as a supplemental form of bonding and nourishment for anywhere from one to three years, depending on a mama's health and energy levels. You'll know that your baby may be ready for solid foods if they have sprouted their first teeth and are showing a strong desire for food, such as interest in the food you are eating. When you choose to introduce solid foods to your baby, Ayurveda suggests doing so in a methodical and harmonious way, to help promote digestive health and prevent food intolerances for the entirety of the baby's life.

When introducing new food, always start with a single ingredient without adding salt or sugar. A grain such as rice or oats is a common choice. The grain can be soaked overnight and then cooked in water at a ratio of 1:10 so that it is very moist and well cooked down. After twenty to thirty minutes of cooking, pour off the water and feed your baby the soft grain. Ensure that it is always made fresh and served warm. Continue with this recipe for five to seven days, looking for any allergic response and seeing how the baby's digestive system responds. After this period, another food can be introduced—for instance, yellow split mung beans—soaked overnight and cooked in the same ratio. Liquidity can be reduced as baby's digestive system adapts, and as they get used to swallowing more dense foods. If you notice signs of constipation, add a little bit of ghee to each meal.

Once baby is digesting grains and legumes efficiently, you can gradually introduce well-cooked vegetables and, finally, fruits. Fruits should always be served at least thirty minutes before or after any other foods in order to digest properly, as they generally do not combine well with other foods in the stomach. Ayurveda also suggests avoiding avocado and banana until the baby is one year old, to avoid the heaviness and potential mucus-forming effects of these fruits. Over time, try to include all six tastes (sweet, sour, salty, pungent, bitter, and astringent) through a diversity of foods as well as spices.

Ysha Oakes's book *Touching Heaven: Tonic Postpartum Care with Ayurveda*, cited in the references section, goes into much more detail on the topic of introducing food to your baby the Ayurvedic way.

BREASTFEEDING CHALLENGES

For some mamas, breastfeeding can be as easy as breathing. For other mamas, or at other times, nursing may be a difficult experience that tests your patience and confidence (and pain tolerance!). Many books on breastfeeding go in depth about the many challenges that may arise, and how to overcome them, so on the following pages I will only mention a few challenges that have simple solutions. If you are struggling with breastfeeding, or need more home remedies, I recommend contacting a lactation specialist or reading the following books: *Ina May's Guide to Breastfeeding* by Ina May Gaskin, *The Womanly Art of Breastfeeding* by La Leche League International, and *The Nursing Mother's Herbal* by Sheila Humphrey.

Establishing a seamless breastfeeding experience begins in pregnancy by nourishing your body with all the care and nutrients it needs to create an abundant and high-quality supply of breast milk for your babe. Massage your breasts regularly (this can be part of your abhyanga) and follow the Ayurvedic nutritional guidelines for diet during pregnancy (in chapter 8) to enhance the quality and quantity of your milk.

The process of labor and birth will also affect your breastfeeding journey. Studies suggest that natural births lead to a higher success rate of breastfeeding because of mother and baby not having any side effects of pain medications. Mamas who initiate breastfeeding during the first "golden hour" after birth tend to notice that their baby will latch naturally and effortlessly. You can also implement the breast crawl, where mama lays her newborn babe on her belly and lets baby root around until they naturally scoot toward the breast and find their latch. Incorporating these simple practices will help to support a happy breastfeeding outcome.

Sometimes mothers, despite all efforts, encounter circumstances where they cannot breastfeed. For such cases, Ysha Oakes's Ayurvedic postpartum care manual includes a cow's milk recipe (see page 264). Baby formula from the store is often difficult to digest, so if you do choose commercial formula for your little one, be sure to buy organic, always serve it warm, and consider supplementing your baby's digestion support in other ways, such as a daily baby massage.

Here are some common breastfeeding challenges and simple solutions to have on hand.

ENGORGEMENT: Engorgement occurs about three days after giving birth, as your milk comes in. You may notice that your breasts become extremely swollen and firm and they might be quite painful. Engorgement can also make it difficult for your babe to latch, which leads to other issues such as a painful latch. When this happens, continue your daily abhyanga, with a focus on massaging the breasts, followed by a warm bath. You can also increase the amount of omega-3 fatty acids in your diet, through foods such as flax oil and walnuts.

For lymphatic drainage, which will relieve the pressure from engorgement, massage your breasts following the arrows on the diagram below.

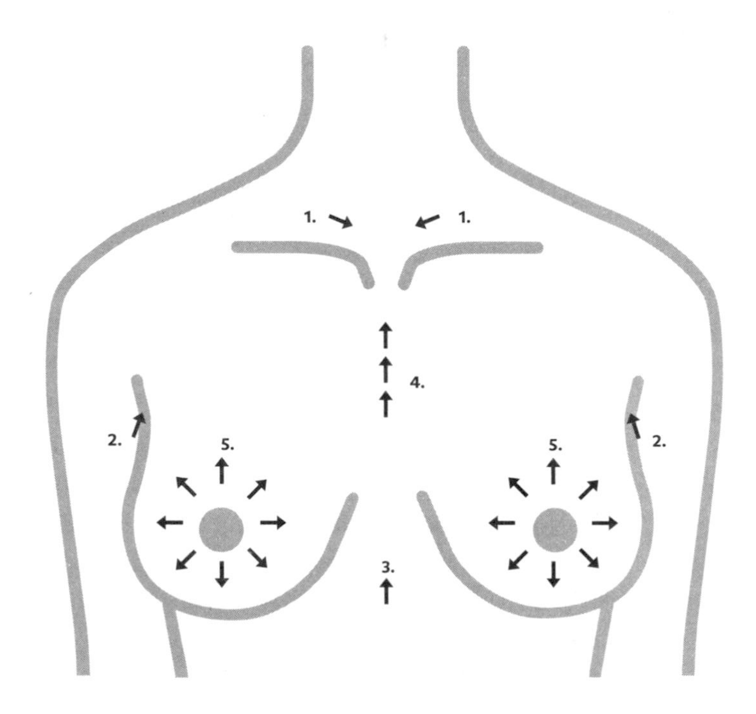

MASSAGE

1. from behind the neck, down the clavicles.

2. up and around the sides of the breasts, through the armpits and toward the chest,

3 and 4. up the center of the sternum and chest, and

5. away from the nipples. Then, lift the breasts away from the chest and gently shake. End your massage by again repeating step 2 and then step 1.

IRRITATED AND SORE NIPPLES: Exposure to sunshine and air is one of the best remedies for irritated and sore nipples. Other treatments include using an herbal salve or oil with St. John's wort, marshmallow root, or calendula lanolin creams (unless you are allergic to sheep's wool). Ghee infused with chamomile and calendula, applied topically, can also provide relief.

LOW MILK SUPPLY: If your breasts do not seem to be supplying sufficient milk, the general Ayurvedic approach will be to focus on hydration and to reduce excess vata by avoiding bitter and astringent foods as well as dry, light, and cold foods. Eat more lactation-enhancing foods such as oats, almonds, cow's milk, garlic, saffron, and ghee. Work to remedy stress and high vata by following the tips at "Postpartum Anxiety and Depression" on page 204). Increase nourishment through warm, oily, and grounding food (follow the Ayurvedic diet guidelines in chapter 8).

Some specific supplements to improve milk supply include sweet water lactation tea (see the recipe on page 288); you can also add a half-teaspoon of blessed thistle or milk thistle, star anise, marshmallow root, or licorice to your sweet water lactation tea on occasion. Include fenugreek in your diet by drinking strong fenugreek tea or using fenugreek as a cooking herb; fennel as a cooking herb also supports lactation. Taking a half-teaspoon of shatavari in the morning and evening will help with low milk supply (but do not take shatavari until ten or more days postpartum to ensure your digestion is strong).

MASTITIS: Mastitis is inflammation and infection of the milk ducts. This happens when a milk duct gets clogged and then leads to an infection. The most common cause of mastitis is when mama does too much too soon. The main remedy is rest, though daily breast massages can also prevent this condition.

If you notice a clogged duct (sometimes you can feel it) do everything you can to mobilize the duct and prevent it from stagnating further. Before nursing, massage the breast with oil using steady and firm pressure, moving from the outside of the clogged duct toward the nipple. You can add warmth by using a heating pad before the massage, or by doing the massage in the shower or bath.

Another option is to have your babe nurse until it unclogs—getting on all fours, hovering over baby as you feed so that gravity can assist the duct in unclogging. If your baby is not willing to nurse that long, use a breast pump. This may prevent the clog from leading to an infection. If an infection does occur, a washcloth or towel soaked in hot water used as a compress can help soothe it. Use a breast pump on the infected breast so that your babe does not drink the infected milk.

Ayurvedic Cow's Milk Formula

For babies who for whatever circumstances are not drinking breast milk, Ysha Oakes offers this recipe for a replacement formula made from cow's milk (from *Touching Heaven: Tonic Postpartum Recipes with Ayurveda*).

Ingredients

2 cups non-homogenized cream-top organic whole milk

2 cups distilled water

⅛ teaspoon turmeric

⅛ teaspoon cardamom

½ tablespoon fennel seed

1 thin slice fresh ginger

⅛ to ¼ cup sucanat (you need much less for older babies)

Instructions

1. Bring all ingredients except sucanat to a boil. Let the boiling milk climb the pot and then lift the pot off the heat so the milk falls; put the pot back on the heat and repeat three times. This makes much smaller, easier-to-digest protein molecules.
2. Add sucanat and immediately turn the heat off.
3. Cover to steep and let cool. Strain, and refrigerate extra. Serve warm, like breast milk is served.

Note that these ingredients were chosen very intentionally. Cow's milk, when properly used, is the most rejuvenative and complete food. Ideally, you will find a source for local, raw cow's milk (from farmers who love and protect their cows for the length of the cow's natural life!) and bring it to a boil three times on the stovetop. If you cannot find raw cow's milk, organic nonhomogenized cream-top whole milk is the next best choice. Anything else will be too highly processed and difficult to digest for both mama and baby. In addition, milk should always be consumed warm. This recipe will not work for all babies, so be sure to keep an eye on your little one's digestion to make sure that it is working for them. You can start with more water and sucanat, slowly decreasing the sucanat and adding more milk as your babe gets older and can digest the milk well.

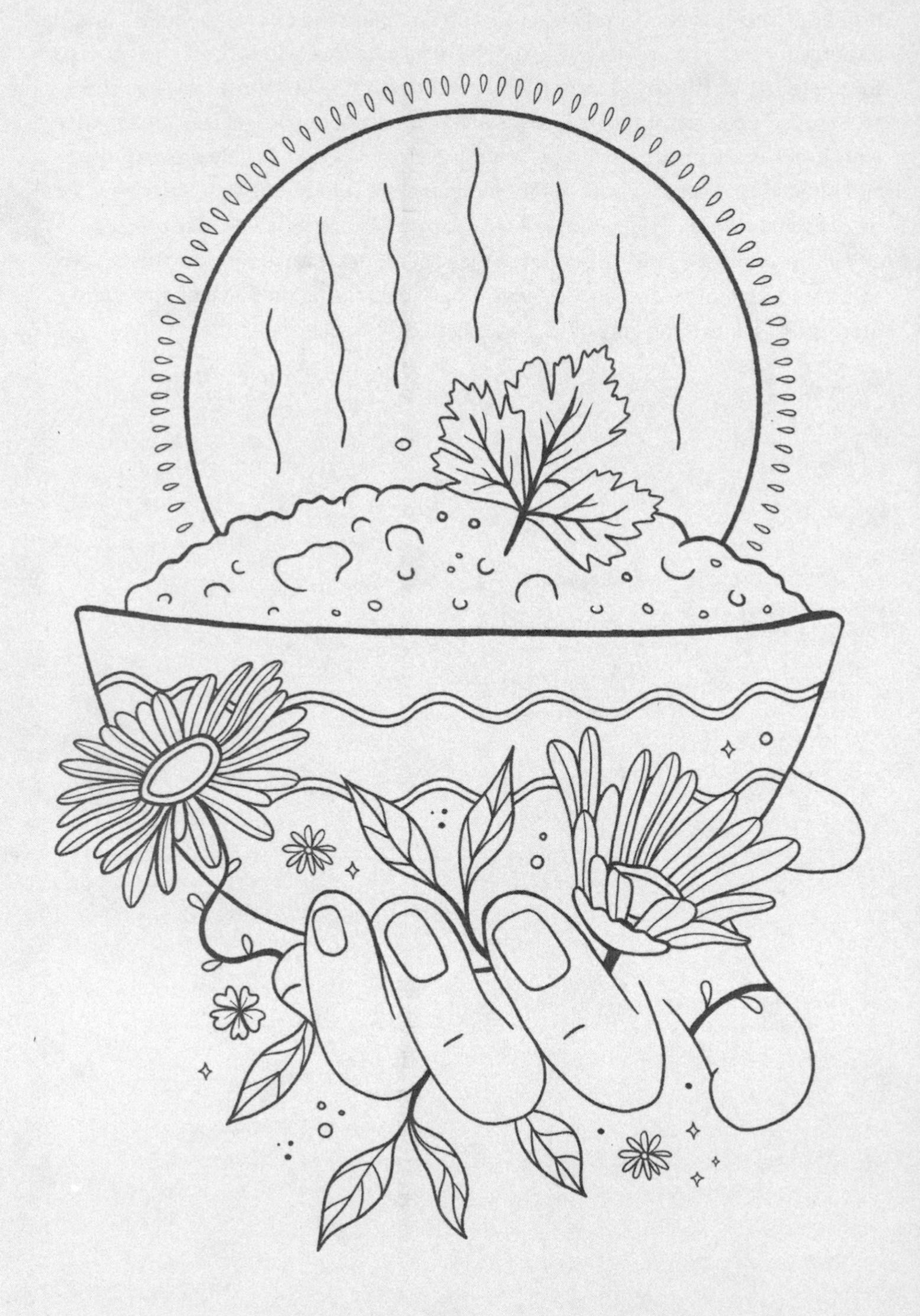

Nutrition and Recipes

· 8 ·

Being an Ayurveda mama means doing everything that you can to nourish yourself and your little babe before conceiving, throughout pregnancy and postpartum, and beyond. When a mama feels confident, she can feel more at ease in her role as a mother. To "mother" means to nourish, and the food that you eat is one of the main ways you will be nourishing you and your little babe.

Many mamas may suddenly feel overwhelmed with the responsibility of having to choose what types of food to favor or avoid during pregnancy and postpartum. What you eat is literally building the tissues of your little one during pregnancy, and your diet postpartum directly affects your baby's mood, skin, and digestion—and thus all other systems in their body. A huge focus in Ayurvedic nutrition is to eat the proper foods at the proper times to ensure that what you eat can be digested, absorbed, and thus easily assimilated into your body.

You know by now that one of the most important factors in pregnancy and postpartum is the pacification of vata dosha. This becomes especially important in your postpartum window as you are rekindling your digestive fire and nourishing your little one in a whole new way.

In this chapter, I share the basic principles around Ayurvedic pregnancy and postpartum nutrition, including why diet is such a pillar of your sacred window and why it is so important to eat simple meals after giving birth. I will then offer some of my favorite recipes to nourish you during pregnancy and to support you postpartum so that you may experience ease in your own body, as well as support your little one in feeling the same.

DIET AND NOURISHMENT DURING PREGNANCY

During pregnancy, diet is the crucial way through which you send nutrients to your little one. The origin of many adult diseases have their roots in the fetal life, so maternal nutrition plays a crucial role in your baby's future health.

The *Charaka Samhita* says that the pregnant woman needs to fulfill three main responsibilities. The first is *swasharirpushti*, nourishment of her own body. The second is *stanyavruddhi*, preparing herself for lactation or milk production. The third is *garbhvruddhi*, nourishment for the development and growth of her little one. In a similar vein, the *Sushruta Samhita* advises: "The essence of the food taken by the mother is divided into three parts—one nourishes her, the other promotes her breast milk, and the third portion nourishes the fetus."

The key word during pregnancy is *nourish*. Nourishment will look different for everyone. The important thing is that you do nourish yourself and avoid extremes that deplete your body. Allow yourself to feed your body in a way that feels deeply satisfying. Trust that when your body is nourished, it knows how to maintain balance regarding weight and general well-being. Your body will work for you when you give it what it needs. In the Ayurvedic approach, nourishment comes not only from a diet that satisfies the body's needs for macro- and micronutrients, but it also requires attention to Ayurvedic basics such as food *quality*, agni, ojas, and balance.

MACRO- AND MICRONUTRIENTS

Your diet should be filled with all essential macro- and micronutrients. As the name implies, macronutrients are needed in larger amounts, as they are the ones that provide energy. There are three macronutrients: carbohydrates, proteins, and fats. Micronutrients are substances such as vitamins and minerals that are needed only in small quantities but are essential for normal physiological functions. The following micronutrients are especially important:

Calcium: important for baby's bones

Folate: to support baby's brain and spinal cord

Iron: to nourish your increased blood volume

Magnesium: to maintain mama's blood pressure and avoid conditions like preeclampsia and eclampsia in later stages of pregnancy

Omega-3 fatty acids: important for brain development of your little one

Vitamin B_{12}: needed for proper brain functioning of both mama and babe

Vitamin C: important for absorption of iron

Vitamin D: helps to absorb the right amount of calcium and phosphate, helping baby's bones, teeth, kidneys, heart and nervous system develop

Zinc: important for baby's immunity

FOOD QUALITY

Ayurvedic tradition advises that pregnant women should favor a (lacto-ovo) vegetarian diet—with healthy fats and protein components from organic raw cheeses, paneer, ghee, milk, and other high-quality dairy—as these foods are nutrient dense and generally lighter and easier to digest than animal meat. A thoughtful diet of vegetarian foods contains all the essential amino acids in simpler and easier-to-digest forms, digestible within six to eight hours. Ayurveda teaches that it is best to avoid nonvegetarian food during this time, as the digestive system slows down and animal meat tends to be more compound and much heavier. A meat-based diet is also considered to be tamasic, carrying a more dulling and dense energy, as well as any of the fear or anxiety that the animal was feeling before death.

Ayurveda recommends *sattvic ahara*: food that is homemade, fresh, made with good thoughts in your mind, and prepared in a clean environment, which will carry sattva—the qualities of clarity, purity, and inner connection—to your baby. Along with this recommendation about preparation comes the emphasis that the main qualities in the food that you eat during pregnancy should be sweet, nourishing, and liquid/watery:

Sweet. The sweet taste is stabilizing, building, and cooling to the body, as well as relieving to thirst and soothing to burning sensations. The sweet taste can be found not only in foods that are obviously sweet—like most fruits and sweeteners—but also in foods like rice, wheat, mung beans, beets, carrots, almonds, milk, and ghee. Eaten in moderation, the sweet taste encourages love, sharing, compassion, and joy.

Nourishing. Eat foods that offer stabilizing sources of energy and deep nourishment for your physical body. Cooked food is generally easier to digest, and thus more nourishing. Generally, these foods will naturally taste sweet. Ideal examples include cooked grains, spiced milk, root vegetables, stewed fruits, soaked nuts, and seeds.

Liquid/watery. Eat foods with generous amounts of high-quality oil or ghee, and be sure to stay hydrated. Drink plenty of fluids, ideally warm or hot, no cooler than room temperature. Favor moist foods like berries, melons, summer squash, and zucchini; oily foods like avocado and coconut; and hydrating preparations such as soups and stews.

AGNI

You can be eating the highest-quality local and organic foods, but if your body isn't able to digest the food properly, then you won't be receiving any nourishment from it. Ayurveda looks at the strength of your agni, your digestive fire, to determine your ability to digest, absorb, and assimilate your food—as well as grow from your life experiences.

SIGNS OF HEALTHY AGNI

- Normal appetite (*Note:* healthy hunger involves lightness, clarity, and a pleasant anticipation of food, but not an urgent need to eat.)
- Clean tongue (no or light coating)
- Appreciation of taste
- Good digestion, balanced metabolism

- Can digest a reasonable quantity of any food without issues
- Proper (and regular) elimination
- Easily maintains homeostasis
- Steady weight
- Sound sleep
- High energy, strong vitality
- Calm mind
- Clear perception
- Courage, lucidity, and intelligence
- Cheerfulness, optimism, and enthusiasm
- Love of life and natural longevity

SIGNS OF IMPAIRED AGNI

The strength of agni is inevitably affected when its qualities are muted by a poor diet, improper food combinations, an unsupportive lifestyle, emotional disturbances, or even damp, rainy weather. If you learn to recognize and quickly address the following signs of imbalances with agni, the effects need not be long-lasting. Otherwise, they will undoubtedly lead to ill health and disease.

- Emotional disturbances, with an increased tendency toward fear, anxiety, anger, confusion, lethargy, or depression
- Low energy, weakness, or fatigue
- Suppressed or overactive appetite
- Indigestion: gas, bloating, constipation, nausea, hyperacidity, loose stools, a sense of heaviness, feeling tired or mentally foggy after meals
- A tendency toward congestion in the sinuses, the lymph, or even the mind

GENERAL AYURVEDIC GUIDELINES TO IMPROVE DIGESTION

Sip on warm water throughout the day.

Drink only a small amount of liquid with your meals (½ cup of warm water) and avoid drinking for at least an hour after eating.

Favor warm or room-temperature beverages over cold or iced.

Eat at regular times each day.

Do not eat anything until your previous meal is fully digested.

Allow lunch to be your biggest meal of the day and dinner to be your smallest meal.

Have your last meal two hours before bedtime.

Eat home-cooked meals (made with love!) as much as possible, rather than going out to eat.

Eat in a calm environment, and when your emotions are calm.

Eat slowly, chewing and tasting your food.

Do not overeat. Eat so that you still feel light after your meal: smaller portions more regularly.

Eat foods that are easy for your body to digest.

Eat freshly cooked food, ideally within two or three hours of when it was prepared.

Avoid reheated or prepackaged foods.

Stay hydrated with mineral-rich water, hydrating teas, fresh food, and juicy fruits.

Sit down while eating.

Eat local and seasonal foods.

OJAS

According to Ayurveda, healthy people have abundant ojas, the vital essence that promotes health, immunity, happiness, and spiritual strength: "It is the ojas which keeps all the living beings refreshed," says the *Charaka Samhita*. "There can be no life without ojas. Ojas marks the beginning of embryo." Signs of abundant ojas are clear radiant eyes, lustrous hair, glowing skin, a strong immune system, a positive outlook on life, joy, mental clarity, and compassion. Signs of depleted ojas are dry skin, cold hands or feet, constipation, anxiety, pain, mental fogginess, negativity, loneliness, and fatigue.

To avoid disruptions in the vital energy of both you and your baby, lean into the ojas-building foods discussed in chapter 4 (see "Building Ojas" starting at page 127), and avoid foods that undermine ojas, such as the following:

canned, processed, and prepackaged foods (these contain color and flavoring agents, preservatives, artificial sweeteners, and chemicals)

frozen foods

tamasic foods

spicy foods

alcohol and caffeine

carbonated beverages

too much of the bitter or astringent tastes

MAINTAINING BALANCE

Each of the five elements found in all things—ether, air, fire, water, and earth—has a specific role in the development of your little one. When you notice symptoms of imbalance such as bloating, acid reflux, constipation, or diarrhea, refer to chapter 1 (and especially the section "Elements and Doshas: Seeking Balance") to find dietary and lifestyle practices that will support you in coming back to a state of ease.

MEALTIME IDEAS FOR PREGNANT MAMAS

Some mamas may feel perfectly fine having three meals per day without any snacks in between. Some mamas might feel that three typical meals are not enough nourishment during pregnancy, and they may end up feeling depleted and exhausted without smaller meals between the main ones. Below are some ideas for your main meals, as well as some simple and nourishing mini-meal ideas for those of you who need more.

FIRST MEAL OF THE DAY, 7–7:30 A.M.

Fresh fruit can be a good way to start the day. Fruits are alkaline and help to reduce acidity and morning sickness. Fruits such as apples, pomegranates, fresh figs, and watermelon also contain iron, necessary for both you and your little one. Bananas contain a lot of potassium, which will help maintain the balance between fluids and electrolytes if you are vomiting. Look for what is fresh, juicy, and local as a guide to what might nourish you most.

Dried fruits and nuts, soaked, are another good option for this time. Organic figs, dates, apricots, raisins, almonds, and walnuts are great choices, as they provide you with magnesium and iron as well as the fat to support your little one's brain development.

A combination of nourishing foods called *panchamrit*—from *pancha*, meaning "five," and *amrit*, meaning "immortal" or "nectar of the gods"—is beneficial to eat in the early morning, before breakfast, to give you energy, nourish the tissues of your body, and reduce fatigue. The five ingredients come together quickly to make a warm, sweet energy booster for mama.

Panchamrit

Ingredients

5 teaspoons milk

2 teaspoons ghee

1 teaspoon raw cane sugar

1 teaspoon honey

1 teaspoon yogurt

Instructions

Warm the milk, ghee, and sugar.

Take off the heat, and add the room temperature yogurt and honey.

Stir it all together, and enjoy!

SECOND MEAL OF THE DAY, 9–10 A.M.

Your main breakfast meal could include one milk product such as fresh yogurt, raw butter, paneer (fresh cheese), or cream-top spiced milk, to supply your body with calcium, vitamin D, and protein. Grain dishes such as *poha* (flattened rice), *upma* (semolina), or porridge made from soaked oats, millet, or rice are other good options, as they provide carbohydrates that will give you good energy and help you feel satisfied.

Sprouts, either roasted in ghee or baked, are a great addition to this meal, as they are a rich source of protein. If you are feeling acidic or nauseated, include breads such as whole-grain or sourdough toast, parathas (Indian stuffed breads), or mung bean pancakes.

THIRD MEAL OF THE DAY, 12–2 P.M.

A good midday meal might include steamed green leafy, local vegetables—to provide vitamin A, vitamin C, vitamin K, folate, iron, and calcium—and dal, which provides the body with necessary protein and calcium. Yellow split mung dal is easiest to digest and the only bean that does not increase vata dosha. Dal will also help to maintain your hemoglobin levels.

Some type of bread with raw butter or ghee can add good carbohydrates, and thus easy-to-use energy, to this meal: options range from an Indian flat bread, such as chapati or roti, to your favorite multigrain or sourdough toast. You can also substitute another grain for the bread, such as rice, millet, barley, or quinoa. In either case, eating a good amount of carbohydrates midday will reduce cravings and acidity, and help you feel more nourished and satisfied.

Add at least 1 teaspoon of ghee to your meal.

ALL-DAY HYDRATION

Lime water provides the body with antioxidants and vitamin C, which supports iron absorption and also serves as a natural antacid. This will also improve your digestion and support hydration. You can add a half-teaspoon of Himalayan or sea salt to increase mineral content.

Buttermilk is incredible for your digestion. It contains vitamin B_{12}, which aids iron absorption as well as reducing acidity and relieving bloating. Try adding a pinch of salt, sugar, black pepper, and cumin powder, a combination that will serve to support your digestion even more. It is best consumed before sundown.

Coconut water helps maintain balance between fluids and electrolytes, and later in pregnancy it will help maintain amniotic fluid levels.

FOURTH MEAL OF THE DAY, 3–5 P.M.

Late afternoon is a good time for snacking on juicy fruits such as oranges, grapes, peaches, and mangos (depending on what is growing locally); the vitamin C in these fruits increases immunity, and the fiber will support elimination. For a more substantial healthy snack, make some dry-fruit laddus to have on hand. Fruit-nut balls will supply you with stable energy, and the dried-fruit laddus in the following recipe are a powerhouse of vital nutrients, protein, and omega-3 fatty acids. They support the development of your baby and keep mama going strong.

Dry-Fruit Laddus

Ingredients

1 cup almonds

1 cup walnuts

1 cup cashews

½ cup sesame seeds

handful of raisins (finely chopped)

1 cup dried apricots (finely chopped)

2 cups seedless dates (finely chopped)

1 cup dried figs (finely chopped)

pinch of cardamom powder

pinch of cinnamon powder

a few drops of vanilla

Instructions

1. In a pan, dry roast the dried almonds, walnuts, cashews, and sesame seeds until they turn golden brown.
2. Mix the nuts in a blender until they are chopped into small pieces.
3. Next, stir the nuts together with the finely chopped dried raisins, apricots, dates, and figs.
4. Add a pinch of cardamom and cinnamon powder and a few drops of vanilla extract; mix thoroughly.
5. Form the mixture into small balls and store in an airtight container.

FIFTH MEAL OF THE DAY, 6–8 P.M.

A substantial meal for the end of the day could include fresh bread with ghee, a blended vegetable soup (for something warm, nourishing, and easy to digest); a grain porridge or rice gruel (which provides hydration and grounding); a seasonal vegetable curry; kitchari; or rice with ghee.

If you are not hungry enough for supper, having a cup of spiced milk is a great option. Milk nourishes all the tissues in your body, as well as the body of your babe. (The *Sushruta Samhita* considers milk to be a complete food, as it contains proteins, fats, calcium, vitamins, and sugar.) Not only is milk capable of nourishing your body, but it also calms your mind. Heating the milk changes its molecular structure and makes it easier to digest, absorb, and assimilate.

Rice Gruel

Ingredients

½ cup basmati rice
1 teaspoon ghee
½ teaspoon cardamom
3 cups milk
½ cup raw cane sugar
Optional: ¼ cup cashews or pistachios
Optional: splash of rose water

Instructions

1. Rinse the rice until the water turns clear. Then soak the rice in water for twenty to thirty minutes. Drain the soaked rice using a colander and set aside.
2. Heat a heavy-bottomed pan on medium heat. Add ghee and cardamom to the pan, then add the soaked and drained rice. Stir the rice with the ghee and cardamom for one or two minutes, stirring constantly until aromatic.
3. Add the milk to the pan and stir well. Set heat to medium-high.
4. Let the milk come to a boil, stirring occasionally so that the milk doesn't stick to the bottom of the pan.
5. Once the milk has come to a boil, lower the heat to low and let the mixture cook for about twenty-five minutes on low heat. Stir every five minutes or so.
6. Add the sugar and optional nuts and cook for an additional five minutes.
7. Bless and enjoy!

GENERAL DIET GUIDELINES FOR PREGNANCY AND THE POSTPARTUM WINDOW

The following tips support you in choosing foods for pacifying the excess vata dosha often prevalent during pregnancy and always present in the postpartum period.

FAVOR WARM OVER COLD

With an eye not only toward temperature but also toward the effect that food has on the body, favor warm over cold: As much as possible, lean toward eating food that is warm in temperature, freshly cooked, and warming to the body. Warm softens and opens the channels in the body, whereas cold constricts. The warm quality of the food can be enhanced by using digestive spices generously. Spices such as ginger, cinnamon, cloves, cumin, black pepper, and mustard seeds all have a warming effect. Try to minimize foods with a cooling effect, such as cold and frozen foods or drinks, raw veggies, and leftovers that have been kept in the refrigerator or freezer.

FAVOR MOIST AND OILY OVER DRY

The Ayurvedic emphasis in pregnancy and postpartum is to nourish and build. To this end, favor moist and oily over dry: Cook everything that you eat with more water than usual so that it is soupy, hot, and moist—making it easier to digest, absorb, and assimilate. Also, plan to add an extra teaspoon of ghee to everything you eat, to keep your tissues nourished and to support digestion and the elimination of toxins. What is more nourishing than being invited to add a generous amount of high-quality oils, raw butter, or ghee to all the warm food you are preparing? The dryness of vata is offset by adding moisture, drinking plenty of fluids (ideally warm or hot—but no cooler than room temperature), and eating foods with more moisture that will add their moisture to your body, such as juicy fruits, avocados, summer squash, soups and stews, and dairy products such as warm milk, raw butter, ghee, and fresh yogurt. Do your best to minimize drying foods like popcorn, crackers, white potatoes, beans, and dried fruits (unless stewed).

FAVOR GROUNDING AND NOURISHING OVER LIGHT

As much as possible, it is best to think in terms of grounding the lightness of vata with sustenance—eating foods that offer nourishment by giving you stable energy. Examples include healthy fats, cooked grains, spiced milk, root veggies, stewed fruits, and soaked nuts and seeds. Lighter foods like raw foods and smoothies as well as stimulants like caffeine and processed sugars should be minimized or avoided because they aggravate vata's need for grounding and stability.

FAVOR SMOOTH OVER ROUGH

Raw veggies (and some fruits!) are considered rough, especially ones that are more fibrous. Even when cooked, there are some foods that will aggravate vata dosha for the same reason; examples of these are kale, broccoli, cauliflower, cabbage, and many beans. This is the main reason why vata, defined by its rough quality, becomes balanced with foods that are smoother, and the guideline for choosing foods during pregnancy and in the weeks after is to favor smooth over rough: Think warm oatmeal, blended soups, spiced milk, and yams, squash, and other root veggies. If you do eat foods that are considered rougher, be sure to add the smooth quality by adding more ghee or oils and add some vata-pacifying spices to make them easier to digest.

DIET AND NOURISHMENT POSTPARTUM

In Ayurveda, digestion is compared to a fire. When the fire is bright and strong, you can digest anything and get energy from it. When the fire is weak, you cannot digest your food no matter how healthy it is, and you experience symptoms like gas, bloating, constipation, and sluggishness.

A mother's choice in foods and how well she digests her food have a big impact on the quality of her breast milk as well as the quality of her rejuvenation, strength, and comfort in the first six weeks after the baby's birth. Mamas who follow the Ayurvedic postpartum diet protocols lose unneeded pregnancy weight easily, have more stable moods and emotions, and have a general sense of stability and well-being. The right food choices will help speed up recovery time; ease cramping; provide deep nourishment; assist in avoiding postpartum depression, anxiety, and depletion; and prevent colic in the baby.

Ayurveda teaches that during labor and birth, the digestive fire goes out completely. The postpartum diet is therefore tailored to rekindle the fire by introducing foods gradually, starting with easy-to-digest, simple, yet nourishing and grounding foods. Almost all cultures from around the world have a traditional "first food" following childbirth that is easy to digest. In

Ayurveda, it is kanji: a watery rice porridge cooked with digestive spices and ghee. Try eating very simple foods for the first three days postpartum, then slowly and gradually add more complex foods as the days go by and your fire rekindles.

In general, during the postpartum window a new mother needs

- an extremely vata-reducing diet (small adaptations can be made to suit mothers who are showing excess pitta or kapha);
- an easy-to-digest diet;
- her agni to be stoked and supported;
- to eat freshly prepared sattvic foods;
- to eat ojas-producing foods;
- to avoid heavy, hard-to-digest, tamasic foods and ama-producing food;
- to favor (generally speaking) ample warmth, oiliness, moisture and love, and to avoid cold, dry, and rough.

In particular, regarding diet, a new mother needs to eat foods that get the bowels moving and encourage easy elimination. She needs nourishment that is energy building and iron rich as well as grounding, and everything she eats and drinks should be warm.

A NUTRITION TIMELINE FOR THE POSTPARTUM WINDOW

During the first ten days after birth, a new mother's diet should be focused on rebuilding her digestive fire and supporting lactation. Everything mama eats should not only be warm but also soupy and oily. Grains and soups should be cooked for a much longer time with much more water than usual—grains should be so soft they look like mush! Vegetables must be used sparingly, if at all, because they are harder to digest and mama just doesn't have the digestive strength to digest them properly yet.

Unless the doctor contraindicates it, 2 or 3 tablespoons of ghee or a suitable substitute such as sesame oil is advised at every meal for mama during the first week after birth, gradually reducing consumption over the six-week period back to the normal amount. If she has liver or gall bladder issues, her doctor must be consulted on the use and amount of fats. (If she had a cesarean birth, use half the amount of ghee or oil, especially until her incision starts to knit together.)

After the first ten days of the postpartum window, the Ayurvedic focus shifts away from rekindling the fire and moves toward rebuilding tissues. A mama should continue eating foods that are oily, soupy, and hot. Grains don't need to be quite as mushy, and it is now safe to introduce thicker stews, soft cheeses, fresh juices, and more vegetables if they are well-cooked and well-oiled.

During the final phase of the postpartum window (weeks 4–6 and after), the Ayurvedic focus is mainly on mama's strong rejuvenation, as well as digestion and lactation. Mama can now gradually eat more complex foods that are still warm or room temperature and easy to digest.

♦

After your forty-two-day postpartum window is complete, you can transition gradually back to your normal diet. Remember to keep eating foods that are warm, cooked, moist, oily, and with good digestive seasonings. Pay attention to the results of adding breads, complex sweets, leftovers, soy, and dairy back into your diet. By consciously and gradually introducing new foods, you will more easily be able to track what works for you and your little hunny, as you both transition out of the nest and into the world outside.

NUTRITION ALTERATIONS FOR KAPHA OR PITTA MAMAS

Kapha or pitta mamas will need to make some alterations to the general guidelines for postpartum nutrition. If you are more kapha, are living in a damp climate, or are experiencing symptoms of excess kapha (see chapter 1), you will need less fats and dairy. If you are more pitta, live in a hot climate, or are experiencing symptoms of excess pitta, you will still need support increasing your digestive strength, but you will need to use more mild spices like fennel, cumin, and coriander rather than really heating spices like dried ginger or cayenne pepper.

FOODS TO AVOID POSTPARTUM

There are specific foods that are contraindicated for postpartum recovery because of their degenerative qualities, or because they are hard to digest. Ysha Oakes's collection of postpartum recipes, *Touching Heaven*, offers a useful outline of foods that postpartum mothers are advised to avoid. The following list is adapted from that book:

Cold foods and drinks. Ice cream, ice, salads, chilled foods and drinks.

Dried foods. Dried fruits (that are not rehydrated by soaking or stewing), crackers, toast, white potatoes, grains such as millet, brown rice and corn, unsoaked legumes, and protein powders.

Heavy foods. Meats; fermented cheeses; homogenized, pasteurized nonorganic milk; sour cream; yogurt; eggs; fried foods; and many types of unsoaked nuts. Eliminate or minimize chicken or fish for two weeks to a month, or more.

Cold milk. Milk digests best when it has been boiled, as boiling simplifies protein molecules, making the milk easier to break down. Warm milk can be used with unsalted grains, in puddings, with sweet taste, and sometimes with dates (which act different from other fruits), or with honey and ginger, cardamom, clove, or saffron. Milk should never be mixed with sour, salty, and astringent tastes, so avoid it with lunch or dinner.

Tomatoes, peas, peppers, sprouts, cruciferous vegetables, and citrus. These foods can create gas for both mother and baby. Tomatoes and citrus can cause rashes for babies, as they are acidic, so avoid them if possible. Also go easy on dark leafy greens during the first postpartum weeks unless you are craving them. After two weeks or so, dark leafy greens can gradually be added to the diet if cooked well with ample oil or water.

Hydrogenated or cooked vegetable oils (trans-fatty acids). Trans fats are a big no. Also, while nursing, it is best not to follow a low-fat diet (unless for medical reasons). Use ghee for all cooking, or use sesame oil if you are vegan for moral or ethical reasons. (Ghee does not contain lactose, so consider using ghee as a source of fat in your postpartum diet, if you normally don't eat dairy because you cannot digest it well.)

Fermented foods and leftovers. All leftovers (cooked food left for longer than six hours) give off their degenerative energy, even those that are normally easy to digest. They slow rejuvenation and often clog digestion and body channels. Make enough food for just lunch and dinner for the family. In addition, avoid fermented foods such as soy sauce, vinegar, pickles, tempeh, miso, most cheeses, and mushrooms.

Honey in cooking. Heating honey is proven to create toxic accumulations over time in the body's channels and around nerves, and it is considered one of the most difficult toxins to remove. Raw honey or honey used in warm (not hot!) beverages is fine.

Leavenings. Yeast, baking powder, and baking soda all strain mama's and baby's digestion and therefore are best avoided.

Touching Heaven also warns that postpartum mothers should cut down on consumption of drying, bitter, and astringent herbs (which may include chamomile, raspberry leaf teas, turmeric, and sage) and should completely avoid coffee, sodas, chocolate, alcohol, garlic (dry, raw, or undercooked), onion, radishes, chilies, and the cabbage family.

All these details aside, Ayurveda says that just as important for digestion as *what* you eat is *how* you eat. As often as possible, have your main meal at noon, do not eat your next meal until your previous one is fully digested, and sit down while eating. Breathe deeply, become present, chew, really taste, and enjoy your food. Let it nourish you and your little one.

MEALTIME IDEAS FOR POSTPARTUM MAMAS

In the weeks postpartum, you can gradually increase the complexity of those very simple first foods recommended after birth, by decreasing soupiness and increasing density as your appetite and capacity to digest food increases. When introducing a new food, be alert to how it affects your digestion. If you feel bloated or gassy, revert to the simpler first foods before trying something else. With each new list, you can include the foods in the previous list.

DAYS 1–5

Breakfast: porridge, soupy oatmeal, cream of rice, Cream of Wheat, kanji—all with adequate spicing, some good-quality fat, and iron-rich sweetener

Savory options: savory kanji

Snack: warm smoothie, stewed dried fruit

Lunch/dinner: vegetable broth or a very light blended vegetable soup

Herbal allies: fenugreek tea, sweet water lactation tea (see page 288 for a recipe), black pepper tea, herbal chai, ginger tea, fennel tea, cinnamon tea, chamomile tea or moon milk tea (see page 306) to soothe your nerves and help you relax into appropriate sleep.

DAYS 5–14

Breakfast: thicker porridge (possibly) and a small amount of soaked nuts or seeds (for instance, walnuts, peeled almonds, pumpkin seeds, sunflower seeds, macadamia nuts, cashews, pecans, hemp seeds), healthy fat and optional warm milk, savory porridge

Snack: same as days 1–5, plus you can add in fresh, sweet, juicy room-temperature fruit (for instance, berries, sweet oranges or mandarins, mangos, peaches, nectarines), almond/date shake

Lunch/dinner: same as days 1–5, but increase complexity—grains cooked with 1:6 grain-to-liquid ratio or a thin, liquid dal

Herbal allies: ginger with lime and salt, sweet water lactation tea, fresh ginger tea or tea bag, fennel tea

GROCERIES FOR DAYS 1–10 POSTPARTUM

Carbohydrates: basmati rice, cream of rice, tapioca, oats, semolina flour, Cream of Wheat

Sugar options: raw cane sugar, date sugar, coconut sugar, molasses, maple syrup, jaggery (Indian molasses sugar)

Fats: ghee, sesame oil (not toasted), olive oil

Proteins: split mung beans, red lentils, nut milks, nonhomogenized whole milk, almonds, cashews (more nuts if you are dairy-free)

Fruits: soaked and dried iron-rich fruits such as dates, apricots, figs, and golden raisins

Sweet juices: apple, white grape, apricot

Vegetables: asparagus, carrots, okra, fresh fennel, dill, cilantro, roasted garlic, fresh fenugreek/methi

DAYS 15–28

Breakfast: same as above (for a savory option: savory porridge made with salt and black pepper), miso soup, dal soup with rice, almond date shake

Snack: same as above plus spiced nuts and seeds, nourishing beverages, lactation cookies

Lunch/dinner: grain cooked in a 1:3 (grain to liquid) ratio (wider variety, still soupy but less so than before), increased complexity in protein sources, increased complexity of meal (protein, grain, vegetables)

GROCERIES FOR DAYS 10–21 POSTPARTUM

Carbohydrates: quinoa, amaranth, unrefined flours, couscous, rice pastas

Fats: high lignan flaxseed oil, raw butter

Proteins: fresh yogurt, ricotta, cottage cheese, paneer, urud dal, roasted tahini

Thickeners: arrowroot powder, kudzu powder

Fruits: apples and pears (cooked), sugar or yellow figs, sweet oranges, sweet berries, limes, avocados

Fruit juices: cherry, peach, apricot

Dried fruits (soaked): cherries, currants, prunes

Vegetables: beets (if lochia has diminished); greens such as chard, kale, or spinach (if craved); sweet potatos or yams; winter squash; pumpkin

DAYS 29–42 AND AFTER

Breakfast: oatmeal, Cream of Wheat, cream of rice, cream of quinoa, barley gruel, sautéed greens

Snack: fresh juicy fruit, cooked fruit, soaked and roasted nuts or seeds with digestive spices

Lunch/dinner: more complex food combinations; wider variety of vegetables, proteins, grains; more complexity in meal components

GROCERIES FOR WEEKS 3–6 POSTPARTUM

Carbohydrates: sprouted bread, whole-grain pastas

Fats: cocoa butter, coconut oil (if mama is not feeling cold)

Proteins: adzuki beans

Fruits: fresh papaya or mango, freshly squeezed orange juice or pineapple juice, tamarind

Vegetables: artichoke, summer squash (chayote, zucchini, yellow), green beans, parsley, parsnips, fresh basil

POSTPARTUM SPICES AND HERBS

The following beneficial spices are good to have on hand to cook with, make teas from, and flavor foods with throughout the entire postpartum window, as they support digestion and/or milk production:

Black pepper: increases internal heat, removes toxins, increases circulation, and supports digestion

Cardamom: helps balance emotions, respiratory function, and digestion

Cilantro: purifies the blood, increases digestion, and supports detoxification

Cinnamon: enhances the quality and quantity of milk, improves digestion

Coriander: eases gastrointestinal discomfort, stimulates appetite, assimilates nutrients, aids in gentle detoxification

Cumin: aids digestion and provides a mild hormonal and cooling support

Fennel: helps lactation and digestion, reduces heat and acidity, and is a gentle diuretic

Fenugreek: supports lactation, rejuvenation, respiration, and digestion; may help the uterus release placental fragments when used in a stronger tea

Garlic (roasted, not raw): supports immunity, digestion, and the circulatory system; is also very grounding, is considered rejuvenating, and supports the quality and quantity of mama's milk

Ginger: offers warmth and grounding along with excellent digestive and respiratory support

Pippali: nourishes the blood, nerves, and reproductive tissues; supports digestion and healthy metabolism

Saffron: increases the medicinal benefits of other herbs and supports reproductive rejuvenation; beneficial for the mind, emotions, and heart

POSTPARTUM MAMA RECIPES

The recipes in the rest of this chapter are some of the main recipes I lived on for my first forty-two days postpartum. Start with three days of just rice porridge (kanji), sometimes using the sweet recipe and other times using the savory digestive spices to add a little bit of variety. Generally, you want to stick to rice kanji until you feel real hunger. After the first few days, slowly introduce other foods, starting with more soupy, blended recipes like the warm oatmeal shake, sweet potato smoothie, or the sautéed and steamed fruits. Then, as you feel your digestion getting stronger, start adding more vegetables and whole foods that require more chewing, like the steamed root veggies or kitchari. In the evenings, have the milk tonic.

Be sure to add things gradually, noticing how your body is able to digest them as well as being aware of how different foods may affect your little one. If you notice your babe has more gas or seems fussier, go back to a few days of just kanji, and then slowly introduce just one recipe at a time to see what may be affecting little babe.

Ghee

Ghee, or clarified butter, is one of Ayurveda's most important contributors to a healthy and strong recovery after birth. It deeply nourishes depleted tissues down to the cellular level and rekindles agni, the fire of digestion. It carries the medicinal qualities of food and herbs that are warmed in it through the tissues, and it also supports mama in making rich milk for her baby, balances her hormones, stabilizes her mood and emotions, remedies constipation, and much more. If you are choosing to not have ghee for physiological or ethical reasons, or if you're experiencing congestion, use sesame oil for cooking instead, as it is gently warming, mildly astringent, antiseptic, and antibacterial.

Ingredients

2 quarts (16 sticks) of organic, cultured, unsalted butter

Instructions

Place butter in a pan on medium-low heat to simmer. As the butter melts, it may look cloudy with foam at the top.

Do not stir the cooking butter.

Continue simmering for twenty to thirty minutes until you see the particulates sink to the bottom of the pan and the foam disappears from the top.

Wait until liquefied butter turns a clear amber color and remove from heat. Let cool and then strain through a cotton cheesecloth. Store in a glass jar.

Dashamula Tea

Dashamula means "ten roots" and is known to be a vata-pacifying, grounding, and nourishing tonic. It will support digestion, balance the nervous system, strengthen the body, and calm the mind. Drink twice a day postpartum; each morning and evening.

Ingredients

1 teaspoon dashamula powder

1 cup water

Instructions

Boil the dashamula in the water until there is only ½ cup of liquid remaining. Drink ½ cup in the morning and repeat in the evening each day for forty-two days.

Sweet Water Lactation Tea

Not only does this tea support healthy lactation and breastfeeding, it also supports digestion and soothes the nerves. The low ratio of herbs to water allows this tea to stay hydrating rather than drying. This recipe by Ysha Oaks is beneficial to drink daily for forty-two days.

Ingredients

1 teaspoon fennel seeds

½ teaspoon fenugreek seeds

4¼ cups water

Instructions

Add spices into boiled water, turn off heat, and steep for fifteen or twenty minutes. Strain and sip warm throughout the day.

CCF Tea

Cumin, coriander, and fennel tea is an Ayurvedic staple. CCF tea supports healthy digestion, absorption, assimilation, elimination, and lactation. It helps the body break down toxins in the gastrointestinal tract, and because it supports agni, the digestive fire, as well as supporting the absorption of nutrients, it is great to sip on before, during, or after meals.

Ingredients

1 teaspoon cumin

1 teaspoon coriander

1 teaspoon fennel

4¼ cups water

Instructions

Boil water, turn down to simmer, and add spices.
Cover and steep for ten minutes. Strain and drink throughout the day.

Garlic Chutney

Garlic supports appetite, digestion, lactation, grounding, and immunity—as long as it is well cooked and properly prepared. Garlic also greatly minimizes the risk of infection and generally speeds up the post-birth recovery process.

This recipe for garlic chutney, from Ysha Oakes's *Touching Heaven*, ensures that the garlic is cooked and the moisture has evaporated, allowing the garlic to release its helpful properties without negative side effects to baby or mother. Mamas can take 1 teaspoon of this chutney with savory meals, beginning three days postpartum, and continue throughout the forty-two days. For example, it can be mixed into a soup broth, rice dishes, or guacamole. Pitta mamas or mamas showing signs of excess heat in body, mind, or emotions should consume this chutney more sparingly.

Ingredients

4 tablespoons ghee

½ cup peeled garlic cloves

1 cup unsweetened coconut, finely shredded

4 tablespoons black peppercorns

½ teaspoon coriander seeds

1¼ teaspoons salt

juice of one lime

Instructions

1. Heat 2 tablespoons of the ghee in a skillet on medium heat and add the garlic cloves. Sauté them on medium heat for about four minutes.
2. When the garlic cloves have cooled, puree the garlic along with the rest of the ingredients in a blender to a fine paste. Add a little water for ease in grinding.
3. Heat the rest of the ghee, add the ground paste, and sauté on medium heat for about twelve minutes.

Herbal Chewing Mix

Build your digestive fire with this simple preparation, another recipe from Ysha Oakes's *Touching Heaven*. Enjoy 1–2 teaspoons after each meal starting three days postpartum, continuing for forty-two days. Chew well for maximum benefit. Keep a day or two's supply of the mixture in a small bowl on your dining table and take some with you to make it available right after a meal. Keep the remaining mix refrigerated. You can experiment with different measures of the ingredients for variety in taste. For a different texture, grind roasted sesame, fennel, and coconut in a coffee grinder.

Ingredients

½ cup fennel seeds

1 cup sesame seeds

2 cups unsweetened coconut flakes

½ teaspoon turmeric

2 teaspoons cardamom

1 tablespoon clove

1 teaspoon ginger

1 teaspoon mineral salt (or black salt if available)

Instructions

1. In a cast-iron pan, toast fennel and sesame seeds until they turn light brown (the sesame seeds will pop, so cover the pan with a splatter screen or glass lid).
2. Add coconut and toast for a few more minutes, until everything turns golden brown; stir constantly to prevent burning.
3. Place the toasted coconut, sesame, and fennel seeds in a bowl.
4. Add the remaining spices and stir well.
5. Let the mixture cool completely before storing in the fridge, keeping out just what you can use in the next day or two.

Hot Milk Tonic

Ayurvedic medicine views milk as uniquely rejuvenative, as milk is valued for its ability to nourish the deepest tissue layers more quickly than any other food. This hot milk tonic will soothe your nerves, encourage healthy digestion and elimination, restore strength and vitality, and build a healthy milk supply. If you can find a local source of raw milk, that is ideal. Otherwise, a cream-top milk from your local health food store is best.

Ingredients

1-inch piece fresh ginger (grated)

1 teaspoon cardamom

1 teaspoon clove buds

1 teaspoon turmeric

1 cinnamon stick

¼ teaspoon black peppercorns

¼ teaspoon fennel seeds

1 cup whole cream-top milk

1 cup water

iron-rich sweetener to taste

Instructions

Bring all ingredients to a boil. Turn down to a simmer and partially cover. Simmer for ten minutes, then remove from the heat. Enjoy every night before bed. Be sure to not mix milk with any salty foods!

Almond Date Shake

This shake made from almonds and dates is a nourishing and delicious ojas-building drink that can be had warm or at room temperature any time of day (or night!).

Ingredients

1 cup raw almonds

4 cups water

6 soaked dates

½ teaspoon cardamom

¼ teaspoon ginger powder

10 saffron threads

Instructions

Soak the almonds overnight and then squeeze the skins off.

Blend the almonds with all other ingredients on high speed for about a minute.

Warm Oatmeal Shake

Oats build ojas and are very nourishing during pregnancy, birth, and postpartum. This warm oatmeal shake can also be used during labor for energy.

Ingredients

4 cups water

½ cup oats (soaked for at least 30 minutes, then rinsed)

½ teaspoon powdered ginger

½ teaspoon cinnamon

½ teaspoon cardamon

pinch of salt

¼ cup soaked cashews

4 tablespoons maple syrup or other iron-rich sweetener (or more, to taste)

1 tablespoon ghee

Instructions

Boil the water, then add oats and spices.

Cook until oats are broken down and the porridge is soupy—about ten minutes.

Pour into the blender. Add cashews and maple syrup and blend on low speed (lightly covered so that the blender doesn't explode from the heat!), and gradually move toward blending on high speed until the mixture is smooth.

Pour the shake into a mug and top with ghee. Enjoy it while it's warm.

Warm Yam Smoothie

Yams are a perfect postpartum root vegetable. They are smooth, building, grounding, and sweet—all qualities that soothe vata dosha. This yam smoothie is warm and blended with nut milk and digestive spices, making it nourishing yet light and easy to digest: the perfect postpartum combination.

Ingredients

1 cup skinned and boiled yams

2–4 Medjool dates, pitted

2 cups water

4 cups fresh almond milk

½-inch chunk fresh ginger (or ¼ teaspoon ginger powder)

½ teaspoon turmeric

pinch of black pepper

1 teaspoon cinnamon

Instructions

Boil the yams and the dates in 2 cups of water; when the yams are soft, remove them along with the dates.

Put the yams and dates in a blender; add almond milk and spices.

Blend until smooth. Enjoy warm.

Kanji: Rice Porridge for Mamas

Rice porridge, also known as kanji or congee, is popular throughout Asia and is the number-one dish for new mothers to eat during the first few days after birth. Traditionally used in both Chinese medicine and Ayurveda, this simple dish contains all the qualities necessary to jump-start postpartum recovery. Hot, soft, oily, sweet, and well spiced, this rice pudding is deeply nourishing as well as comforting. It not only soothes the nerves, but it also nourishes the tissues, stimulates digestion, and rebuilds the blood. Kanji is medicine for mamas!

You can gradually decrease the amount of water in this kanji recipe as your digestive capacity increases.

*Ingredients**

½ cup basmati rice

8 cups water

½ cup sucanat (iron-rich sugar)

¼ cup ghee

1 teaspoon ginger powder

½ teaspoon cinnamon powder

½ teaspoon cardamom powder

½ teaspoon clove powder

¼ teaspoon black pepper

¼ teaspoon turmeric powder

**Note:* If you are craving salty, you can use the same spice blend as in the kitchari recipe instead of the sweet spices listed here after three days postpartum.

Instructions

Rinse rice several times until the water runs clear. Bring water to a boil and add rice. Reduce heat to a simmer. Cook with the lid off, stirring occasionally for several hours. It is important to cook this dish long enough so that the rice actually breaks down and loses its form—it works great in a slow cooker! (Add all ingredients to the slow cooker and cook on low for eight hours.) When the rice begins to thicken, add sugar, spices, and ghee. When the consistency is gelatinous, take the kanji off the heat and serve hot with a spoonful of ghee on top.

Nourishing Oatmeal

Oatmeal is grounding, nourishing, and soothing for the nervous system—all desirable qualities to cultivate after the intensity of birth. Its vata-soothing properties promote postpartum healing and restoration. Oatmeal can be a bit heavy, so this recipe lightens it up with some warming spices like cinnamon, ginger, and nutmeg to make it easier to digest. Ground flax seeds and dates will further oatmeal's rejuvenative and lactation-boosting properties. It needs to be liquidy, slimy, and smooth to have the desired effects of being digestible and calming.

Ingredients

¾ cup oats (soaked in water for at least 30 minutes)

3 cups water (or substitute 1 cup of the water with 1 cup of milk for added nourishment)

1 tablespoon ghee

½ teaspoon cinnamon powder

¼ teaspoon ginger powder

⅛ teaspoon nutmeg powder

5 dates, chopped

⅓ cup coconut sugar or maple syrup

¼ cup ground flax seeds

Instructions

Add oats, water, ghee, and spices to a pot and bring to a boil.

Turn down to medium-low heat, add the dates, and simmer for ten minutes. Cook until soft and soupy.

Take the pot off the heat and add the sweetener and ground flax seeds.

Iron-Rich Dal

Mung bean soup is the perfect addition to a postpartum diet. This dal is easy to digest, highly nourishing, and gives strength to the recovering mama. In combination with beets—root veggies that are rich in iron—the result is the perfect grounding and nourishing postpartum soup. You can make a thinner soup by using a smaller amount of beans at first, and gradually increase to the full amount as your digestive capacity increases.

Ingredients

⅔ cup yellow split mung beans

5 cups water

1½ cups cubed beets

1 teaspoon cumin

1 teaspoon coriander

2 tablespoons lime juice

salt and pepper to taste

Instructions

Soak yellow split mung beans overnight. Drain and rinse the beans.

Boil the beets, beans, and spices in 5 cups of water until the beans soften and start to separate (about forty-five minutes). Add lime juice. Season with salt and pepper to taste.

Optional: Blend it all up! Be careful blending hot liquids, as the blender might explode! Start with the vent open on super-low speed, then gradually turn the speed up until it is at its highest. Blend until smooth.

Kitchari

Kitchari is a complete food that's easy to digest and gives strength and vitality while nourishing all the tissues of the body. Kitchari is tridoshic (balancing for all body types) and literally the perfect meal! The marriage of white basmati rice (unhulled, so it's easier to digest than other grains) and split mung beans (the one legume that won't cause intestinal discomfort) provides the ten essential amino acids our body craves, forming a complete plant-based protein. You will receive fiber and nutrients from the vegetables in this recipe and medicinal qualities from your spices.

Its digestibility makes kitchari an excellent meal for postpartum healing. When you first introduce kitchari postpartum, cut back on the rice and mung beans (perhaps starting with a quarter-cup of each, rather than the suggested two-thirds) to make for a soupier kitchari. Gradually increase the amount as mama's digestion increases.

Ingredients

⅔ cup basmati rice

⅔ cup split yellow mung dal, soaked for four to eight hours

about 6 cups water

1½ cups assorted vegetables

2 tablespoons ghee

½- to 1-inch ginger root, chopped or grated

1 teaspoon coriander powder

1 teaspoon cumin powder

½ teaspoon mustard seeds

½ teaspoon turmeric powder

¼ teaspoon black pepper

½ teaspoon asafetida (Hing)

½ teaspoon fennel seeds

handful fresh cilantro leaves

salt to taste

Instructions

Wash rice and soaked mung beans in two changes of water.

Add the beans to about 6 cups of water and cook for twenty minutes on a low boil.

Add the rice and simmer covered until it becomes soft, about thirty more minutes. While the rice and beans are cooking, prepare the veggies, cutting them into bite-sized pieces.

Add the vegetables to the cooked rice and mung bean mixture and cook twenty minutes longer.

In a separate saucepan, sauté the seeds in the ghee until they pop. Then add the other spices. Stir together to release the flavors.

Stir the sautéed spices into the cooked mung bean, rice, and vegetable mixture. Add chopped fresh cilantro and salt to taste (avoid salt until after three days postpartum in the case of swelling; avoid cilantro until after two weeks postpartum).

Steamed Veggies with Tahini Sauce

Steaming or boiling is the best way to have your veggies postpartum, as these methods add liquidity that helps to balance the dry quality of vata. I prefer steaming, as the veggies do not lose as many of the nutrients into the water as they do when boiled. Any root vegetable can be used in this recipe (besides white or red potatoes), as root veggies are very grounding for a postpartum mama. Tahini (sesame seed paste) is delicious and rich with calcium—a critical postpartum nutrient, especially for nursing mamas. This veggie and tahini combination is best served after two or three weeks postpartum.

Ingredients

For the steamed veggies:

½ cup cubed yams

½ cup peeled, cubed beets

½ cup chopped fennel bulb

½ cup cubed zucchini or asparagus

For the tahini sauce:

⅓–½ cup tahini

½ small lime, juiced

2 bulbs roasted garlic

water as needed

salt and pepper, to taste

Instructions

Add sufficient water to the steamer and insert the steamer basket, making sure that the water is below the steamer basket.

Place yam and beets into the steamer basket. Cover with lid, and steam the root vegetables over medium heat for twenty to twenty-five minutes.

Add fennel and zucchini to the steamer basket and steam until all vegetables are very soft.

Separately, blend all ingredients for tahini sauce, adding water 1 tablespoon at a time until the sauce reaches the desired consistency.

Serve veggies topped with as much tahini sauce as desired.

Sautéed and Stewed Apples

A cooked apple serves as a gentle daily cleanse for the digestive system. It supports regularity, strengthens digestion, lowers acidity and excessive hunger, boosts immunity to prevent most colds and flus, and is a simple and delicious way to start the day.

Apples are best eaten starting seven to ten days postpartum. Prior to that, stewed dried fruits that are rich in iron (such as raisins, dates, and prunes) are recommended. You can follow this apple recipe and substitute iron-rich fruits for the apples.

Ingredients

1 large apple
1 tablespoon ghee
3–5 saffron threads
1 teaspoon cardamom
3 cloves
½ teaspoon fennel seeds
3 soaked dates (optional)
3 soaked prunes (optional)
¼ cup water

Instructions

Peel the apple and cut it into bite-sized pieces.

In a pan, add ghee with saffron, cardamon, cloves, and fennel seeds.

Sauté the spices in the ghee for about two minutes to enhance flavor and extract their medicinal potency.

Add the apples, stirring them occasionally as you let them sauté for three minutes. (*Optional:* sauté dates or soaked prunes along with the apples.)

Add ¼ cup of water and then cover until the apples are soft and transparent.

Tahini Cookies

Sesame is revered in Ayurveda as an ojas builder and breast milk enhancer; its naturally balanced composition of qualities makes it a tonic for increasing strength and immunity. High in healthy fats from the oily sesame seeds, tahini paste nourishes and strengthens nervous, muscle, and fat tissue. Because tahini is also high in calcium, it supports the maintenance of bone strength. Its earthy quality and magnesium content help soothe and relax tension in the muscles, allowing you to unwind after a period of stress. Enjoy these tahini cookies throughout pregnancy. Resume this nutrient-filled treat again after two weeks postpartum.

Ingredients

1 cup tahini
2 cups oat flour
1 cup sucanat
2 tablespoons yogurt or apple sauce

¼ teaspoon salt

½ teaspoon cinnamon

½ teaspoon ginger powder

2 teaspoons black and white sesame seeds, plus extra for topping

1 tablespoon shatavari powder(optional)

Instructions

Mix all ingredients together, adding one at a time in the order listed.

Make little balls with the batter and gently flatten with a fork on a greased cookie sheet, leaving space between.

Bake at 350 degrees Fahrenheit for twelve to fourteen minutes and let them cool completely.

Mama Jill's Cookies

This is a delicious, nourishing cookie recipe from my sister's husband's mama. Enjoy throughout pregnancy and after six weeks postpartum.

These cookies are the perfect ojas booster! My family uses husked almond flour and ghee to nourish the tissues and maple syrup to nourish vata dosha. Feel free to play with added ingredients such as dates instead of the chocolate chips, black sesame seeds, and nuts!

Ingredients

¼ cup coconut oil or ghee

¼ cup date sugar or maple syrup

1 spoonful yogurt (vegan is fine too!)

1½ cups almond flour

2 tablespoons coconut flour

½ teaspoon baking soda

½ teaspoon sea salt

½ cup chocolate chips

Instructions

Mix wet ingredients in one bowl, dry ingredients in another, then mix together.

Spoon dough out onto a baking tray in small scoops.

Bake at 350 degrees Fahrenheit for nine to twelve minutes.

My little love,
Every moment with you is so, so precious.
I am seeing how time moves so quickly
as I watch you shift and change and grow each day.
Your smile lights up my life.
The new little sounds you make;
your wiggles and squirms;
your beautiful blue eyes;
the way you look at the world
gives me a clearer perspective
of the newness,
the presence,
the gifts
of each moment.
You are this precious little soul
that has somehow been entrusted in our care,
and it is the greatest privilege I've ever had:
to get to love you.
You are the smallest you will ever be, in this moment.
The joy and the heartache that comes with loving you so much.

It is the sweetest experience: getting to be your mama.
Thank you,
for being the easiest thing to love.

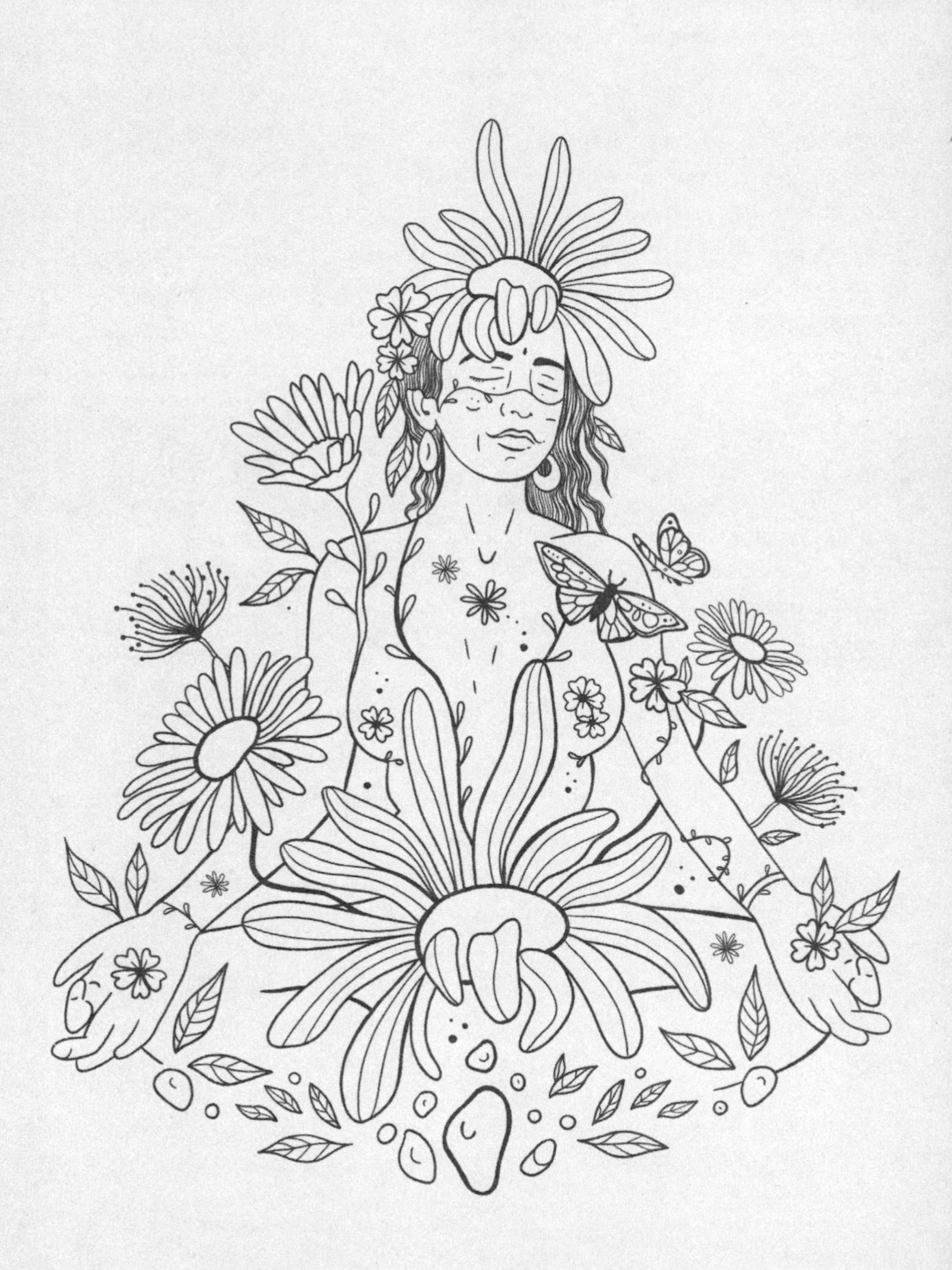

Beneficial Herbs and Essential Oils

· 9 ·

The medical model of care has given us ways to treat acute conditions, but allopathic medicine often leaves us with a trail of side effects that may complicate our situation even more. Pharmaceuticals treat symptoms but often don't address the root cause of an imbalance, meaning that we become dependent on using these medicines in order to feel okay. Natural plant-based medicine helps to ease the discomfort of symptoms while simultaneously treating the root cause of the imbalance, leading to sustainable health and healing in the body and mind.

Using herbs and oils as part of your daily routine, as outlined in this chapter, will bring astounding abundance into your life, as that is the energy of Mama Nature. She helps you to heal in a holistic way, nourishing your mind, body, and emotions. Not only will the plants discussed in the next pages deliver their medicine into the tissues of your body, but their energetic blueprint also leaves a mark on your energy field. Think of each plant as a personality; as you spend time with them each day you will begin to develop a relationship and understand the energetic qualities of each.

Ayurvedic plant-based remedies can support you in the journey of motherhood, whether you are using these botanicals to prepare your womb for conception, to address occasional or acute imbalances during pregnancy, or for supporting healthy lactation, balanced mood, and restful sleep postpartum. The chapter also discusses oil remedies for labor and birth, and then for supporting your little one as you welcome them into the world.

In addition to the herbs cited in this chapter, you can refer back to Krsna Jivani's "Light on the Sacred Window" in chapter 6 (see the sidebar on page 191), along with "Postpartum Spices and Herbs" in chapter 8 (see page 285), for other staple herbs that are highly recommended postpartum.

HERBAL ALLIES FOR PREGNANCY AND THE POSTPARTUM WINDOW

The herbs described below are safe during pregnancy and breastfeeding and can be made into teas to be consumed daily or as needed. Drinking herbal teas during pregnancy is an easy way to boost nutrients so that you can grow a healthy babe. During the postpartum period, herbal support can provide nourishment for your body to heal; teas should be made with a ratio of 1 teaspoon of herbs to 8 cups of water to keep their hydrating properties. If you are using the powdered form of the herbs, especially for the roots, you can make a decoction by boiling 1 teaspoon of the powder in 2 cups of water and boiling until you have just one cup of water left.

ASHWAGANDHA ROOT

Ashwagandha root is a rejuvenative and an adaptogen—it helps the body adapt to stress and intense changes. The word *ashwagandha* translates as "strength of a horse"—ashwaganda is renowned for its ability to enhance strength and vitality. It also supports healthy sleeping patterns, reduces stress, and supports the immune system and the health of the reproductive systems for both men and women.

FENNEL SEED

Fennel is medicine for the gastrointestinal tract, easing cramping, gas, and bloating. In addition to its many digestive benefits, fennel seed has been used for boosting fertility, alleviating water retention, and facilitating a healthy supply of breast milk in nursing mamas.

GINGER

Ginger's warm, soothing qualities make it one of the most well-known medicinal plants. Celebrated not only for its spicy flavor that stimulates the palate and supports digestion, ginger also offers relief for expectant mamas by easing morning sickness and nausea.

NETTLES

Nettle contains a rich supply of vitamins and minerals and is a powerful support for the nervous system. From an Ayurvedic perspective, nettle serves as a nourishing and rejuvenative tonic—particularly for the kidneys and adrenals. The herb increases ojas (vitality), making it useful for mamas who need extra nourishment during pregnancy and breastfeeding—but nettles have astringent properties, so new mamas should wait at least six weeks postpartum to resume nettles in their diet.

OATSTRAW

Oatstraw is an incredible herb for soothing the nervous system (similar to oats) and is thus a perfect tonic for pacifying vata. Rich in calcium, magnesium, and B vitamins, it is a nutritive tonic for the whole body. Make oatstraw into a tea whenever you feel fatigue, nervous exhaustion, anxiety, stress, low energy, unsettled sleep, or insomnia. Oatstraw is the perfect herbal ally during pregnancy and in your first forty-two days after giving birth.

RED RASPBERRY LEAVES

Throughout history, herbalists and midwives have turned to red raspberry leaf tea to ease discomfort during menstruation, pregnancy, and labor. As a mineral-rich remedy, red raspberry leaf is especially valuable in the last two or three months of pregnancy, because of its ability to strengthen the uterus prior to giving birth. Many mamas continue to drink red raspberry leaf tea after childbirth because of the way it helps restore the reproductive system and continues to nourish.

ROSE

Rose—whether it be petals used in teas or rosewater for drinks and flavoring—is medicine for the heart and mind. Rose will support mama in processing her emotions so that they are well digested and integrated into her being. Rose also brings the energetic experience of feeling God's grace in our lives, and thus a feeling that life is happening *for* you, not *to* you.

SHATAVARI

The literal translation of *shatavari* is "she who possesses one hundred husbands." Shatavari is an adaptogen—it helps the body adapt to its circumstance, bringing the body back into a state of balance, whether that means resisting stress when needed, giving energy when depleted, or increasing milk supply based on the baby's need. It has been used in Ayurveda for thousands of years to support female reproductive and maternal health.

Shatavari is helpful in regulating menstrual cycles because it supports estrogen and the luteinizing hormone—the hormone responsible for triggering ovulation, crucial for conceiving. Postpartum (after 10 days or so to assure the digestive fire is strong), shatavari can help to increase milk supply, reduce stress, balance hormones, rebuild strength and vitality, and boost immunity.

Note: Shatavari is contraindicated if the mother has any history of high estrogen conditions such as fibroid tumors, cysts, polyps, or reproductive cancers. In this case, guduchi is a recommended replacement for shatavari, as an herb that will strengthen the uterus during pregnancy without affecting estrogen levels.

Blue Lotus for New Mothers

Blue lotus (*Nymphaea caerulea*) has been known since ancient Egyptian times as the "flower of intuition." It was traditionally used for its meditative qualities that aid in Third Eye intuition and lucid dreaming. Although there is no reference to blue lotus that I am aware of in Ayurveda, it has become one of my main herbal allies as a new mother.

Blue lotus has the power to cool the nervous system and relax the entire body. As a sedative and a nervine, it provides a calming, euphoric feeling. It can be a wonderful aid for sleep and stress (hello, motherhood!). Some people may experience it as deeply relaxing, while others experience it as a mild stimulant.

Blue lotus has the intelligence to provide what is needed for a new mother. How we experience the effects of plants often reflects the profile of the plant itself. In this case, the plant that is used to enhance intuition in the recipient itself in turn uses intuition to serve the one who takes it.

Blue lotus is believed to bring insight, release of fear, and connection with the cosmos. I love this herb for new mothers because it provides a feeling of calm, centered, meditative relaxation that is greatly needed throughout motherhood. It can help to promote restful sleep, calm anxiety, strengthen breast tissue, uncover the root of your depression, release the worries in your mind, relieve pain and muscle spasms (such as afterpains and cramping), connect to your "motherly instincts," and much more.

Blue lotus is traditionally an aphrodisiac, used to support fertility and conception. But its use is dangerous during pregnancy; only use it prior to conception, during postpartum, and throughout motherhood.

See the pages that follow for two of my blue lotus milk tea recipes, along with recipes for two ready-to-use herbal tea blends to keep on the shelf.

—Krsna Jivani, clinical herbalist

Mama's Mood Tea 1

You can drink this tea as your daily pick-me-up—it boosts dopamine levels in the brain and gives sustainable energy. Omit the jasmine green tea in the early postpartum period or when you are choosing not to consume caffeine. I find jasmine green tea to have a gentle, uplifting, energizing effect that keeps me in balance while still providing the daily energy I need!

Ingredients

1 teaspoon jasmine green tea

1 teaspoon rose petals

1 teaspoon mucuna powder

1 teaspoon brahmi

1 teaspoon blue lotus (omit during pregnancy)

1–3 tablespoons (to taste) honey

milk or nut milk

Moon Milk Tea

During the postpartum window, drink this tea before bed for a deep, relaxing sleep. *Note:* if you are co-sleeping with your babe, be cautious of overdoing sleep aids. If you sleep too deeply, sharing a bed can be dangerous for your newborn. Use your motherly intuition to do what is best for you and your babe.

Ingredients

1 teaspoon blue lotus (omit this ingredient during pregnancy)

1 teaspoon rose

1 teaspoon chamomile

1 teaspoon passionflower (use sparingly during pregnancy)

1–3 tablespoons (to taste) honey

milk or nut milk to taste

Instructions for Both Teas

Bring a pot of water to almost boiling on the stove.

Leaving out the rose, honey, and milk, steep all the other ingredients in the near-boiling water for five to seven minutes.

Remove the pot from the stove, add the rose petals, and steep for three minutes.

Strain out the tea leaves and petals.

Once the tea is cooled enough to sip, add honey (as honey should not be heated).

Enjoy warm, adding milk to taste if you wish (if you are using cow's milk, boil the milk with a pinch of cardamom before adding it).

The following recipes suggest blends you can make to have ready-to-use herbal elixirs on the shelf.

Mama's Mood Tea 2

This variation on Mama's Mood Tea leaves out the blue lotus but adds ginger, shatavari, and maca. Like the blue lotus version, it boosts dopamine levels in the brain and gives sustainable energy—it can be taken as an aphrodisiac during preconception, to boost mood during pregnancy, and to regulate mama's hormones postpartum.

Ingredients (makes 7–8 servings)

1 tablespoon rose petals or powder

1 tablespoon mucuna powder

1 teaspoon dried jasmine flowers

1 tablespoon dried ginger or powder

1 tablespoon shatavari

1 tablespoon maca

1 tablespoon vanilla powder

Mood Milk Tea 2

This variation on Moon Milk Tea leaves out the blue lotus but adds ginger and ashwaganda. It can be taken during pregnancy and postpartum to ease anxiety and aid with sleep.

Ingredients (makes 3–6 servings)

1 tablespoon rose petals or powder

1 tablespoon chamomile

1 tablespoon ginger powder

1 tablespoon passionflower (use sparingly during pregnancy)

1 tablespoon ashwagandha

Instructions (for Both Teas)

Mix the herbs and store these tea blends in a jar in your pantry. Use 1 tablespoon of the desired tea steeped in boiled water or simmered in hot milk as desired. After steeping or simmering in your water or milk, let the elixir cool down enough to sip and then add 1 tablespoon of honey, or to taste. (Do not add honey to boiling hot water or milk, as honey becomes toxic when heated.) Enjoy your elixir or milk tonic while it's warm.

These tea blends are made with potent herbs, so take them only one to three times per week rather than daily. You can also alter the recipes by omitting various herbs and picking and choosing others to add, switching it up every time you make it.

ESSENTIAL OILS FOR SUPPORT AND HEALING

Mama earth has given us everything that we need to be healthy and to heal.

Our world and our food are laden with chemicals. Over one hundred thousand children in the United States get sick every year from the chemicals in house cleaners alone. These are toxins that we consciously invite into our homes. The smell after cleaning your bathroom that makes it feel "clean"? Those are the chemical constituents of toxic cleaners entering into your nose, and thus into your bloodstream, transferring into every organ of your body within minutes. Essential oils work the same way, though instead of having negative side effects, each and every oil carries side benefits that will help your body heal.

Essential oils can be used to make your own nontoxic house cleaners. They can be used to make your own natural bath salts, as well as hair and skincare products, and they can treat chronic and acute health conditions. They are scientifically proven to heal tissues and organs, they have powerful effects on your mind and your mood, and they may even mend broken hearts.

Essential oils always seemed a little "woo-woo" to me. As far as I knew, they were something you used for relaxation or to make your home smell pleasant. Little did I know, essential oils are mama earth's most potent form of medicine. One drop of peppermint oil is equivalent to the medicinal compounds found in 28 cups of peppermint tea! They are the volatile compounds (meaning they evaporate quickly—and are absorbed into the skin just as quickly) found in the bark, resin, seeds, stems, flowers, roots, and leaves of plants, as well as in the skin of citrus fruits.

Each plant, and thus each oil, has distinctive qualities and healing properties. They are a secondary metabolite of the plant, meaning they are not needed for the plant's survival but are there to fend off predators and other threatening influences. They support the entire plant's system, enabling it to thrive. When humans use them, they support us in the same way.

QUALITY IS EVERYTHING

Because essential oil regulation is limited and standards are minimal, many botanical oil companies can advertise that their oils are 100 percent pure but, in fact, they may be full of chemical additives and fillers used in order to save money and time. Unfortunately, when proper testing measures are not taken, it is impossible to ensure that an essential oil is truly "pure." For effective healing to take place, it is important to only use unprocessed oils that are sourced directly from mama nature with nothing added—*especially* when using these oils as a pregnant mama or for your babe.

doTERRA is a company that I have grown to love and feel completely comfortable advocating for. They have trusted alliances with honest growers and distillers. They have searched the world for the plants with the most therapeutic compounds. They have strict standards that verify the purity of each batch, along with third-party testing to guarantee transparency. To ensure that each bottle of essential oil is pure and free from contaminants or synthetic fillers, doTERRA created the Certified Pure Therapeutic Grade protocol. The oils and blends that I suggest below are all from doTERRA and can be ordered through the link provided in the resources section of this book.

APPROACHES FOR USING OILS

For acute conditions, essential oils can be used every twenty minutes until symptoms subside, then used every two to six hours as needed. For ongoing conditions, use two times per day as preventive medicine, typically in the morning and the evening.

You can access the healing properties of essential oils three main ways: aromatically, topically, and internally. When essential oils are used *aromatically*, they are inhaled, absorbed through the respiratory tract and lungs, and then circulated through your bloodstream. Aromatic oils can be used in a scent diffuser, or you can inhale the scent from your cupped hands or directly from the oil bottle. Your nose is the most direct route to your brain, which makes the aromatic use of oils one of the fastest ways to alter your mood. The scent travels from your olfactory nerve to your limbic system, and once in the limbic system it triggers a response in your brain based on memories and experiences, offering immediate benefits that can be uplifting, renewing, soothing, calming, or energizing.

To use oils *topically*, you put the oils directly on your skin or diluted in a carrier oil; the oil gets absorbed into your bloodstream and circulates around your entire body within minutes. (*Note:* There are some "hot" oils—such as oregano, cassia, clove, thyme, and cinnamon—that you should never apply directly onto your skin without a carrier oil.) The tissues and the organs then absorb what they need, whether it is the plant medicine or the energetic quality of the plant, such as "calm" or "energize." When using essential oils for your little one, always dilute 1 drop of oil per 1 tablespoon of a carrier oil such as olive, sweet almond, sesame, or coconut oils.

You can apply oil topically to any area of pain or concern (dilute as needed), or apply more generally under the nose, at the back of neck, to forehead, or to wrists. To affect the entire body, apply oil to the bottoms of feet, spine, or navel. Add a warm compress or massage into tissues to drive the oils deeper, if you wish. You can also add 6–8 drops of essential oils to bath salts before adding them to your bath.

Pure essential oils can also be taken *internally*: remember that oils are what give plants and fruits much of their flavor. Because our bodies are already designed to metabolize and process plants and fruits, we are consequently equipped to metabolize essential oils (when taken in appropriate doses), which have higher concentrations of the natural compounds. When taken internally, the oils are absorbed into systemic circulation via the digestive tract. As lipid-soluble compounds, essential oils can easily be transported to all the body's organs, even the brain. *Note:* Not all essential oils are safe for internal use, and I only advocate the use of doTERRA's essential oils internally.

To use an oil internally, put a drop under your tongue, hold for a few seconds, and then swallow. You can also dilute a drop of oil by adding it to a teaspoon of honey, and then adding that to warm water. To send the oil directly to your digestive system, put a drop of oil in an empty veggie capsule and swallow.

MAMA MUST-HAVES

The next few pages provide an outline of the oils that I would personally suggest to have on hand for common conditions that a pregnant, birthing, and postpartum mama might experience, as well as essential oil solutions for your babe.

PREGNANCY

Copaiba. Take 1 drop under the tongue morning and evening for headaches and nervous system support.

doTERRA DigestZen blend. Take 1 drop internally when needed to relieve nausea and morning sickness, as well as indigestion.

Lemon. Use aromatically to help with nausea and for its energizing and uplifting effect.

Frankincense. Take internally to tone and strengthen the uterus, and for its emotional effect of calming the nervous system (helping us to "be here now").

Peppermint. Apply topically for headaches, sore muscles, and tension; inhale as an aromatic to relieve indigestion and nausea; use for cooling if you are feeling overheated.

LABOR

Lavender and clary sage. Diffuse lavender and clary sage together to promote relaxation and stabilize contractions.

Lavender and frankincense. Lavender and frankincense, used topically with a carrier oil, can be used to promote skin integrity of the perineum throughout the birthing process. They can be applied topically toward the end of pregnancy and during birth to help prevent tearing.

Peppermint. Peppermint has the ability to stimulate the central nervous system, offering profound effects on mood. Diffuse to give energy and to ease any anxiety.

Ylang ylang. Ylang ylang is a feminine, floral scent. It reduces stress, muscle tension, and pain. Ylang ylang contains a naturally occurring substance called linalool that reduces anxiety. During labor, ylang ylang can be diffused or placed in a carrier oil for massage.

Cardamon. Traditionally, Ayurveda recommends that a birthing mother inhale the smoke of cardamom and calamus during labor. This can be inhaled as an incense, or the room can be filled with these scents by using a diffuser. Cardamon particularly is a warming and powerful vata pacifier that eases cramping, helps with nausea, and reduces pain.

POSTPARTUM

doTERRA Balance blend. Created with the purpose of grounding the body, mind, and emotions, doTERRA Balance is formulated with emotionally beneficial oils that work together to create a sense of calmness, stability, and well-being. Diffuse or apply topically to the bottoms of your feet.

doTERRA Serenity blend. doTERRA's Serenity is medicine for the nervous system. It is a restful blend that helps reduce stress and promotes deep sleep and relaxation for mama and baby. Diffuse it as desired, and apply topically to the bottoms of your feet.

NEWBORN

DigestZen blend. Diluted with a carrier oil, DigestZen can be massaged clockwise on baby's belly and spine if they are experiencing any discomfort due to colic or gassiness.

Lavender. Lavender is amazing to diffuse at nighttime to support little babe's rest, as well as to create an association with scent and sleep. You can put a drop in baby's massage oil anytime to support rest and relaxation. Lavender also helps to relieve skin irritations, including cradle cap, diaper rash, and heat rash.

Melaleuca. Melaleuca, more widely known as tea tree, is medicine for skin infections and rashes. It also boosts your little one's immune system and improves blood and oxygen circulation. Apply topically mixed with a carrier oil.

Roman chamomile. Babies who have trouble sleeping can benefit from the natural soothing effects of chamomile, an oil that is traditionally used to treat insomnia. Together with lavender, chamomile can also relieve symptoms of colic, and its soothing and anti-inflammatory properties make it valuable as a treatment for skin conditions.

Rosewood. Rosewood is said to protect baby's energetic field; use it in a diffuser throughout the day and night

ESSENTIAL OIL SOLUTIONS FOR PREGNANCY

The following are essential oil solutions for common conditions during pregnancy. Whereas the oils listed above are ones that I would suggest every mama have on hand, the ones below are suggested on a case-per-case basis and to be used as needed.

EDEMA/SWELLING: During pregnancy, the extra fluid in the body and the pressure from the growing uterus can cause swelling (*edema*) in the ankles and feet—and it can even show up in other parts of the body. Use the following oil blends to increase blood and lymphatic flow and reduce the discomfort associated with edema.

Edema Massage Oil

3 drops ginger
2 drops cypress
2 drops lavender
2 teaspoons carrier oil such as almond, coconut, or sesame oil

Combine oils with 2 teaspoons of carrier oil and massage onto legs and feet, toward the heart.

Edema Foot Soak

Bowl of hot water
1 teaspoon Epsom salt
1 drop cypress essential oil
1–2 drops lemon or grapefruit oil

Stir oils into the Epsom salt, then add to hot water.
Soak feet for ten or fifteen minutes.

BALANCE METABOLISM, RELIEVE SUGAR CRAVINGS, SUPPORT APPETITE, AND SUPPORT BODY ACCEPTANCE

Grapefruit, doTERRA Slims and Sassy blend, or kumquat. Use aromatically.

FATIGUE

doTERRA Motivate, Citrus Bliss, or Passion blends. Use aromatically or apply topically.

Basil. Use aromatically or apply topically.

Lemon or peppermint. Use aromatically.

GESTATIONAL DIABETES

Cinnamon, coriander, or cassia. Use aromatically or apply topically.

HEADACHES

Copaiba and frankincense. Take internally.

Peppermint. Use aromatically; apply topically to temples, forehead, and the back of your neck; or put a drop on your thumb and press to the roof of your mouth as far back as you can for fifteen seconds.

HEARTBURN

DigestZen blend, peppermint, or ginger. Apply topically directly onto your breastbone; take 1 drop internally.

Cardamom. Take internally or apply topically.

ITCHY SKIN

Roman chamomile, blue tansy, or lavender. Take internally or apply topically.

JOINT PAIN

Turmeric and copaiba. Take internally or apply topically.

doTERRA Deep Blue blend. Apply topically.

NAUSEA

DigestZen blend, peppermint, or lemon. Take internally, diffuse, or apply topically.

Ginger. Take internally.

PREECLAMPSIA

Marjoram or frankincense. Use aromatically, apply topically, or take internally.

PRETERM LABOR

Lavender. Rub 1–3 drops on your belly.

SLEEPLESSNESS

Serenity blend, lavender, vetiver, or Roman chamomile. Use aromatically or apply topically.

INDUCTION (AT FULL TERM)

Myrrh and clary sage. Apply 1–2 drops to your wrists and abdomen, as well as inside your ankle bones to induce labor or if labor has begun and then stalled.

Stretch Mark Blend

5 drops lavender
5 drops myrrh
5 drops helichrysum
10 ml carrier oil

Mix the oils into the carrier oil and massage onto your belly, thighs, lower back, and breasts.

ESSENTIAL OIL SOLUTIONS FOR LABOR

Essential oils can be incredibly supportive during labor and the birth of your babe. Whether you are looking for general support in creating an ideal birthing environment or are in need of specific solutions to something that is arising, the following list is for you.

OVERALL SUPPORT FOR AN OPTIMAL LABOR

Lavender, basil, clary sage, geranium, or ylang ylang.
Diffuse or apply topically

doTERRA ClaryCalm blend or Peace blend. Use aromatically.

According to Ayurveda, you should inhale cardamom, kustha, vacha, and chitrak during active labor and the pushing stage.

BLEEDING

Geranium, helichrysum, or myrhh. Apply topically on tummy (can be used for postpartum bleeding as well).

NERVOUSNESS AND STRESS

Basil, frankincense, or lavender. Apply topically or use aromatically.

Balance blend or Serenity blend. Apply topically or use aromatically.

CONTRACTIONS OR STALLED LABOR

Clary sage and myrrh. Apply topically to belly, ankles, and wrists.

Cinnamon, fennel, jasmine, or lavender. Use aromatically.

LOW CONFIDENCE

Basil, clary sage, marjoram, lavender; doTERRA Balance blend, Motivate blend, or Serenity blend. Use aromatically.

PAIN MANAGEMENT

Cardamom, basil, cypress, lavender, or marjoram. Apply topically or use aromatically.

doTERRA Deep Blue blend. Apply topically.

OVERHEATING

Peppermint, eucalyptus, or wintergreen. Apply topically.

PERINEUM PREPARATION

Frankincense, geranium, lavender, Roman chamomile, or sandalwood. Apply topically.

TENSION

Clary sage, geranium, lavender, magnolia, or neroli. Use aromatically or apply topically.

ESSENTIAL OIL SOLUTIONS FOR THE POSTPARTUM WINDOW

The following oils will support mama and babe postpartum, whether it be to enhance their environment, stabilize mood and emotions, or support major or minor imbalances that are arising.

Uplifting Diffuser Combinations

1 drop rose + 1 drop wild orange + 3 drops sandalwood

1 drop lavender + 3 drops grapefruit + 1 drop ylang ylang

MOOD ENHANCER

Vetiver, jatamamsi, clary sage, frankincense, geranium, bergamot, sandalwood, rose, or any citrus/conifers. Use aromatically.

AFTERPAIN/UTERINE CRAMPING WHILE NURSING

Cardamom, bergamot, clary sage, frankincense, or doTERRA Deep Blue blend. Apply topically.

CONSTIPATION

DigestZen blend, fennel, or ginger. Take internally or apply topically.

HEMORRHOID RELIEF

Balance blend, turmeric, clove (diluted). Apply topically, directly on affected area.

LOW MILK SUPPLY

Fennel or rosemary. Apply fennel or rosemary topically to breasts; take fennel internally.

MASTITIS

Lavender. Apply topically.

Thyme or oregano. Take internally (diluted or in a veggie capsule).

Peppermint. Take internally or apply topically.

DRY, CRACKED, OR SORE NIPPLES

Helichrysum or lavender. Apply directly to nipples to invite healing and elasticity.

OVERSUPPLY OF MILK

Peppermint. Take internally.

Basil. Apply topically on breast(s) (specifically for engorgement).

POSTPARTUM DEPRESSION

Elevation blend, frankincense, melissa, or Citrus Bliss blend. Apply topically under nose and on ears.

doTERRA Cheer blend. Use aromatically or topically.

Frankincense, rose, or clary sage. Apply topically or take internally.

SLEEP

Jatamamsi. Apply topically to the back of the knees and the bottom of the feet.

Valerian. Use aromatically.

Lavender, Roman chamomile, or blue lotus. Use aromatically with a diffuser in the bedroom or apply a portion of a drop to the back of the neck, temples, and heart before bed.

TEARING, INFLAMMATION, AND SORENESS

Frankincense, helichrysum, myrrh, or lavender. Apply any, or all, topically.

Frankincense, melaleuca, and lavender. Apply topically in a sitz bath, as a perineal spray, or with frozen feminine pads (see instructions below).

Sitz Bath Blend or Frozen Feminine Pads

Warmth is generally recommended for postpartum healing, but if there is inflammation and pain, these frozen feminine pads will offer great relief. If there is no pain, you can use this blend in warm water as a sitz bath or perineal spray.

1 bottle witch hazel

Herbal bath blend (see page 92)

4 drops lavender

4 drops melaleuca

2 drops frankincense

aloe vera gel

1. Prepare the herbal bath blend as a strong tea.
2. Mix into a spray bottle with half herbal tea blend and half witch hazel.
3. Add essential oils. Shake to mix.
4. Cut large menstrual pads into thirds, and spray the mixture onto the pads.
5. Pour aloe vera gel down the center of each pad and freeze them.
6. Put any remaining solution in a peri bottle to apply as needed.
7. Use these frozen pads following labor to heal perineal tissues or stitches.

ESSENTIAL OIL SOLUTIONS FOR BABY

When using essential oils for baby topically, always dilute 1 drop of essential oil to 1 tablespoon of a carrier oil.

COLIC

DigestZen or Tamer blend. Apply topically on baby's spine and tummy (clockwise motions).

Fennel. Apply topically on baby's spine and tummy.

Roman chamomile, doTERRA Serenity or Adaptiv blends, or ylang ylang. Apply topically.

CRADLE CAP

Lavender, melaleuca, sandalwood, or frankincense. Apply topically.

CRYING

doTerra Serenity blend, Peace blend, Tamer blend, Roman chamomile, or lavender. Use aromatically or apply topically.

JAUNDICE

Frankincense, lemon, or geranium. Apply topically.

REFLUX

doTERRA DigestZen or Tamer blends, fennel, lavender, peppermint, or Roman chamomile. Apply topically.

TEETHING

Copaiba, Roman chamomile, or lavender. Apply topically on jawline or use aromatically.

THRUSH

Spikenard, clary sage, arborvitae, or melaleuca. Apply topically.

Diaper Rash Cream

5 drops lavender

4 drops melaleuca

½ cup raw coconut oil

Melt coconut oil in a glass cup using the double-boiler method. Add essential oils and stir. Store in a sealable glass container and leave in a cool place. Apply as needed.

Waking up with you each morning
has easily become the most special part of my day.
Your smile;
your giggles and wiggles;
your beautiful little voice that's starting to make so many new sounds;
the way you look at the wall,
the shadows,
and out of the window in so much awe;
your sweetness.
Your incredible sweetness
makes life so, so sweet.
How odd it would be
to wake up without your dark blue eyes looking for mine.
Or the late nights I lie awake just looking at you, thinking how incredibly beautiful you are.
How odd it would be to not walk miles and miles with you every day,
to not sit on the back porch and watch you look in such wonder at the world all around.
You're still so new,
though how odd it would be
to have a life without you now
. . . where just a few months back I had no idea what it would be like
with you here.

You're this precious little soul.
I still don't feel like you're mine,
and I pray that it stays like that.

I'm here to serve you, little love.
To help you remember God;
to help you remember who you *really* are.

And for now I'll love you like my son,
like my little buddy,
my dear most friend,
my little companion.
Not mine,
but God's—
Entrusted in my care
for this little bit of time.

I pray to love you like the precious soul that you are,
inside this tiny, cute, and round little body.

It is the perfection of motherhood actually,
and such a grace-filled spiritual path:
to see the soul within you,
to see God within your heart,
and to serve you,
selflessly,
like every mother does—
Knowing that you're not mine,
but eternally His.
And I get to care for you
for this short little time.

You've awakened within my heart
a love I've never known,
and you've pulled out of me
an ability to care
in ways I never knew I was capable of.

Thank you, little love.

Epilogue

AND BEYOND

You've got this, mama. Motherhood is the most beautiful, powerful, transformational, hardest, and most meaningful thing you will do in your life.

With every stage comes new challenges and new joys. Every baby is so different, and you are blessed with your little angel who will support you to grow in the most profound and important ways.

You'll learn what you need to learn, as you need to learn it. Trust that.

You have everything that you need to mother your little one.

As the saying goes: the days may be long, but the years fly by. Savor your moments. Be as present as you can. Love them with everything that you have and everything that you are. Work on yourself, keep growing—do the best that you can and keep trying to be better—and the fruits will show up in who your little one is, and who they become.

You are doing the most valuable work.

I see you. I honor you. I am here for you.

In service and gratitude,
Dhyana

Online Resources

The following list of websites are online services and products available from the author and book contributors.

AyurvedaMamaBox.com

An online shop with everything you need for preconception, pregnancy, birth, and the postpartum window. Purchase single items, specialty and gift boxes, or subscribe to receive a box each month with essentials for nourishing yourself and your little one—specific to your month of motherhood. Here you'll find herbal remedies specifically for preconception, pregnancy, birth, and postpartum, as well as for your continued journey through motherhood. The site also offers Ayurvedic training and consultations.

AyurvedaHealthRetreat.com

Come experience anywhere from three to twenty-eight days of a personalized Ayurvedic Pancha Karma retreat.

theSisterScience.com

Online, self-paced Ayurveda trainings and courses, as well as access to my online community, Soul Space. Through all of our offerings, we are dedicated to supporting your journey to total wellness, so that you may feel truly inspired in living your most fulfilling life, every moment of every day.

my.doterra.com/dhyanamasla

My online shop offering essential oils from doTERRA. I'll be notified when you use this link to purchase your oils and will email free access to my online Essential Education course with any purchase.

♦

The following are online shop recommendations and resources for your Ayurvedic care.

banyanbotanicals.com

An online shop offering traditional Ayurvedic herbs and oils, herbal-infused ghees, chyavanprash, and more.

innersunandmoon.com/directory

A directory of certified Ayurvedic postpartum doulas.

mountainroseherbs.com

An online shop offering organic herbs, spices, and botanicals.

References and Suggested Reading

A. C. Bhaktivedanta Swami Prabhupāda. *Bhagavad-Gita As it Is.* Alachua, FL: Bhaktivedanta Book Trust, 1997.

A. C. Bhaktivedanta Swami Prabhupāda. *Srimad Bhagavatam, Third Canto.* Alachua, FL: Bhaktivedanta Book Trust, 1988.

Blossom, Scott. "Intro to Ayurveda: Understanding the Three Doshas." *Yoga Journal*, January 21, 2021.

Collins, Faith. *Joyful Toddlers and Preschoolers: Create a Life That You and Your Child Love.* Chino Valley, AZ: Hohm Press, 2017.

Frawley, David, and Vasant Lad. *The Yoga of Herbs.* Twin Lakes, WI: Lotus Press, 1993.

Gaskin, Ina May. *Ina May's Guide to Breastfeeding.* London: Pinter and Martin, 2009.

——. *Ina May's Guide to Childbirth.* London: Ebury, 2008.

——. *Spiritual Midwifery.* Summertown, TN: Book Publishing Company, 2002.

Gerber, Magda. *Dear Parent.* Los Angeles, CA: Resources for Infant Educators (RIE), 2003.

Humphrey, Sheila. *The Nursing Mother's Herbal.* Minneapolis: Fairview Press, 2003.

Kitzinger, Sheila. *The New Experience of Childbirth.* London, UK: Orion Publishing Group, 2004.

Knost, L. R. *The Gentle Parent.* Saint Cloud, FL: Little Hearts Books, LLC, 2013.

——. *Two Thousand Kisses a Day*. Saint Cloud, FL. Little Hearts Books, LLC, 2013.

La Leche League International. *The Womanly Art of Breastfeeding.* London: Pinter and Martin, 2010.

Lad, Vasant. *Textbook of Ayurveda: Fundamental Principles.* Vol. 1. Albuquerque: Ayurvedic Press, 2002.

Leboyer, Frédérick. *Birth without Violence.* Rochester, VT: Inner Traditions International, 2009.

Liedloff, Jean. *The Continuum Concept.* New York: De Capo Press, 1986.

Oakes, Ysha. *Touching Heaven: Tonic Postpartum Care with Ayurveda.* Vols. 1 and 2. Sacred Window Studies, 2012. https://sacredwindowstudies.com/product/recipes-and-routines.

Rafael, Terra. *Ayurveda for the Childbearing Years: A Primer.* London: Lulu.com, 2009.

Reddy, Kumuda, Linda Egenes, and Margaret Mullins. *For a Blissful Baby: Healthy and Happy Pregnancy with Maharishi Vedic Medicine.* Delhi: New Age Books, 2004.

R. K. Sharma Bhagwan Das. *Caraka Samhita.* Varanasi, India: Chowkhamba Sanskrit Series Office, 2016.

Romm, Aviva. "Hypothyroid Testing: The Six Labs You Need." avivaromm.com/hypothyroid-testing-need-know.

——. *Natural Health after Birth.* Rochester, VT: Inner Traditions/Bear and Company, 2002.

Rosenberg, Marshall. *Nonviolent Communication.* Encinitas, CA: Puddle Dancer, 2003.

Rothman, Barbara Katz. *A Bun in the Oven.* New York: New York University Press, 2016.

Sacinandana Swami. *The Living Name.* Pinner, London: Saranagati Publishing, 2018.

Siegel, Daniel J. *Parenting from the Inside Out.* New York: J. P. Tarcher/Putnam, 2003.

Srila Gopala Bhatta Gosvami. *Sat Kriya Sara Dipika.* Mayapur, India: The Bhaktivedanta Academy, 1999.

Swami, Radhanath. *The Journey Within.* San Rafael, CA: Mandala Publishing, 2016.

Teitelbaum, Marianne. *Healing the Thyroid with Ayurveda.* Rochester, VT: Inner Traditions/Bear and Company, 2019.

Weed, Susun. *Wise Woman Herbal for the Childbearing Year.* Woodstock, NY: Ash Tree Publishing, 1996.

Weschler, Toni. *Taking Charge of Your Fertility.* New York: William Morrow/HarperCollins, 2015.

Wolf, David. *Relationships That Work: The Power of Conscious Living.* San Rafael, CA: Mandala, 2008.

Index

A

A. C. Bhaktivedanta Swami Prabhupada, 72–73, 232
abhyanga
 for colic relief, 250
 contraindications, 211
 after C-section, 215
 in daily routine, 65
 in early labor, 129, 151
 instructions, 66–67
 for newborns, 246–47, 252, 255
 oils for, 66, 198
 postpartum, 180–81, 202, 205, 207, 214
 during pregnancy, 90, 110
 for vata balancing, 22
acid reflux/heartburn, 98–99, 110
 in newborns, 252–53, 319
 pitta imbalance and, 24
adoption, 216–18
adrenaline, 121, 151
affirmations, 131
agni, 54
 after childbirth, 179, 279–80
 after C-section, 214
 healthy, 270–71
 impaired, 271
 in postpartum, 200–201, 202
 supporting, 127, 213
air element, 15, 17, 18–19, 174, 201
alfalfa juice powder, 127
Allison, Jenny, *Golden Month*, 171
almond flour, 298
almond milk, 215–16, 292
almond oil, 310, 313
almonds, 99, 102
 Almond Date Shake, 291
 Almond-Date Laddus, 215–16
 Dry-Fruit Laddus, 276
 for lactation, 260, 263
 for ojas building, 95, 128
 powdered, 56, 69
alternate-nostril breathing (*nadi shodhana*), 104
 benefits, 22
 instructions, 22–23
 postpartum, 210–11
ama (toxins), 112, 179, 201, 212, 280
amalaki (aka amla, Indian gooseberry), 58, 59, 99, 102
amniotic fluid, 95, 144, 146, 147
anemia, 24, 99–100, 127
anxiety, 76
 about childbirth, 116, 121, 165
 agni impairment and, 271
 body therapies for, 66, 181
 essential oils for, 311
 and health, overall, 8, 11, 12
 herbs for, 58, 100, 200, 212, 303–4, 305, 307
 lack of sleep from, 207
 ojas depletion and, 272
 postpartum, 175, 192, 195, 204–6, 209
 vata imbalance and, 19, 20, 62, 94, 155
apana vata, 95, 102, 120, 123, 154–55, 175
aphrodisiacs, 57, 305, 307
apples, 273, 285
 sauce, 297–98
 Sautéed and Stewed Apples, 123, 296–97
apricots, dried, 273, 276, 284
arborvitae oil, 319
arnica tablets, 177, 215
artava dhatu, 87
asafetida (Hing), 294–95
ashoka, 55, 199, 217
ashwagandha
 in basti, 125
 description, 302–3

Mood Milk Tea 2, 307
postpartum, 181, 205, 207, 208, 210
preconception, 57
during pregnancy, 100
transdermal, 209
asparagus, 284, 296
association, power of, 72–73
asthi dhatu, 86
attachment (*raga*), 10–11, 12, 34, 38
auric field, 192, 238, 242
aversion (*dvesha*), 10–11, 12, 34, 38
avocado, 128, 260–61, 270, 278, 285
awareness, 12, 37
and breath, connection between, 96, 210
of fetus, 85
for healing, 229
during labor, 159–60
spiritual, 78–80
Ayurveda
on gestation, imprinting in, 2
goal of, 14, 16
on health, overall view of, 8–9, 98
on newborns, 238, 240, 244–45
nutritional focus of, 267–68
as personalized science, 15
on postpartum, 185, 191–92
as science of life, 7–8
Ayurvedic postpartum doulas, 181, 183, 197, 203, 206, 211, 212
Ayurvedic practitioners, consulting, 17, 62, 147, 206, 211

B

babies
constitution of, 72
essential oils for, 310, 319–20
unborn, reflecting on, 142–43
in womb, 73, 103
See also newborns
baby showers, 197–98
bala, 125, 181, 205, 207
bananas, 260–61, 273
basal body temperature, 62–63
basil
fresh, 285
oil, 313, 315, 316, 317
basmati rice
kanji, 292–93
kitchari, 294–95
Rice Gruel, 277
basti (warm oil enema), 125, 129, 151, 181, 202, 206
baths. *See* herbal baths; sitz baths
bedtime, 21, 66, 207
beets, 99, 100, 270, 285
Iron-Rich Dal, 294
Steamed Veggies, 296
belly wrapping
after delivery, 153–54
instructions, 182
postpartum, 180, 197, 202, 207, 215
bergamot oil, 317
Bhagavad Gita, 71, 80, 81, 159
Bhakti tradition, 10
birth plans, 128–29
delivery, 130
for labor, 129–30
pain coping techniques, 132–33
partner/support person's responsibilities, 131–32, 133–34
birth stories
author's daughter, 161–67
author's son, 156–61
peace with, 214
sacredness of, 142
birthing, 149–50
catching baby, 135, 153, 161, 163
considerations for, 115–18
daily rituals to prepare for, 123–24
"en caul," 144
ideal, envisioning, 128
locations for, 119–21
as natural, 142, 164
nourishment immediately after, 153
positions, 108, 130, 133, 163
premature, 95
shoulder dystocia, 156
support during, 148
type of, breastfeeding and, 261
Birthing Ayurveda blog, 127
birthing centers, 121, 147
birthing partner roles, 148, 150, 152, 154, 156

black pepper/peppercorns, 21, 28, 104
  Garlic Chutney, 289
  Hot Milk Tonic, 290–91
  for postpartum, 179, 212, 275, 278, 283, 286, 292–93, 294–95
Blackwell, Sarva, 174, 182, 217
Blossom, Scott
  on kapha, 26–27
  on pitta, 23–24
  on vata, 19
blue lotus, 206, 306
  description, 305
  essential oil, 318
blue tansy oil, 314
bodily tissues (dhatus)
  of embryo, 85
  nourishing, 259, 281
  types, 54
bodily urges, suppressing, 95
body
  Ayurvedic view of, 9–10
  after childbirth, 175
  emotions in, 226
  identifying with, 41
  knowing of, 142, 164
  memory of, 2–3
  nourishment and, 268
  postpartum care of, 180–81, 196
  surrendering, 191
body time (*kayakalpa*), 192
Brahma Samhita, 80
brahmi (a.k.a. water hyssop), 58, 100
  infused oil, 152, 181, 182, 204, 205, 207
  in teas, 208, 306
brain
  formation, 1–2, 86
  neuroplasticity of, 45
  support for, 58
brain fog, 58, 208
Braxton-Hicks contractions, 143–44, 146, 165–66
breastfeeding, 174, 258–59, 261, 280
  antigalactogogues, 254
  Ayurvedic guidelines on, 240
  breast milk, quality of, 278
  challenges in, 195, 262–64
  essential oils for, 317
  frequency, 244, 253
  golden hour and, 151, 154
  hypothyroidism and, 209
  lactation herbs, 180, 199, 202, 212, 213, 263
  list of essentials for, 241, 242
  nipple soothing oil, 198
  oversupply, 252–54, 317
  partner's support during, 187
  rasa dhatu nourishment during, 259–60
  spitting up, 243–44, 252–54
  transitioning from, 260–61
  vata balancing in, 259–60
buttermilk, 98, 275

C

caffeine, 76, 272, 278
  breast milk and, 249, 250, 251
  conception and, 54, 57
  in kapha, balancing, 28
  in pitta imbalance, 25
  sleep and, 207
  thyroid and, 209
  in vata imbalance, 20, 21, 124
calendula, 92, 181, 198, 199, 204, 263
cardamom
  in baby formula, 264–65
  black, roasted, 106
  essential oil, 130, 136, 151, 153, 311, 314, 316, 317
  Herbal Chewing Mix, 289–90
  Hot Milk Tonic, 290–91
  during labor, 153, 311, 315
  for ojas building, 56, 69
  for postpartum, 208, 282, 286, 291, 292–93, 296–97
  powder, 215–16, 276, 277
  during pregnancy, 87, 98
cashew milk, 131
cashews, 128, 276, 277, 284, 291–92
cassia oil, 310, 313
celibacy, 94
ceremonies and rituals
  for baby's five senses, 88–89
  blessing way, 197–98
  garbhadhana-samskara (conception), 59, 67–69
  jata karma (birth), 168
  nama karana samskara (name-giving), 234

newborn's welcome bath, 245
niskaraman samskara (welcoming baby), 220–21
postpartum, 184
simantonnayana (hair parting), 113
śosyantī homa (safe delivery), 138
cervix
dilation of, 147, 148, 162
incompetence of, 95
position and texture of, 64
"ripening" of, 144
cesarean birth, 211
belly wrapping and, 182
consent instructions, 136
ghee use and, 280
postpartum after, 213–16
chamomile, 100, 198, 210
in baths, 92, 199, 250
in ghee, 263
in teas, 208, 249, 283, 306, 307
See also Roman chamomile
channels, 96, 112, 113, 211
Charaka Samhita, 68, 268, 272
chickpea flour, 247–48, 256
chitrak, 153, 179, 212, 315
chocolate chips, 298
choice
balance and, 16
conscious, 11–12, 37
ignorance in, 13
in responding, 226–29
sense control and, 40–41, 77
chyavanprash, 58, 99
cilantro, 284, 286, 295
cinnamon, 56, 76, 278
essential oil, 310, 313, 315
Hot Milk Tonic, 290–91
for postpartum, 215–16, 283, 286, 291–92, 293–94
Tahini Cookies, 297–98
Warm Yam Smoothie, 292
circadian rhythms, 64
clary sage oil, 311, 314, 315, 316, 317, 319
cleanliness, 43, 75
in baby products, 255
in food preparation, 81, 270
cleanses, 54–55, 98
climate, 15–16, 21, 25, 28
clove, 56, 278, 282, 292–93, 296–97
essential oil, 310, 317
Herbal Chewing Mix, 213, 289–90
Hot Milk Tonic, 290–91
coconut, 215–16, 270, 289–90
flour, 298
milk, 247–48
oil, 254, 255, 285, 298, 310, 313, 320
sugar, 284, 293–94
water, 101, 107, 131, 156, 256, 275
colic, 249–50, 319
comfrey, 198, 199
communication
breastfeeding as, 258–59
conscious, 51
effective, 47–48
by newborns, 240–41
with newborns, 230–32, 236
compassion, 42, 75
ahimsa and, 37–38
in mothering, 229–30, 231
in postpartum, 194
self-knowledge and, 45
Sri Radha as embodiment of, 232
conception
Ayurvedic ideal, 31
building health prior to, 4
constitution at time of, 15
doshas and, 61, 84
menstrual cycle tracking and, 62–64
preparation for, 31–33
timing, 59
conditioned responses, 225–26, 231
conditioned worldview, 227
congestion, 27, 101, 271
consciousness, 33–34
in childbearing, 1–2, 3–4
in embryo, 85
entering matter, 31
in marma therapy, 211
nourishing, 80
preconception, 36
uplifting, practices for, 42
constipation, 101–2
of newborns, 250–51
postpartum, 203–4, 209
relief from, 127, 317
contentment, 43–44

contractions
- in active labor, 147
- in early labor, 146–47
- essential oils for, 315
- massages between, 152
- pitta support during, 156
- planning for, 130, 131
- position during, 159–60, 162
- in pushing stage, 149
- resting between, 129
- stimulating, 127, 203
- timing, 129, 157, 158–59
- in transition stage, 148
- vata support during, 151, 155
- *See also* Braxton-Hicks contractions

cooling breath (*sitali*), 26, 104, 107
copaiba oil, 311, 313, 314, 319
coriander, 179, 199
- essential oil, 313
- for postpartum, 281, 286, 289, 294–95
- in teas, 55, 99, 202, 214, 288

cortical stimulation, reducing, 155
cortisol, 91
cradle cap, 254–55, 319
cravings, 85, 86, 275, 313
crowning, 124–25, 130, 149, 160, 162
crying, 2
- colic and, 249–50
- essential oils for, 319
- postpartum, 211
- reasons for, 238
- responding to, 235

cumin, 21, 56, 179, 275, 278
- for postpartum, 199, 281, 286, 294–95
- in teas, 55, 99, 202, 249, 288

cypress oil, 313, 316

D

dairy, raw, 260
dal
- Iron-Rich Dal, 294
- yellow split mung dal, 260, 274–75, 294, 295

dashamula, 197, 200. *See also under* herbal teas
date sugar, 284, 298
dates, 56, 95, 99, 102, 127, 197, 260, 282, 297
- Almond Date Shake, 291
- Almond-Date Laddus, 215–16
- Dry-Fruit Laddus, 276
- Nourishing Oatmeal, 293–94
- during pregnancy, 127, 128, 152, 273
- Warm Yam Smoothie, 292

decision-making, 11, 14, 37
depression, 76
- agni impairment and, 271
- consulting professional for, 206
- essential oils for, 317
- hyperthyroidism and, 209
- kapha imbalance and, 27, 62
- over loss of child, 217
- postpartum, 175, 192, 195, 204–6, 209
- during pregnancy, 105
- self-care for, 66

desire
- of baby and mama, connection between, 86, 106
- being controlled by, 40
- consciousness and, 33–34

Devani, Vrinda, 127
dhatus. *See* bodily tissues (dhatus)
diabetes, gestational, 103–4, 119, 127, 313
diapers
- changing, 239
- diaper rash, 255–56
- Diaper Rash Cream, 320

diet
- dosha fluctuation in, 15–16
- kapha in, 28–29
- pitta in, 25–26
- postpartum, 179
- preconception, 54, 56–58
- role of, 14
- vata in, 20–21
- vegetarian and meat-based, differences in, 269–70
- *See also* foods; meals; nourishment

digestion
- Ayurvedic guidelines for, 271–72
- bodily tissues and, 54
- importance of, 112
- lime water for, 275
- of mama and baby, connection between, 248, 249
- *See also* agni

digestive spices, 21, 95, 112, 213, 303
digestive system, 14, 199, 260
dinacharya, 64–66
discipline, 231–32
disease
  causes of, 10–11, 74, 96
  fetal origins of, 268
  three causes of, 13
Divine
  grace, 83, 304
  offering to, 80–81
  surrendering to, 45–46
  will, 34, 165
doshas
  balancing, 16–17
  elements of, 15, 17
  in first trimester, 84–85
  fluctuation of, 15–16
  sex and, 93–95
  translation of term, 16
  weight gain and, 111
  See also individual dosha
doTERRA essential oil blends, 309
  Adaptiv, 319
  Balance, 311, 315, 316, 317
  Cheer, 313
  Citrus Bliss, 313, 317
  ClaryCalm, 315
  Deep Blue, 314, 316, 317
  DigestZen, 311, 312, 314, 317, 319
  Elevation, 317
  Motivate, 313, 316
  On Guard, 123
  Passion, 313
  Peace, 315, 319
  Serenity, 312, 314, 315, 316, 319
  Slims and Sassy, 313
  Tamer, 319
Douillard, John, 96
Dustan baby language, 240–41
dysfunction, cycles of, 2, 3, 12

E

earth element, 15, 17, 26
ectopic pregnancy, 20
edema (swelling), 103, 108, 312
  Edema Foot Soak, 313
  Edema Massage Oil, 313
eggs (ovum), 32, 62, 84
elements, five, 15, 17, 273. *See also individual element*
elimination, 271
  Ayurvedic and Western views, comparison of, 250–51
  of newborns, 243
  postpartum, 280
  support for, 101–2, 179, 215
emotions and feelings
  of baby in womb, 47
  breath and, 96–97
  changing, 12, 52
  children's, holding space for, 227, 236
  in early labor, 146
  fickleness of, 44
  identifying with, 41
  nesting and, 122
  noticing, 225–26
  postpartum, 181, 211
  during pregnancy, 85, 105
  regulating, 231
  rose and, 304
  sadhaka pitta and, 217
  water element and, 91
endometriosis, 208
environment
  baby in womb and, 80
  for birthing, 116, 120, 130
  dosha fluctuation in, 15–16
  for newborns, 172, 228–29, 248
  in postpartum, 178, 187, 238
  preconception, 32–33
  rajasic, 76
  sattvic, 75
  sensitivity during pregnancy, 86
  spiritual, 82
episiotomy, 135, 145
Epsom salts
  in baths, 92, 103, 107
  Edema Foot Soak, 313
  Epsom Salt Soaks, 199
essential oils
  for house cleaning, 122–23
  purity of, 309
  uses for, 308
  ways to use, 309–10
  See also under individual herbs

estrogen, 57, 58, 106, 304
ether element, 15, 17, 18–19, 211, 228
eucalyptus oil, 101, 123, 316
exercise
in daily routine, 65
for kapha balance, 28–29
pitta and, 25
for pitta balance, 25–26
during pregnancy, 95–97
for vata balance, 21–22

F

fall, 19, 21, 61
fathers, 79, 113, 129. *See also* birthing partner roles
feeling (sense of touch), 75, 76, 77
fennel, 260, 294–95, 296–97
in baby formula, 264–65
bulb, 296
description, 303
essential oil, 315, 317, 319
Herbal Chewing Mix, 289–90
Hot Milk Tonic, 290–91
for postpartum, 197, 199, 260, 286, 288
fenugreek
fresh, 284
for postpartum, 197, 199, 260, 263, 286
in teas, 180, 202, 212, 283, 288
fermented foods, 282
fertility, 32, 55, 56, 58, 62–64, 303, 305
fetus, 31, 85–86, 217, 218, 268
fibrocystic breast disease, 208
figs, 273, 276, 284, 285
fire element, 15, 16, 17, 23–24
flax
oil, 262, 285
seeds, 293–94
fluid retention, 27, 111, 214
folic acid deficiency, 100
foods
during birthing, 131
colic and, 249
cooked, benefits of, 270
for lactation enhancement, 259–60, 263
preparing Ayurvedic view of, 80
quality of, 269–70
rajasic, 76
real hunger for, 112
sattvic, 75, 81
solid, for newborns, 260–61
tamasic, 77
tridoshic, 294–95
forgiveness, 50–51
formula, baby
Ayurvedic Cow's Milk Formula, 264–65
need for, 261–62
frankincense oil, 254, 311, 313, 314, 315, 316, 317, 318, 319
free birthing, 161, 165
fruits, 273, 275
dried, when to avoid, 282
Dry-Fruit Laddus, 276
for lactation, 260
for newborns, 260

G

garlic, 76, 213, 263
Garlic Chutney, 289
roasted, 260, 284, 286, 296
when to avoid, 249, 283
Gaskin, Ina May
Ina May's Guide to Breastfeeding, 261
Ina May's Guide to Childbirth, 116, 119, 120, 153
generosity, 25, 26, 42, 232
geranium oil, 315, 316, 317, 319
Gerber, Magda, *Dear Parent*, 231
ghee, 278
Almond-Date Laddus, 215–16
instructions, 287
kanji, 292–93
for lactation, 260
neem, 204, 254
panchakola, 130, 137, 153, 179, 212
Panchamrit, 274
postpartum, 280, 282, 289, 291–92, 293–95, 296–97
during pregnancy, 127
Rice Gruel, 277
shatavari, 87, 207
ginger, 303
Edema Massage Oil, 313
essential oil, 314, 317
fresh, 264–65, 294–95
Herbal Chewing Mix, 289–90
Hot Milk Tonic, 290–91

for postpartum, 286, 291, 293–94
powder, 56, 199, 215–16, 291
Tahini Cookies, 297–98
in teas, 55, 103, 106, 180, 283, 284, 307
Warm Yam Smoothie, 292
God, 10, 52, 232–33
golden hour, 150–51, 261
goldenseal, 245
grapefruit oil, 123, 313, 316
gratitude, 39, 42, 47, 80, 81, 125, 259
green tea, jasmine, 306
greens, leafy, 100, 260, 274, 282
grief, 175–76, 217
guduchi (heart-leaved moonseed), 58, 305
guests (in postpartum), 178, 186
guilt, 231–32
gum acacia resin, 215–16
gunas, twenty, 18. *See also* maha gunas

H

hair loss, 204, 209
headaches, 62, 99, 108, 311, 313
heart
formation, 86, 217
of mothers, 218–19
of newborns, 243
heat rash, 254, 256, 312
helichrysum oil, 214, 315, 317, 318
hemorrhoids, 24, 181, 198, 200, 204, 317
herbal baths
ashoka, 55, 217
Ayurvedic Baby Soap, 247–48
for colic relief, 250
essential oils for, 310
guidelines for, 92
labor and, 151
for newborns, 244–45
postpartum guidelines, 181, 199–200
during pregnancy, 91
herbal chewing mix, 213, 289–90
herbal teas, 302
CCF tea, 55, 103, 180, 202, 288
for colic, 249–50
dashamula, 179–80, 202, 205, 208, 212, 214, 287–88
herbal blends, 198–99
during labor, ratio for, 152
Mama's Mood Tea 1, 306
Mama's Mood Tea 2, 307
Moon Milk Tea, 306
Moon Milk Tea 2, 307
sweet water lactation tea, 212, 263, 288
hibiscus, 200, 207, 256
home birth, 120, 163
benefits of, 153
hospital transfer plan, 133
VCI and, 163, 164–67
homeopathic treatments, 177, 215, 250
honesty, 38, 42, 45, 75
honey, 56, 61, 274, 310
in baths, 92
heating, toxicity of, 282
during labor, 130, 131, 132, 137, 153
during pregnancy, 85, 274
in teas, 306, 307
hormones
balancing, 204, 213
imbalances in, 57
kapha and, 26
mood swings and, 104–5
hospital birth, 121
Ayurvedic packing list, 136–37
plan for, 133–36
reasons for, 163–64
restrictions during, 152, 153
vata excess in, 154–55
when to leave, 147
hot packs, 181
house cleaner, DIY, 122–23
Humphrey, Sheila, *Nursing Mother's Herbal, The*, 261
hydration
congestion, 101
foods for, 57, 270
during labor, 148, 152, 155, 156
low milk supply and, 263
in postpartum, 179, 187, 201–2, 204
during pregnancy, 275
for vata balance, 112, 278
hypertension, 103, 104, 108
hyperthyroidism, 209–10
hypoglycemia, 156
hypothyroidism, 208–9

I

imbalance
causes of, 11, 12
chronic, 98
correcting, 14, 16
defining, 15
treating root of, 301
immunity/immune system, 55, 65, 208, 272
abhyanga for, 66, 181
baby's, 246, 258, 269
baths for, 91
digestion and, 14
herbal support, 58, 213, 303
vata and, 19
indigestion, 24, 146, 271, 311. *See also* acid reflux/heartburn
induction, labor, 145, 314
inflammation, 24, 58, 65, 86, 181, 263, 318
informed consent, 133–34
intention, 91, 184
in childbearing, 1–2, 3–4
in conception, 32, 33, 67–68
early labor, setting, 146
in mothering, 228–29
in parenthood, 79
in sexual desire, 41
interventions, 116, 120, 121, 128, 134, 135
intuition, 194, 243, 305
iron anemia, 100
irritability, 16, 24, 62, 104–6, 202, 206–7, 256

J

jaggery, 56, 284
jasmine, 75, 207, 306, 307
jasmine oil, 126, 151, 198, 315
jatamamsi oil, 317, 318
Jivani, Krsna, 305
Journey Within, The (Radhanath Swami), 81
Judith, Anodea, *Eastern Body, Western Mind*, 1

K

kalala, 84–85
Kali-Santarana Upanishad, 83
kanji, 153, 280, 283, 292–93
kapha
balancing, 28–29
constitutions, 94
diabetes and, 103–4
imbalances, 27–28, 62, 112
overview, 26–27
postpartum, 203, 281
during pregnancy, 86–87
kirtan, 75, 78, 83, 89, 158
kitchari
in home cleanse, 55
instructions, 294–95
Kitzinger, Sheila, *Experience of Childbirth, The*, 115
Knost, L. R., 236
Krishna, 157–58, 159, 232
kumquat oil, 313
kustha (costus root), 153, 315

L

labor
active, 147–48
early, 146–47
essential oils for, 311, 315–16
herbs for, 304
in hospital birth, planning, 135
kapha during, 156
messages about baby during, 148
nourishment during, 152–53
pain reduction during, 125
pitta during, 155–56
placenta phase, 150
planning for, 129–30
preterm, 95, 314
pushing stage, 149
slowing or stopping, 120, 131
terms for, 143–45
transition stage, 148–49
vata during, 20, 154–55
visualizing, 124
lactation specialists, 249, 253, 254, 261
Lad, Vasant, 7
lavender, 198, 199, 200, 210
after C-section, 214
Diaper Rash Cream, 320
Edema Massage Oil, 313

essential oil, 252, 311, 312, 314, 316, 317, 318, 319
Stretch Mark Blend, 315
law of conservation of mass, 9
leavenings, avoiding, 283
Leboyer, Frédérick, *Birth without Violence*, 124
leftovers, 278, 281, 282
legs, restlessness of, 110
lemon balm, 208, 210
lemon oil, 107, 123, 311, 313, 314, 319
lemons, 55
licorice, 99, 124, 198, 199, 263
life, six symptoms of, 9–10, 31
lifestyle
for balancing pitta, 25–26
for balancing vata, 21–22
of father, preconception, 32
during pregnancy, recommendations, 93–95
role of, 14
sedentary, 28, 77
like increases like, opposites balance, 18, 60, 61, 100
limbic system, 309
limes, 65, 99, 275, 284, 285, 289, 294, 296
linden, 126, 151, 200
lochia, 174, 179, 200, 202, 285
love, 3, 229
ahimsa and, 37
in baby massage, 247
commitment and, 52
of God and mothers, 232–33
in mothering, 224, 228–29
for newborns, 173–74, 196
preconception, 35
responding from, 230–32
Sri Radha as embodiment of, 232
surrender and, 46
for unborn child, 137
unconditional, 4, 142, 174, 187–89
lunar cycles, 62
luteinizing hormone, 304
lymphatic system, 27, 66, 85, 103, 246, 262, 271, 312

M

maca, 207, 307
macro- and micronutrients, 269
magnesium, transdermal, 207, 209, 210
magnolia oil, 316
maha gunas, 18, 71, 73–78
maha mantra, 83–84, 158
Maharishi Ayurveda, 31
majja dhatu, 86
mamsa dhatu, 85
mantra meditation, 42, 83–84
maple syrup, 56, 284, 291–92, 293–94, 298
Marginal Cord Insertion, 163
marjoram oil, 314, 316
marma therapy, 79, 110, 211, 214, 215
massage
for babies, 187, 247, 254
breast, 261, 262–63, 264
head and foot, 110
perineal, 124–25
scalp, 204
See also abhyanga
matter, 8
as always changing, 41–42
consciousness entering, 31
five elements in, 15
identifying with, 9, 10–11
maha gunas and, 78
as spiritual, 78–80
meals
Ayurvedic guidelines for, 271–72, 283
for postpartum, 283–85
during pregnancy, 273–77
regularity in, 112, 179
timing and amounts, 65
meda dhatu, 86
meditation, 25, 43, 64, 68, 75, 86, 92. *See also* mantra meditation
melaleuca (tea tree) oil, 312, 318, 319, 320
melissa oil, 317
Melnick, Narelle, 141
menopause, 208
menstruation, 57, 62, 208, 304
microcosm-macrocosm, 60
midwives and doulas, 62
author's experiences with, 162, 165
communicating with, 147
newborns and, 243, 251
roles of, 152–53, 156

milk, 215–16, 276
Ayurvedic Cow's Milk Formula, 264–65
in baby soap, 247–48
cold, 282
cow's, 260, 265
Hot Milk Tonic, 290–91
Panchamrit, 274
tonic, 180, 207, 208, 252
mind
as always changing, 12
identifying with, 41, 44
maha gunas and, 74
noticing, 225–26
nourishing, 80
understanding nature of, 8
mirror metaphor, 34
miscarriage, 20, 94, 102–3, 208, 216–18
mood
balancing, 213
essential oils for, 317
postpartum disorders, 204–6
mood swings, 104–6, 206–7
morning sickness, 24, 106–7, 303
mornings, daily practices for, 64–65
Mother Earth (Bhumi), 232
Mother Teresa, 224
motherhood
boundaries in, 230–31
reflections for, 228
as spiritual practice, 225–27, 231, 236–37, 321
transition to, 141–42, 161, 172–74, 192–93
two hearts in, 218–19
universal principles, 194
mucuna, 206, 207, 306, 307
mucus plug, 144, 146, 159
mustard seeds, 278, 294–95
myrrh oil, 314, 315, 318

N

nadi shodhana. *See* alternate-nostril breathing
Natural Health after Birth (Romm), 210
nature, 14, 90–91
nausea, 95
agni and, 271
essential oils for, 311, 314
herbs for, 303
in labor, 149
pitta imbalance and, 24, 62
postpartum, 206
during pregnancy, 97, 108, 274
vata imbalance and, 19
See also morning sickness
neroli oil, 316
nervous system, 90–91
abhyanga for, 66
herbs for, 198, 212, 303–4, 305
imprints on, 2–3
kapha and, 26
of newborns, 192, 238
parasympathetic, activating, 21
vata and, 100
yoga for soothing, 208
nesting, 121–22, 157, 194, 196
nettles, 100, 109, 204, 303
newborns, 192, 223–25, 238
basic needs, 239–40
common challenges, 249–54
essential oils for, 312
in hospital births, 136
immediately following birth, 150–51
list of essentials, 241–42
loving, 232–33, 235, 256–58
mother's health and, 248
needs of, responding to, 230–32
normal occurrences, 243–44
nourishment for, 239–40
oiling head and feet, 154
sense of self, 172
skin changes, 254–56
solid foods for, 260–61
niyamas, five
ishvarapranidhana, 45–46
purpose of, 36–37
santosha, 43–44
saucham, 43
svadhyaya, 45
tapas, 44–45
nonattachment, 41–42
nonviolence, 37–38, 75
nourishment
Ayurvedic and Western views, differences in, 71–72
Ayurvedic basics of, 268–73
importance of, 267

kapha and, 26
preconception, 33, 85
See also under birthing; labor; newborns; pregnancy
nutmeg, 56, 110, 206, 207, 293–94

O

Oakes, Ysha, 171, 186. See also *Touching Heaven*
oat flour, 297–98
oats, 260, 263, 274, 284
colloidal, 92
Nourishing Oatmeal, 293–94
Warm Oatmeal Shake, 291–92
oatstraw, 100, 200, 303–4
oil pulling, 65
ojas
abstinence and, 55
abundant and depleted, signs of, 272
building, 95, 102, 127–28, 215–16, 280, 291, 303
diminishing, 56–57
foods that undermine, 272
between mama and baby, 154
Ojas Milk, 56
sex and, 94, 128
in third trimester, 87, 123
oregano oil, 310, 317
Osho, 172
ovaries, 53–54, 208
ovulation, 62–63
oxytocin, 127, 150

P

panchakarma, 54–55
panchamrit, 273–74
parenthood, 11, 12, 14, 46, 47, 53
partnership
celibacy in, 94–95
conscious, 3–4
explorations for, 53
in postpartum period, 185–88, 189
in preconception, 46
separation and, 117–18
passionflower, 208, 306, 307
pediatricians, 243, 244, 249, 251, 252
pelvis, 102, 107–8, 181
peppermint, 76, 254
peppermint oil, 101, 123, 308, 311, 313, 314, 316, 317, 319
perineum
during birthing, 149
cleaning, 180
essential oils for, 316
massage, 124–25, 145
softening, 126
pippali, 179, 212, 286
pitta
balancing, 25–26
digestive problems and, 98–99, 106, 107
imbalances, 24–25, 58, 62
during labor, 155–56
of newborns, 248, 256
overview, 23–24
postpartum, 202, 281, 289
sadhaka, 217
placenta
delivery, 150
previa, 95, 147
PMS, 208
poppy seeds, 207
postpartum, 238
asking for help, 182–84, 195
checklist, 177
diet and nourishment for, 277–79, 280–81, 286–87
doshas and, 17
essential oils for, 311–12, 316–18
foods contraindicated for, 281–83
four pillars of care for, 177–82
Frozen Feminine Pads, 318
grocery lists, 284, 285
herbal support for, 179–80, 212–13, 283, 284
imbalances in, common, 203–10
meal train, 89, 197
partners during, guidance for, 185–88
practices to support healing, 210–11
preparing for, 195–200
support during, 197–98
vata in, 20, 61–62, 259
See also under meals; sacred window
Prabhupada, Srila, 34
prakruti, 15, 16, 17
prana (life force), 32, 56, 96, 211

pranayama, 42
  during late pregnancy, 128
  postpartum, 210–11
  for sattva, increasing, 75
  ujjai, 208, 210, 211
  See also alternate-nostril breathing; cooling breath
prasadam (spiritual food), 80–81, 138
prayers
  to baby in womb, 79–80
  in conception ritual, 68
  maha mantra, 83–84
  for name-giving, 234
  for safe delivery, 138
  for welcoming baby to world, 220–21
preconception, 20
  daily rituals for, 123–24
  time for ("season"), 32–33
preeclampsia, 108–9, 127, 314
pregnancy, 33
  diet and nourishment for, 85, 86, 87, 126–27, 277–79
  doshas and, 17
  early loss, 102–3
  energy levels during, 121
  essential oils, general, 311
  essential oils by condition, 312–15
  herbs for, 302–5
  imbalances common in, 97, 98–102, 103–11
  kapha in, 27
  mother's happiness in, importance of, 47, 72, 106
  pitta in, 24
  sattvic lifestyle during, 77
  self-care practices for, 90–92
  senses during, 73
  support during, 2, 46
  three main responsibilities during, 268
  vata in, 20
  See also under meals; *individual trimesters*
presence, 3, 12
  while breastfeeding, 258–59
  while eating, 54
  in mothering, 224, 231, 239
  during pregnancy, 2
progesterone, 106
prolactin, 151
Puranans, 232

R

Radha, 232
raisins, 99, 273, 276, 284, 297
rajas, 73, 74, 76
rakta dhatu, 85
rasa dhatu, 85, 259–60
red raspberry leaf, 126, 199, 304
relationships
  commitment in, 51–52
  communication in, 51
  conflict in, 46–48
  real health and, 8
  trust in, 48–51
  See also partnership
reproductive system, 32, 199, 303, 304
reproductive tissues, 54, 55, 56–58, 59, 87
Rescue Remedy Back Flower Essence, 177
rice. *See* basmati rice
Roman chamomile, 252, 312, 314, 316, 318, 319
Romm, Aviva, 120, 134, 210
rose, 75, 188, 194
  in baths, 92, 126, 151, 184, 199
  description, 304
  essential oil, 68, 125, 152, 198, 313, 316, 317
  for newborns, 256
  postpartum, 181, 182, 200, 205, 207
  Sun-Cooked Ayurvedic Rose Petal Jam, 217–18
  in teas, 208, 306, 307
rosehips, 99
rosemary, 76, 199
rosemary essential oil, 101, 317
Rosenberg, Marshall, *Nonviolent Communication*, 51
rosewater, 69, 89, 106, 156, 247–48, 304
rosewood oil, 136, 312
Rothman, Barbara Katz, *Bun in the Oven, A*, 116

S

Sacinandana Swami, *Living Name, The*, 84
sacred window, 171
  author's experience, 196
  beauty in, 184

end of, 189–90, 220–21
greatest need during, 174
poem for, 175–76
traditional practices, 172, 191–92
saffron, 207, 282
for lactation, 260, 263
for ojas-building, 56, 69, 215–16
for postpartum, 286, 291, 296–97
sage, 181, 199, 254, 283. *See also* clary sage oil
samskaras. *See* sensory impressions (*samskaras*)
sandalwood, 75
essential oil, 68, 316, 317, 319
powder, 247–48, 256
sat-chit-ananda, 10
sattva, 213
increasing, 75
mind of, 36–37, 58
in postpartum, 192, 197, 210, 280
during pregnancy, 72, 86
qualities and characteristics, 73, 74
signs of, 75
sattvic ahara, 270
Schott, Lelia, 223
seasons
dosha fluctuation in, 15–16
ritucharya and, 60–61
selflessness, 233
self-realization, 36, 43
senses
consciousness and, 33–34
controlling, 39–41, 45
doshas and, 16, 25
misusing, 13
overstimulating, 21
sensory impressions (*samskaras*), 41, 42, 72, 85
sesame oil, 197, 207
for babies, 154, 246, 250, 255
for basti, 125, 181
cooking/eating, 280, 282, 284, 287
infusions, 198, 205
for massage, 22, 29, 124–25, 151, 152, 155, 181, 313
for oil pulling, 65
for stretch marks, 182
for yoni picchu, 126
sesame seeds, 56, 128, 260
Dry-Fruit Laddus, 276
Herbal Chewing Mix, 213, 289–90
See also tahini
sexual desire, regulating, 41
sexual intercourse
apana vata and, 102
Ayurvedic guidelines for, 68–69
ojas and, 94, 128
preconception, 55
during pregnancy, 93–95
shatavari
for acid reflux, 99
contraindications, 58, 305
descriptions, 213, 304
in ghee, 87, 207
for lactation, 260, 263
powder, 215–16, 297–98, 307
preconception, 58
shilajit, 58
showers, 29, 43
shukra dhatu, 87
sitali. *See* cooling breath
sitz baths, 87, 126, 318
skin
healthy fats for, 110
herbal baths for, 91
itchy, essential oils for, 314
of newborns, 244, 245, 254–56
pitta imbalance and, 24
skin-to-skin contact, 150
sleep
co-sleeping with baby, 306
difficulties in, 109–10
essential oils for, 314, 318
excess, from kapha imbalance, 27
herbs for, 303
of newborns, 240, 243
newborn's and mother's, 251–52
pitta and, 66
postpartum, 207–8
during pregnancy, positions for, 93
sleep apnea, 110
snacking, 21, 65

soul, 42, 81
ahimsa and, 37
conception and, 32
maha gunas and, 78
of newborns, 233
nourishing, 4, 80
presence of, 9–10
study of, 8
sounds
for baby in womb, 78, 80
maha gunas and, 75, 76, 77
spiritual vibrations, 83–84
sperm, 32, 54, 57, 63
spikenard oil, 319
spiritual people, associating with, 82
spiritual traditions, 38, 42
spirituality, 8, 32, 35, 52, 78–80, 233
spring, 27, 28, 60
sprouts, 274, 282, 285
Śrīla Gopāla Bhaṭṭa Gosvāmī, *Sat Kriya Sara Dipika*, 138
Srimad Bhagavatam Canto, 59
stillbirth, 216–18
stress hormones, 33, 57, 151
stretch marks, 110–11, 182, 315
sucanat, 56, 264–65, 292–93, 297–98
sugar, 19, 275
avoiding, 28, 105, 215, 278
cane, 56, 274, 277
cravings, reducing, 313
for newborns, 260
options, 284
rapadura, 215–16
turbinado, 217–18
summer, 23, 25, 61
surrogacy, 216–18
Sushruta Samhita, 85, 100, 268, 276
svastha, 9, 14
swaddling, 252
Swami, Radhanath, 42, 81, 157–58
symphysis pubis dysfunction (SPD), 107–8

T

tahini
Tahini Cookies, 297–98
Tahini Sauce, 296
tamas, 73, 74, 76–77
tastes, six, 261
celebrating, 88–89
seasons and, 60, 61
sweet, 270
Teitelbaum, Marianne, *Healing the Thyroid with Ayurveda*, 210
tests and procedures, 119, 134, 162–63
thyme oil, 310, 317
thyroid, 204, 208–10
time of day, 16
tongue scraping, 65
Touching Heaven (Oakes), 215, 261, 281–82, 283, 289
travel, 84, 178, 206
trimester, first
imbalances during, 97, 100
miscarriage in, 102–3
overview, 84–85
vata in, 20
trimester, second
overview, 85–86
pitta in, 24
trimester, third, 86–87
hair-parting ritual, 113
imbalances during, 97, 107, 108–9
kapha in, 27
pain reduction during, 125
triphala, 58
true Self, 13, 44, 45, 64, 83, 233
trust
in birthing process, 122, 128–29, 142, 160, 162
in relationships, 48, 49–51
turmeric, 56, 104, 264–65
avoiding, 283
essential oil, 314, 317
Herbal Chewing Mix, 289–90
Hot Milk Tonic, 290–91
kanji, 292–93
kitchari, 294–95
Warm Yam Smoothie, 292

U

umbilical cord
bathing and, 245
ceremony for cutting, 168
massage and, 247
when to cut, 154

Upanishads, 10
uterus
 involution of, 203
 irritable/exhausted, 155
 preconception influences on, 32
 strengthening, 57, 58, 212, 304, 305

V

vacha (calamus root), 153, 315
vaginas
 during birthing, 149
 bleeding from, 95
 oiling, 151
 tissues of, preparing for birth, 123, 126
valerian, 208, 318
values
 choice based on, 12
 guilt and, 231–32
 living in alignment with, 38–39
vanilla, 207, 276, 307
vata
 balancing, 21–23, 66
 in breastfeeding, 263
 depression and, 217
 imbalances, 20–21, 62, 94, 100, 204
 during labor, excess, 154–55
 nesting as, 122
 overview, 18–19
 pacifying, foods/herbs for, 277–79, 303–4
 postpartum, 174–75, 180, 201–2
 preconception, 57
 during pregnancy, 17, 20, 86–87, 90
 sleep and, 109
 stabilizing, 64, 126
 vitiated, eliminating, 125
 weight gain and, 111–12
 See also apana vata
Vedas, 10, 11–12, 232–33
Vedic tradition
 parameters in, 36
 rituals, 138, 168, 220–21, 234
vegetables
 Kitchari, 294–95
 Steamed Veggies, 296
 when to avoid, 282
 See also individual vegetables
vegetarian diet, 269
Velamentous Cord Insertion (VCI), 163, 164–65
vernix, 135, 244
vetiver oil, 314, 317
vitamin B (various forms), 57, 109, 210, 269, 275
vomiting
 by newborns, 243–44, 252
 during pregnancy, 97, 106, 108, 149, 273

W

walking, 22, 79, 84, 87, 90–91, 178
walnuts, 56, 262, 273, 276, 284
water breaking, 144, 146, 147
water element, 15, 17, 23–24, 26–27, 91
Weed, Susan, *Wise Woman Herbal for the Childbearing Year*, 109, 256
weight gain, 27, 111–13, 209
Western/allopathic medicine, 14, 71, 301
Williamson, Marianne, 1
winter, 19, 21, 60, 61
wintergreen oil, 316
witch hazel bark, 181, 200
Wolf, David B., *Relationships That Work*, 51
Womanly Art of Breastfeeding, The (La Leche League International), 261

Y

yamas, five
 ahimsa, 37–38
 aparigraha, 41–42
 asteya, 39
 brahmacharya, 39–41
 purpose of, 36–37
 satya, 38–39
yams, 128, 279, 285
 Steamed Veggies, 296
 Warm Yam Smoothie, 292
yarrow, 181, 198, 199
Yasoda, 232
yeast infections
 from kapha imbalance, 27
 in newborns, 255, 256
ylang ylang oil, 151, 311, 315, 316, 319
yoga nidra, 104, 208

yoga practices
  for apana vata, 102
  and Ayurveda, relationship between, 8
  gentle, 26, 42
  hatha, 22
  for kapha balance, 29
  during pregnancy, 79, 84, 85, 87, 95–97
  prenatal, 86
  weight gain and, 112
Yoga Sutras (Patanjali), 36
Yoga tradition, 2
yogurt, 56, 99, 105, 250, 278, 282
  in cookies, 297–98
  Panchamrit, 274
yoni picchu, 87, 126

Z

zucchini, 270, 285, 296

About the Author

Dhyana was born to a family of Bhakti yoga practitioners, with the practices and teachings of Ayurveda woven seamlessly throughout her life. Growing up around her family's retreat center (www.AyurvedaHealthRetreat.com), she was trained in all the healing modalities that are offered there and witnessed, firsthand, the profound healing that happens when the principles of Ayurveda are applied in one's daily life.

She is a certified Ayurveda health counselor and educator, specialized in guiding groups and individuals on transformative and healing journeys. Through her yoga and Ayurveda trainings as well as her online community, Soul Space, she empowers countless individuals to become healers in their own homes and to live a life of real meaning.

She lives in Alachua, Florida, with her beautiful family.